SECOND EDITION

STUDY GUIDE AND REVIEW MANUAL OF THE

Human Nervous System

KEITH L. MOORE, PH.D., F.I.A.C.

Professor of Anatomy
Associate Dean, Basic Sciences
Faculty of Medicine
University of Toronto
Toronto, Ontario
Canada

EWART G. BERTRAM, PH.D.

Department of Anatomy
Faculty of Medicine
University of Toronto
Medical Sciences Building
Toronto, Ontario
Canada

MURRAY L. BARR, M.D.

Professor Emeritus of Anatomy
452 Old Wonderland Road
London, Ontario
Canada

W. B. SAUNDERS COMPANY   **1986**

PHILADELPHIA   LONDON   TORONTO   MEXICO CITY   RIO DE JANEIRO   SYDNEY   TOKYO   HONG KONG

W. B. Saunders Company: West Washington Square
                          Philadelphia, PA 19105

Library of Congress Cataloging in Publication Data

Moore, Keith L.
   Study guide and review manual of the human
nervous system.

   Designed to accompany: The human nervous system
Murray L. Barr.
   1. Neuroanatomy--Examinations, questions, etc.
2. Anatomy, Human--Examinations, questions, etc.
I. Bertram, Ewart G.   II. Barr, Murray Llewellyn,
1908-   .   III. Barr, Murray Llewellyn, 1908-
Human nervous system.   IV. Title.   [DNLM 1. Nervous
System--anatomy & histology--examination questions.
WL 101 B268h 1974 Suppl.]
   QM451.B27 1983 Suppl.   611'.8   85-11805
   ISBN 0-7216-1524-4

Listed here is the latest translated edition of this book together
with the language of the translation and the publisher.

Japanese (1st Edition) - Ishiyaku Publishers, Inc., Tokyo, Japan

Study Guide and Review Manual
of the Human Nervous System   ISBN 0-7216-1524-4

Last digit is the print number: 9 8 7 6 5 4 3 2 1

PREFACE

The encouraging acceptance by students of the first edition of
this Study Guide indicates that it has fulfilled a useful purpose. The
publication of a fourth edition of *The Human Nervous System* by Barr and
Kiernan, and a new *Atlas of the Human Brain and Spinal Cord* by Bertram
and Moore, has made revision of this study guide necessary.

Many of the questions and notes have been rewritten, some
illustrations have been modified, and a few new ones have been added to
reflect the improved understanding of connections in many parts of the
nervous system.

Although the questions and explanations are primarily anatomical,
functional aspects are referred to and examples of clinical conditions
are given. Because of the curtailment of time available for studying
neuroanatomy, there is a trend to teach only those aspects that are
useful in clinical practice. Students naturally wish to know how much
their teachers expect them to know.

Because of the complex nature of the nervous system, most students
find neuroanatomy difficult. The objectives listed at the beginning of
each chapter in this Study Guide define what students should know about
neuroanatomy before they begin their clinical studies. The objectives
are based on our view that it is neither necessary nor desirable to
expect first year students to master more than the essentials of the
vast amount of knowledge on the nervous system that exists. By
restricting the amount of formal instruction to basic neuroanatomy and
by formulating instructional objectives, students are afforded the
opportunity of acquiring additional knowledge in their clinical years
from special lectures, case studies, and by interaction with their
colleagues.

Because multiple-choice examinations are commonly used and are
formidable even to the best prepared, commonly used types of question
have been developed around each region of the nervous sytem. Many
questions have been developed to exemplify important concepts and
clinical applications of neuroanatomy. Questions related to *clinical
problems* requiring neuroanatomical knowledge for their solution are
used frequently. All questions are intended for those wishing to test

the state of their knowledge and to improve their skills with multiple-choice examinations.

Because we have attempted to establish what aspects of neuroanatomy are important for every student to know, we should appreciate receiving constructive criticism from neuroanatomy teachers about the instructional objectives and questions. We want the questions and answers to be free of ambiguity and representative not only of the important aspects of neuroanatomy, but also of the high standards of education.

We are grateful to Harper and Row Publishers Inc. for permitting us to use many illustrations from The Human Nervous System (Barr and Kiernan) and to the Williams and Wilkins Company for letting us use several photographs from An Atlas of the Brain and Spinal Cord (Bertram and Moore). Although these are the main reference books for this Study Guide, students who use other textbooks and atlases should also find this learning aid useful.

We are grateful to Marion Moore, B.A. who did the word processing of this book in preparation for its photo-offset printing. Her exceptional skills in set-up and design are obvious.

Toronto and London
Ontario, Canada   *The Authors*

This study guide is designed to help you study and later review your knowledge of THE HUMAN NERVOUS SYSTEM by providing objectives and various types of multiple-choice question.

The questions are not intended to be a substitute for careful study of your textbooks, but they should enable you to detect areas of weakness and afford you the opportunity of correcting the defects in your knowledge. Although answers to these questions are explained and notes are given, you should consult your textbooks freely for further information. Through discussion of your areas of weakness with your colleagues and instructors, you can improve your ability to do the things listed as objectives at the beginning of each chapter.

To use this Study Guide most effectively, we suggest that you:

1. *Read the objectives listed at the beginning of the region or system you plan to study.*

2. *Carefully read the appropriate chapters in your reference books and study the photographs and drawings in your atlas.*

3. *Attempt to answer the multiple-choice questions. The knowledge required to answer the questions indicates how much are you expected to know in order to fulfill the objectives. The test questions are similar to those used in various board and medical school multiple-choice examinations, and are designed to be answered at the rate of about one every 45 seconds.*

4. *As you complete each set of questions, check your answers. If any of your answers are wrong, read the notes and explanations carefully and study the appropriate material and illustrations in your reference books, before proceeding to the next set of questions.*

5. *If you get 80 percent or more of the questions correct on the first trial, or during a subsequent review, you have performed very well and should have no difficulty answering similar questions based on these objectives.*

6. *When you have completed the study of a region or system, e.g., the brain stem, attempt the review examination on this region or system at the end of the book. If the level of your performance is not superior, determine where your knowledge is defective and review this material before attempting the examination at a later date.*

To our wives and grandchildren

CONTENTS

PART ONE REGIONAL ANATOMY

PART TWO *THE SYSTEMS*

REFERENCE BOOKS FOR THIS STUDY GUIDE

Barr, M.L. and Kiernan, J.A.: The Human Nervous System. An Anatomical
   Viewpoint. 4th ed. Philadelphia, Harper and Row Publishers, Inc.,
   1983.

Bertram, E.G. and Moore, K.L.: An Atlas of the Human Brain and Spinal
   Cord. Baltimore, Williams & Wilkins Company, 1983.

Moore, K.L.: Clinically Oriented Anatomy, ed. 2, Baltimore, Williams
   & Wilkins Company, 1985. Chapter 7.

Moore, K.L.: The Developing Human. Clinically Oriented Embryology.
   3rd ed. Philadelphia, W. B. Saunders Company, 1982. Chapters 4
   and 18.

Moore, K.L.: Before We Are Born. Basic Embryology and Birth Defects.
   2nd ed. Philadelphia, W. B. Saunders Company, 1983. Chapters
   5 and 17.

PART ONE

Regional Anatomy

ONE

Early Development of the Nervous System

OBJECTIVES

BE ABLE TO:

* Discuss the origin of the nervous system using simple diagrams to illustrate the neural plate, neural groove, neural folds, neural tube, and neural crest.

* Make simple sketches showing the development of neurons and neuroglial cells.

* Construct and label diagrams illustrating the adult derivatives of the walls and cavities of the forebrain, midbrain, and hindbrain.

* Explain the embryological basis of anencephaly and the various types of spina bifida.

FIVE- CHOICE COMPLETION QUESTIONS

DIRECTIONS: Each of the following questions or incomplete statements is followed by five suggested answers or completions. SELECT THE ONE BEST ANSWER OR COMPLETION in each case and underline the appropriate letter at the right.

----

1. Each of the following statements concerning the mesencephalic flexure of the embryonic brain is false EXCEPT:

   A. It is a pronounced ventral bend in the developing mid-brain region during the fourth week
   B. It separates the mesencephalon from the diencephalon
   C. It indicates the region where the neural tube bends in a dorsal direction
   D. It separates the midbrain from the metencephalon
   E. It causes the roof of the rhombencephalon to become very thin   A B C D E

SELECT THE ONE BEST ANSWER OR COMPLETION

2. The rostral and caudal neuropores normally close during the _____ week of human development.

   A. third   D. sixth
   B. fourth   E. seventh
   C. fifth   A B C D E

3. The pons and cerebellum of the mature brain are derived from the walls of the

   A. myelencephalon   D. diencephalon
   B. metencephalon   E. telencephalon
   C. mesencephalon   A B C D E

4. Growth and differentiation of the neural tube are greatest in the _____ portion.

   A. middle   D. lateral
   B. caudal   E. cranial
   C. cervical   A B C D E

5. Which of the following terms is used for both a primary and secondary brain vesicle?

   A. Myelencephalon   D. Diencephalon
   B. Metencephalon   E. Telencephalon
   C. Mesencephalon   A B C D E

6. Which structure is NOT a derivative of the diencephalon?

   A. Thalamus   D. Neurohypophysis
   B. Epithalamus   E. Hypothalamus
   C. Corpus striatum   A B C D E

7. Which of the following regions is the least differentiated component of the central nervous system?

   A. Myelencephalon   D. Mesencephalon
   B. Spinal cord   E. Diencephalon
   C. Cerebrum   A B C D E

8. Which region of the embryonic brain undergoes the most differentiation during development of the human brain?

   A. Myelencephalon   D. Telencephalon
   B. Metencephalon   E. Diencephalon
   C. Mesencephalon   A B C D E

4

9. Which structure listed below is NOT derived from the telencephalon?

   A. Cerebral hemisphere
   B. Corpus striatum
   C. Medullary center
   D. Insula
   E. Thalamus

   A B C D E

10. Anencephaly, a malformation exhibiting markedly defective brain development, most likely results from failure of the

    A. bones of the cranial vault to develop fully
    B. rostral neuropore to close normally
    C. prosencephalon to divide into two secondary brain vesicles
    D. neural folds to form in the rostral region of the embryo
    E. mesencephalic flexure to form in the midbrain region

    A B C D E

ANSWERS, NOTES, AND EXPLANATIONS

1. A The mesencephalic (cephalic) flexure is a ventral bend that occurs in the midbrain or mesencephalic region as the brain grows rapidly during the fourth week. A similar bend, the cervical flexure, occurs at the junction of the developing myelencephalon and the spinal cord. For illustrations and more information on the flexures of the developing brain, see Chapter 18 in the 3rd edition of The Developing Human or Chapter 17 in the 2nd edition of Before We Are Born (Moore).

2. B Fusion of the neural folds to form the neural tube begins in the midregion of the embryo early in the fourth week and proceeds in both cranial and caudal directions. The neural folds at the open ends of the neural tube (rostral and caudal neuropores) fuse around the middle of the fourth week. The rostral neuropore closes about two days before the caudal neuropore. *Failure of the neuropores to close normally results in severe neural tube defects.*

3. B The pons and cerebellum develop from the walls of the metencephalon, the fourth secondary brain vesicle. The cavity of the metencephalon becomes the superior portion of the fourth ventricle, part of the ventricular system of the brain.

4. E Growth and differentiation are greatest in the cranial or rostral portion of the neural tube, from which the large and complex brain develops. The Latin word rostrum means "beak". Rostral refers to structures in the cranial end that are near the nose region.

5. C The mesencephalon, one of the three primary vesicles, does not divide into secondary vesicles during the fifth week and so its name

does not change. The mesencephalon of the mature brain is also called the midbrain.

6. C The diencephalon of the mature brain consists of the thalamus, epithalamus, hypothalamus, and subthalamus. It is derived from the prosencephalon of the embryonic brain. The diencephalon forms the central core of the cerebrum. The *corpus striatum*, a large mass of gray matter, forms from the telencephalon.

7. B The spinal cord is the least differentiated component of the neuroaxis or central nervous system; that is, it is the least modified portion of the embryonic neural tube. The primitive segmental arrangement of the spinal cord is reflected in the 31 paired spinal nerves, each of which is attached to the cord by a dorsal sensory root and a ventral motor root.

8. D The telencephalon, represented by the massive cerebral hemispheres, undergoes the most differentiation during development of the mature brain. Most of the cerebral cortex is neocortex (G. neos, new + L. cortex, bark) which provides areas for all modalities of sensation, exclusive of smell, and special motor areas.

9. E The thalamus is a derivative of the diencephalon; however both the diencephalon and telencephalon are derivatives of the primary brain vesicle, known as the prosencephalon or forebrain.

10. B Anencephaly results when the rostral neuropore fails to close around the twenty-fourth day of development. This leads to failure of the cerebral hemispheres to form normally. As a result the cranial vault does not develop. The incidence of anencephaly is about 1:1000 births. As the exposed brain and membranes (meninges) are highly susceptible to infection, these infants rarely live very long after birth.

M U L T I - C O M P L E T I O N   Q U E S T I O N S

DIRECTIONS: In each of the following questions or incomplete statements, *one or more* of the completions given is correct. At the lower right of each question, underline A if 1, 2, and 3 are correct; B if 1 and 3 are correct; C if 2 and 4 are correct; D if only 4 is correct; and E if all are correct.

----

1. The walls of the prosencephalon give rise to the

    1. thalamus   3. hypothalamus
    2. cerebrum   4. corpus striatum   A B C D E

	A	B	C	D	E
	1,2,3	1,3	2,4	only 4	all correct

2. Correct statements about the developing nervous system in-clude:

    1. The brain and spinal cord form from the neural tube
    2. Nerve cells are derivatives of the neuroectoderm
    3. Growth and differentiation are greatest in the rostral portion of neural tube
    4. The primary brain vesicles form toward the end of the third week of development   A B C D E

3. The cavities of the embryonic brain vesicles give rise to the

    1. lateral ventricles in the cerebral hemispheres
    2. cerebral aqueduct of the midbrain
    3. third ventricle in the diencephalon
    4. central canal in the spinal cord   A B C D E

4. Embryological names of brain vesicles commonly used to describe parts of the adult brain include:

    1. Prosencephalon   3. Metencephalon
    2. Diencephalon   4. Mesencephalon   A B C D E

5. Parts of the brain NOT derived from the telencephalon include:

    1. Thalamus   3. Cerebellum
    2. Cerebral hemisphere   4. Corpus striatum   A B C D E

6. The cerebral hemispheres are derived from the

    1. diencephalon   3. metencephalon
    2. mesencephalon   4. telencephalon   A B C D E

7. Secondary brain vesicles contributing to formation of the brain stem include:

    1. Myelencephalon   3. Mesencephalon
    2. Metencephalon   4. Diencephalon

8. The cavity of the rhombencephalon becomes the

    1. lateral ventricle   3. third ventricle
    2. cerebral aqueduct   4. fourth ventricle   A B C D E

9. Congenital malformations resulting from a neural tube defect include:

    1. Spina bifida   3. Myeloschisis
    2. Anencephaly   4. Microcephaly   A B C D E

A	B	C	D	E
1,2,3	1,3	2,4	only 4	all correct

10. The diencephalon of the embryonic brain is represented in the
mature brain by the

1. thalamus
2. epithalamus

3. hypothalamus
4. subthalamus   A B C D E

ANSWERS, NOTES, AND EXPLANATIONS

1. E <u>All are correct</u>. The prosencephalon (forebrain vesicle) divides
into two secondary brain vesicles, the diencephalon and telencephalon.
The diencephalon develops into the thalamus, epithalamus, hypothalamus,
and subthalamus. The telencephalon gives rise to the cerebral
hemispheres, consisting of the olfactory system, corpus striatum,
cerebral cortex, and medullary center.

2. A <u>1, 2, and 3 are correct</u>. The brain and spinal cord develop from a
thickened area of embryonic ectoderm, the neural plate. A neural
groove develops in the midline of this plate that is flanked by neural
folds which begin to fuse early in the fourth week. By the end of the
fourth week, three primary brain vesicles are present: prosencephalon
(forebrain), mesencephalon (midbrain) and rhombencephalon (hindbrain).

3. A <u>1, 2, and 3 are correct</u>. The cavities of the embryonic brain
vesicles give rise to the lateral ventricles, the third ventricle, the
cerebral aqueduct, the fourth ventricle, and the central canal of the
caudal medulla oblongata. The central canal of the spinal cord, like
the ventricles of the brain, is derived from the lumen of the neural
tube but does not originate from the cavity of any of the brain
vesicles.

4. C <u>2 and 4 are correct</u>. The embryological terms *diencephalon* and
mesencephalon are retained to designate parts of the adult brain. The
diencephalon forms the central core of the cerebrum. The mesencephalon
undergoes less change than any other part of the brain, except the
caudal part of the hindbrain. In the adult brain, the mesencephalon is
usually called the midbrain.

5. B <u>1 and 3 are correct</u>. The *thalamus* is a derivative of the
diencephalon, not of the telencephalon, and the *cerebellum* is derived
from the metencephalon. The telencephalon gives rise to the cerebral
hemispheres. The corpus striatum, which has motor functions, is *a mass
of gray matter in the base of the cerebral hemisphere*.

6. D <u>Only 4 is correct</u>. The cerebral hemispheres are derived from the
telencephalon. The telencephalon undergoes the greatest development
of the brain as it forms the cerebral cortex, corpus striatum, and
medullary center.

7. A <u>1, 2, and 3 are correct</u>. The brain stem consists of three parts:

a) the *medulla*, a derivative of the myelencephalon; b) the *pons*, derived from the metencephalon; and c) the *midbrain*, a derivative of the mesencephalon.   Although each of these regions has special features, they have certain fiber tracts in common and each region includes nuclei of cranial nerves.

8. D <u>Only 4 is correct</u>. The cavity of the *rhombencephalon* is converted into the *fourth ventricle*, which is bounded by the medulla, pons, and cerebellum. The central canal of the closed portion of the medulla is also derived from the cavity of the hindbrain vesicle or rhombencephalon.

9. A <u>1, 2, and 3 are correct</u>. Failure of the rostral neuropore to close results in *anencephaly*, a severe brain malformation which occurs about once in 1000 births. It is characterized by absence of forebrain derivatives. Failure of the caudal neuropore to close results in *myeloschisis*, a severe form of *spina bifida and spinal cord abnormality. Spina bifida occulta is a defect of the vertebral arch only* and usually is of no clinical significance.

10. E <u>All are correct</u>. The diencephalon of the embryonic brain retains its original name in the mature brain. The four components of the brain derived from the embryonic diencephalon are: the thalamus, epithalamus, hypothalamus, and subthalamus.

F I V E -C H O I C E   A S S O C I A T I O N   Q U E S T I O N S

DIRECTIONS: Each of the following groups of questions consists of a numbered list of descriptive words or phrases accompanied by a diagram with certain parts indicated by letters, or by a list of lettered headings. For each numbered word or phrase, SELECT THE LETTERED PART OR HEADING that matches it correctly and insert the letter in the space to the right of the appropriate number. <u>Each lettered heading may be selected once, more than once, or not at all.</u>

A. Telencephalon

B. Myelencephalon

C. Mesencephalon

D. Metencephalon

E. Diencephalon

1. ____ Thalamus

2. ____ Olfactory bulbs

3. ____ Cerebellum

4. ____ Midbrain

5. ____ Hypothalamus

ASSOCIATION QUESTIONS

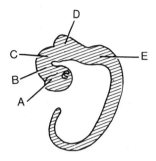

7. ____Primordium of pons

8. ____Gives rise to thalamus

9. ____Forms medulla

10. ____Metencephalon

11. ____Gives rise to cerebral hemispheres

12. ____Its cavity becomes the cerebral aqueduct

(From Moore, K.L.: The Developing Human, 3rd ed., Philadelphia, W.B. Saunders Co., 1982)

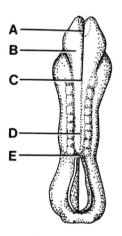

13. ____Defective closure of it results in anencephaly

14. ____Caudal neuropore

15. ____Neural fold

16. ____Gives rise to part of spinal cord

17. ____Forms part of telencephalon

18. ____Defective closure of it results in spina bifida

(From Moore, K.L.: Before We Are Born, 2nd ed., Philadelphia, W.B. Saunders Co., 1983)

ANSWERS, NOTES, AND EXPLANATIONS

1. E The thalamus, represented bilaterally, is derived from the embryonic diencephalon. The thalamus is the largest component of the mature diencephalon and is subdivided into several nuclei on the basis of its fiber connections and sequence of phylogenetic development.

2. A   The olfactory bulbs are the first parts of the olfactory system to develop. They first appear as hollow outgrowths from the developing cerebral hemispheres which develop from the telencephalon.

3. D   The cerebellum, like the pons, is derived from the metencephalon. The cerebellum, which has motor functions, is especially large in the human brain.

4. C   The midbrain is derived from the mesencephalon, the second of the three primary vesicles. It is morphologically the most primitive of the brain vesicles.

5. E   The hypothalamus is derived from the diencephalon of the embryonic brain. The hypothalamus is the principal autonomic center of the brain and as such has an important controlling influence over the sympathetic and parasympathetic divisions of the autonomic nervous system.

6. D   The pons is derived from the metencephalon. Along with the medulla and midbrain, the pons forms part of the brain stem. The pons (L. bridge) is the part of the brain stem which lies between the medulla and midbrain. Because fibers enter into the cerebellum from its basal aspect, the pons appears to constitute a bridge between the right and left halves of the cerebellum.

7. D   The primordium of the pons is the metencephalon, the fourth brain vesicle. This secondary brain vesicle also gives rise to the cerebellum. Primordium means the first trace of an organ or structure.

8. B   The thalamus is derived from the diencephalon, the second brain vesicle. The diencephalon of the mature brain consists of four parts: thalamus, epithalamus, hypothalamus, and subthalamus. Each part is represented bilaterally and differs in structure and function.

9. E   The myelencephalon, the most caudal of the embryonic brain vesicles, develops into the medulla (medulla oblongata) and its cavity forms the inferior part of the fourth ventricle.

10. D   The metencephalon, the fourth embryonic brain vesicle, is derived from the rhombencephalon or hindbrain vesicle. It gives rise to the pons and cerebellum of the mature brain.

11. A   The telencephalon, the most rostral brain vesicle, gives rise to the cerebral hemispheres consisting the olfactory system, corpus striatum, cerebral cortex, and medullary center.

12. C   The cavity of the mesencephalon is converted into the cerebral aqueduct of the midbrain, a canal connecting the third and fourth ventricles.

13. C   Defective closure of the rostral neuropore would most likely result in anencephaly in which there is markedly defective development of the brain, together with absence of the bones of the cranial vault.

11

14. E The caudal neuropore is an opening in the embryo leading from the lumen of the neural tube to the exterior. It normally closes around the end of the fourth week.

15. B The neural folds in the cranial region fuse to form three primary brain vesicles by the end of the fourth week.

16. D The neural tube in this region of the embryo forms the spinal cord. Its lumen becomes the central canal of the spinal cord.

17. B The neural folds in this region fuse to form the primary brain vesicle known as the prosencephalon or forebrain. It divides into two secondary brain visicles (telencephalon and diencephalon).

18. E Failure of the caudal neuropore to close by the end of the fourth week results in a severe defect of the vertebral column and spinal cord, known as spina bifida with myeloschisis. Defective development of the nerves to the sphincters of the urinary bladder and anal canal and to the lower limbs is associated with this type of spina bifida.

TWO

Cells of the Central Nervous System

OBJECTIVES

BE ABLE TO:

* Discuss the configuration of a neuron, adapting it to the specialized role of receiving stimuli and transmitting a nerve impulse to other neurons or effector cells.

* Discuss the intrinsic structure of neurons, including their organelles and inclusions.

* Describe the major responses of nerve cell bodies and axons (together with their sheaths) to interruption of axons, and name the main staining techniques that are used to demonstrate these responses.

* Discuss the location of synapses on neurons and illustrate the ultrastructure of the end-bulb type of synapse as seen with the electron microscope.

* Discuss the various types of neuroglial cell according to structure and function.

FIVE-CHOICE COMPLETION QUESTIONS

DIRECTIONS: Each of the following questions or incomplete statements is followed by five suggested answers or completions. SELECT THE ONE BEST ANSWER OR COMPLETION in each case and underline the appropriate letter at the right.
---

1. Which of the following constituents of a nerve cell is responsible for propagation of a nerve impulse?

    A. Nissl substance
    B. Golgi apparatus
    C. Surface membrane
    D. Neurofibrils
    E. Mitochrondria

    A B C D E

SELECT THE ONE BEST ANSWER OR COMPLETION

2. The nucleus of large neurons is typically

   A. vesicular   D. pyknotic
   B. eccentric   E. irregular
   C. oval-shaped   A B C D E

3. Section of the axon of a large motor neuron results in one
   of the following changes in its cell body:

   A. Disappearance of synaptic end-bulbs
   B. Dispersal of Nissl substance
   C. Total dissolution within a few days
   D. Shrinkage within a few days
   E. Prompt removal by neuroglial cells   A B C D E

4. White matter is so named because of the appearance created
   by

   A. abdundant pale-staining cells
   B. dendritic processes of neurons
   C. small nerve fibers lacking sheaths
   D. myelinated axons
   E. neuroglial elements   A B C D E

5. Which of the following neuronal components is nonliving
   cytoplasmic material?

   A. Neurofibrils   D. Golgi apparatus
   B. Mitrochondria   E. Lipofuscin
   C. Nissl substance   A B C D E

6. Myelin sheaths in the central nervous system are formed by

   A. Schwann cells
   B. astrocytes
   C. oligodendrocytes
   D. fibroblasts
   E. resting nicroglial cells   A B C D E

7. Wallerian degeneration of myelinated nerve fibers in the
   central nervous sytem is characterized by

   A. degeneration of axis cylinders and myelin sheaths
   B. continued conduction along intact but atrophied nerve
      fibers
   C. degeneration of myelin sheaths only
   D. degeneration of axis cylinders only
   E. eventual regeneration of the nerve fibers A B C D E

14

SELECT THE ONE BEST ANSWER OR COMPLETION

8. Which characteristic applies to Nissl substance?

    A. The amount is in inverse proportion to the size
       of the neuron
    B. Being acidophilic, it is stained by dyes such as
       eosin
    C. It is uniformly distributed throughout the cell
       body and axon
    D. It consists of granular endoplasmic reticulum
       and has basophilic properties
    E. No comparable substance occurs in any other type
       of cell in the body   A B C D E

9. Melanin pigment is present in

    A. the substantia nigra   D. Purkinje cells
    B. spinal ganglia   E. sympathetic
    C. lower motor neurons   ganglia   A B C D E

10. Synaptic end-bulbs are NOT characterized by the presence of

    A. synaptic vesicles
    B. mitrochondria
    C. interneuronal continuity
    D. a neurotransmitter substance
    E. a synaptic cleft   A B C D E

11. Which statement is most applicable to astrocytes?

    A. They are the same in white matter and gray matter
    B. They are connective tissue cells derived from mesoderm
    C. They are involved in neuronal circuitry
    D. They are not present in the cerebral cortex
    E. Their processes terminate on small blood vessels   A B C D E

12. The full complement of neurons is essentially established
    by the

    A. third fetal month   D. age of puberty
    B. time of birth   E. twentieth year
    C. tenth year   A B C D E

ANSWERS, NOTES, AND EXPLANATIONS

1. C Excitation, inhibition, and propagation of a nerve impulse are
   surface membrane phenomena. The cell membrane is semipermeable in that
   it allows diffusion of some ions, but restricts others. In the resting

state the membrane is disproportionately permeable to K^+ ions. These ions diffuse from the cytoplasm, in which they are in high concentration, to the external surface of the cell membrane. In this way the external surface acquires a resting potential with the inside of the cell about -80mV with respect to the outside. During excitation, when the membrane potential has been reduced by about 10mV-15mV to threshold value, there is a sudden functional alteration in the membrane, characterized by a selective increase in permeability to Na^+ ions being relatively high externaly. This causes a reversal of charge and creates a local action potential. Once generated the action potential is self-propagated along the membrane by local circuits of electrical current. This is the *nerve impulse*.

2. A Large neurons contain a spherical <u>vesicular nucleus</u> in which the chromatin is finely particulate. The large nucleus has a smooth contour, a prominent nucleolus, and is usually located in the center of the cell body.

3. B. Dispersal of Nissl substance (material), or <u>chromatolysis</u>, begins in motor neurons about two days after axon interruption and reaches a maximum at about three weeks. The cell body becomes more rounded in contour and slightly swollen, but the synaptic end-bulbs on its surface are not materially affected. Typically there is an eventual restoration, or nearly so, of the normal appearance of the cell body. Some types of neuron are more severly affected and they may even degenerate completely following section of their axons.

4. D The only neuronal elements in white matter are nerve fibers, a large proportion of which are <u>myelinated axons</u>. The lipoproteins of myelin sheaths are responsible for the whitish appearance that led to the term white matter.

5. E <u>Lipofuscin</u> (lipochrome) is a nonliving pigment or cytoplasmic inclusion. It is more common in some types of neuron than in others and the amount of pigment increases with age.

6. C Oligodendrocytes in the brain and spinal cord, like neurolemmal or Schwann cells in peripheral nerves, are responsible for forming myelin sheaths. The myelin sheaths consist of layers derived from the surface membranes of these cells.

7. A Interruption of myelinated nerve fibers causes <u>degeneration of the axis cylinders and myelin sheaths</u> distal to the site of injury. Nerve conduction therefore soon ceases. There is no effective regeneration in the central nervous system comparable to that which occurs under favorable circumstances in peripheral nerves.

8. D Nissl substance (material) consists of <u>granular endoplasmic reticulum which has basophilic properties</u> by virtue of the RNA in the ribosomes. Nissl substance occurs in clumps (Nissl bodies), and is more abundant, the larger the neuron. It is the counterpart in neurons of the basophilic substance (ergastoplasm or chromidial substance) in certain other types of cell, e.g., those composing pancreatic acini.

9. A Melanin-containing cells are particularly characteristic of the substantia nigra, a large nucleus with motor functions in the midbrain. The pigment may be an inert by-product of the sequence of chemical transformations that includes dopamine, a neurotransmitter substance.

10. C There is no continuity between neurons at synapses, but rather contiguity with synaptic clefts about 20 m wide intervening between the pre- and post-synaptic membranes. The axon terminals have mitochondria and synaptic vesicles which contain and release the neurotransmitter substance.

11. E Astrocytes occur throughout the central nervous system, the protoplasmic variety in gray matter and the fibrous variety in white matter. They are of ectodermal origin and their processes terminate on small blood vessels (especially capillaries) and adjacent to neurons. The gliofilaments in astrocytes may provide physical support for neurons and they may assist in the exchange of certain metabolic substances between blood and neurons.

12. B The full complement of neurons is nearly established in full-term newborn infants. Some increase in the population of small neurons occurs during infancy.

MULTI - COMPLETION QUESTION

DIRECTIONS: In each of the following questions or incomplete statements, *one or more* of the completions given is correct. At the lower right of each question, underline A if 1, 2, and 3 are correct; B if 1 and 3 are correct; C if 2 and 4 are correct; D if only 4 is correct; and E if all are correct.

---

1. Severe damage resulting from trauma to a fiber tract in the spinal cord, or disease at some point along its course, is followed by

   1. regeneration after a year
   2. no significant regeneration
   3. degeneration beginning after a month
   4. removal of debris by phagocytic cells   A B C D E

2. Synaptic end-bulbs are, or may be, situated on

   1. other end-bulbs   3. the cell body
   2. the axon hillock   4. dendrites   A B C D E

	A	B	C	D	E
	1,2,3	1,3	1,4	only 4	all correct

3. Which cells are known as Golgi type 1 neurons?

   1. Lower motor neurons
   2. Large pyramidal cells
   3. Purkinje cells
   4. Stellate cells   A B C D E

4. The sex chromatin in humans is

   1. demonstrable in many cell types in normal females
   2. limited to nerve cell nuclei of normal females
   3. a heteropyknotic X chromosome
   4. a non-sex specific chromatin mass   A B C D E

5. Staining methods for revealing the configuration of nerve cells and their processes include:

   1. Nissl method
   2. Hemotoxylin and eosin
   3. Weigert method
   4. Golgi method   A B C D E

6. The ventricles of the brain are lined by

   1. squamous epithelium of mesodermal origin
   2. a thin layer of collagen fibers
   3. ependymal epithelium composed of several layers of cells
   4. ependymal epithelium composed of a single layer of cells   A B C D E

7. Structures related to synaptic transmission include:

   1. Dendritic spines
   3. End-bulbs of Held-Auerbach
   3. Surface membrane
   4. Neurofibrils   A B C D E

8. Protein synthesis to maintain a nerve cell and its processes is most closely associated with

   1. mitrochondria
   2. neurofibrils
   3. Golgi apparatus
   4. Nissl substance   A B C D E

9. Which of the following are NOT cytoplasmic organelles?

   1. Golgi apparatus
   2. Melanin
   3. Nissl substance
   4. Lipofuscin   A B C D E

10. Cell types NOT part of the reticuloendothelial system of the body include:

   1. Oligodendrocytes
   2. Ependymal cells
   3. Astrocytes
   4. Microglial cells   A B C D E

A	B	C	D	E
1,2,3	1,3	1,4	only 4	all correct

11. Neuroanatomical methods based on axoplasmic transport
    include:

    1. Autoradiographic method
    2. Silver degeneration method
    3. Horseradish peroxidase method
    4. Deoxyglucose method   A B C D E

12. Substances used to block synapses when tracing pathways
    in the CNS include:

    1. Radioactively labelled 2-deoxyglucose
    2. Horseradish peroxidase
    3. Osmium tetroxide
    4. Nicotine   A B C D E

ANSWERS, NOTES, AND EXPLANATIONS

1. C 2 and 4 are correct. Degeneration of the nerve fibers distal to the
    lesion, which are separated from their cell bodies, begins within a few
    days and progresses rapidly. The debris is removed by phagocytes,
    mainly microglial elements. The affected region is converted to a form
    of scar tissue by astroglial proliferation. Although effective
    regeneration occurs in some lower animals, it is restricted in mammals
    to some sprouting from the central ends of interrupted fibers. *There
    is no convincing evidence of clinically significant fiber regneration
    in the human spinal cord.*

2. E All are correct. Details on synaptic end-bulbs vary according to
    their location in the central nervous system and the type of neuron.
    In motor neurons of the spinal cord, for example, the synaptic recep-
    tive area includes dendrites and the cell body. End-bulbs may also be
    present on the axon hillock and the proximal portion of the axon before
    the myelin sheath begins. In some locations, end-bulbs may be apposed
    to axon terminals in an end-bulb to end-bulb relationship. Axoden-
    dritic synapses are usually excitatory, whereas the others (especially
    axoaxonic synapses) are likely to be inhibitory. Other synaptic con-
    figurations are characteristic of certain locations, as in the basket-
    like arrangement of axon terminals which surround the cell bodies of
    Purkinje cells in the cerebellar cortex.

3. A 1, 2, and 3 are correct. Golgi type 1 neurons are large and have
    long processes. Stellate cells in the cerebral cortex, typical of
    Golgi type 11 neurons, are small cells with several short dendrites.

4. B 1 and 3 are correct. The sex chromatin represents one of the XX sex chromosome pair of females in a heteropyknotic and generally inert state, as opposed to the other X chromosome and the 44 autosomes which are euchromatic and genetically active. Sex chromatin can be identified in the nuclei of cells of many human tissues of females, the requirement being that the nuclei are reasonable vesicular, i.e., do not have a dense chromatin pattern. The nuclei of many cells of males with the Klinefelter syndrome also contain sex chromatin.

5. D Only 4 is correct. The *Golgi method*, in which blocks of tissue are immersed in a silver nitrate solution following fixation in a solution of potassium dichromate, stains the cell body and processes of neurons a brownish-black color. Nerve cell bodies are stained by the Nissl method and by hematoxylin and eosin, whereas the Weigert method stains only myelin sheaths.

6. D Only 4 is correct. The ventricles and the central canal of the spinal cord are lined by ependymal epithelium, the cells of which are in a single layer and range, according to their location, from flattened to columnar in shape. The ependymal epithelium is of ectodermal origin.

7. A 1, 2, and 3 are correct. Dendrites of some types of nerve cell have many protuberances (spines or gemmules) which make synaptic contact with passing axons or axon terminals. Synaptic end-bulbs (end-bulbs of Held-Auerbach) are a rather typical form of axon terminal and the pre- and postsynaptic membranes are specialized local modifications of the surface membranes. Although the role of neurofibrils is unclear, there is no evidence that these delicate filaments in the cytoplasm have any direct relationship with nerve impulse transmission.

8. D Only 4 is correct. *Nissl substance* (ribosomes of granular endoplasmic reticulum) contains RNA and is involved in the synthesis of proteins to replace those degraded as a normal event in living cells. The axon, typically the longest neuronal process, receives replacement proteins through axoplasmic flow from the cell body or perikaryon.

9. C 2 and 4 are correct. *Melanin and lipofuscin are pigments* and therefore are nonliving cytoplasmic inclusions. The Golgi apparatus and Nissl substance are organelles, i.e., specialized forms of living cytoplasm.

10. A 1, 2, and 3 are correct. The only cellular elements in the central nervous system that belong to the reticuloendothelial system are reactive microglial cells. When a pathological situation requires it, these cells, derived from monocytes, enter the nervous system by migrating from the lumina of normal blood cells. The *reactive microglial cells are like other phagocytic macrophages.* Comparable cells include histiocytes of connective tissue and Kupffer cells in the liver.

11. B 1 and 3 are correct. Tracing methods based on degenerating axons are not used much nowadays. They have been replaced by more sensitive techniques that reveal both the cells of origin and the sites of termination of axons. Both the autoradiographic and horseradish peroxidase methods are based on axoplasmic transport.

12. D Only 4 is correct. *Nicotine* has been used to block synapses and thereby establish their location, especially in autonomic ganglia.

F I V E - C H O I C E   A S S O C I A T I O N   Q U E S T I O N S

DIRECTIONS: Each group of questions below consists of a numbered list of descriptive words or phrases accompanied by a diagram with certain parts indicated by letters, or by a list of lettered headings. For each numbered word or phrase, SELECT THE LETTERED PART OR HEADING that matches it correctly and insert the letter in the space to the right of the appropriate number. Each lettered heading may be selected once, more than once, or not at all.

A. Centrosome   C. Lipofuscin   E. Nuclear membrane

B. Mitrochondria   D. Nissl substance

1. ____ Related to the aging process

2. ____ Granular endoplasmic reticulum

3. ____ Inconspicuous or absent in neurons

4. ____ Has pores closed by thin diaphragms

5. ____ Important in the energy-producing reaction in cells

6. ____ Concerned with synthesis of enzymatic and structural proteins

ASSOCIATION QUESTIONS

A. Astrocyte   C. Ependymal cells   E. Oligodendrocytes

B. Reactive microglia   D. Macroglia

7.   ____Form the lining epithelium of the ventricles

8.   ____Produce and maintain myelin sheaths in the central nervous
         system

9.   ____Have processes attached to blood vessels

10. ____Astrocytes and oligodendrocytes

11. ____May form a special kind of scar tissue

12. ____Are reticuloendothelial cells

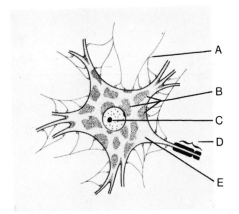

13. ____Lipoprotein membrane
         system

14. ____Axon terminal branch

15. ____Axon hillock

16. ____Nucleolus

17. ____Basophilic clumps

18. ____Conducts nerve impulses

(From Barr, M.L. and Kiernan,J.A.:
The Human Nervous System, 4th ed.,
1983. Courtesy of Harper & Row,
Publishers, Inc.)

ASSOCIATION QUESTIONS

A. Axon reaction   C. Nissl method   E. Weigert method

B. Marchi technique   D. Golgi method

19. ____Uses basic aniline dyes

20. ____Stain for normal myelin sheaths

21. ____Chromatolysis

22. ____Silver staining

23. ____Stain for degenerating myelin sheaths

ANSWERS, NOTES, AND EXPLANATIONS

1. C Traces of lipofuscin (lipochrome) pigment appear in nerve cells of spinal and sympathetic ganglia and in some cells of the spinal cord and medulla, among other sites, at about the eighth year. The yellow-brown granules become more numerous with increasing age and are usually abundant in elderly persons.

2. D Nissl substance, as seen with the light microscope, corresponds with the granular endoplasmic reticulum observed with electron microscopy. Virtually all cells contain this basophilic material in amounts ranging from scanty to abundant.

3. A The centrosome is inconspicuous or absent in mature cells, although it is present in their developmental precursors. This observation is no doubt related to the inability of nerve cells to divide because the centrosome, which includes a pair of centrioles, is important in mitosis.

4. E Pores in the nuclear membrane, even though closed by thin diaphragms, probably enhance the permeability of the membrane and hence the exchange of certain chemical substances between the nucleoplasm and the cytoplasm.

5. B Mitochondria are universal components of body cells which *contain enzymes of importance in metabolic processes*, including respiratory and phosphorylating enzymes of the Krebs citric acid cycle.

6. D Nissl substance, the granular endoplasmic reticulum, is concerned with protein synthesis mainly because of the RNA contained in the

constituent ribosomes. The ribosomes participate in the synthesis of structural and enzymatic proteins. This accounts for the abundance of Nissl substance in large neurons which have considerable cytoplasm to maintain in the long processes of the cell.

7. C A single layer of ependymal cells (epithelial cells) lines the ventricles of the brain. The free surface is ciliated in most locations and processes from the deep surface intertwine with those of astrocytes to form a delicate layer known as the internal limiting membrane.

8. E Formation and maintenance of the myelin sheath in the form of a variable number of layers of cell membrane is a function of oligodendrocytes in the central nervous system, just as it is a function of neurolemmal or Schwann cells in peripheral nerves.

9. A Processes of astrocytes, both fibrous astrocytes in white matter and protoplasmic astrocytes in gray matter, terminate on capillaries, arterioles, and venules as foot-plates or perivascular feet.

10. D Astrocytes and oligodendrocytes are sometimes combined under the heading of macroglia to distinguish them from the smaller microglia or microglial cells.

11. A Areas of degenerated nervous tissue, e.g., those following Wallerian degeneration, are likely to be converted into a special form of scar tissue by astroglial proliferation.

12. B The mesodermal origin and ameboid and phagocytic properties of reactive microglial cells under pathological conditions form the basis for considering them as a component of the reticuloendothelial system of the body.

13. D The myelin sheath consists of lipid and protein layers. This lipoprotein membrane system is derived from the plasma membrane of oligodendrocytes in the central nervous system and from neurolemmal (Schwann) cells in peripheral nerves.

14. A An axon of a neuron divides terminally and its branches may be directed toward several neurons. Each branch forms the axonal part of a synapse (or synapses), often in the form of end-bulbs or boutons terminaux.

15. E The axon hillock, which is devoid of Nissl substance, is at the periphery of the perikaryon from which the axon originates. The perikaryon is the cytoplasm of the nerve cell body.

16. C All nerve cell nuclei contain a nucleolus. They are especially prominent in large nerve cells (e.g., Golgi type 1 neurons) because of the role of the nucleolus in the synthesis of RNA and the role of the DNA in the synthesis of cytoplasmic proteins.

17. B The Nissl substance is usually disposed in clumps called Nissl bodies. They are basophilic because of the RNA they contain.

18. A Of all the components of a nerve cell, only the surface membrane, including that of the terminal branches of the axon, propagates the nerve impulse.

19. C The Nissl staining method uses basic aniline dyes, such as cresyl violet, toluidine blue, and thionine. Cellular components containing ribose nucleic acid (RNA) or desoxyribose nucleic acid (DNA) react to the Nissl stain. Nissl stains demonstrate nuclei, nucleoli, and Nissl substance.

20. E In the Weigert method, blocks of tissue are treated in a solution of potassium dichromate and sections cut from them are stained with hematoxylin. *The Weigert method is a classic stain for white matter.* Myelin sheaths are stained darkly, hence a degenerated fiber tract appears as a pale area in Weigert-stained sections.

21. A Chromatolysis is the dispersal of clumps of Nissl substance into finer particles. It is a characteristic component of the reaction of a nerve cell to an interruption of its axon (axon reaction).

22. D In staining nerve cells by the Golgi method, pieces of nervous tissue are fixed in a potassium dichromate solution, treated in a silver nitrate solution, and sectioned. The Cajal, Bielschowsky, and Bodian staining methods also employ silver compounds to stain nerve cells.

23. B The Marchi technique is based on treating nervous tissue with osmium tetroxide and potassium chlorate simultaneously. *Particles of degenerating myelin are stained black*, but normal myelin is not. The method is therefore useful in tracing a degenerating fiber tract in the central nervous system.

THREE

The Peripheral Nervous System

O B J E C T I V E S

BE ABLE TO:

* Make a schematic drawing to show the components of a spinal nerve between the first thoracic or second lumbar segments.

* Describe the structure, distribution, and function of general sensory endings or receptors and make simple drawings of them.

* Give an account of the histological features of ganglia, especially the sensory ganglia on dorsal spinal nerve roots.

* Describe the histology of peripheral nerves, identifying the types of their constituent fibers on a structural and functional basis.

* Discuss how an axon or axis cylinder acquires its sheaths.

* Describe a motor end-plate, using a simple illustration.

F I V E - C H O I C E   C O M P L E T I O N   Q U E S T I O N S

DIRECTIONS: Each of the following questions or incomplete statements is followed by five suggested answers or completions. SELECT THE ONE BEST ANSWER OR COMPLETION in each case and then underline the appropriate letter at the right.

---

1. Which of the following constitutes a sheath surrounding a bundle or fascicle of nerve fibers?

    A. Axolemma
    B. Endoneurium
    C. Perineurium

    D. Neurolemma
    E. Epineurium

    A B C D E

2. Which statement about pacinian corpuscles is correct?

    A. They are delicate touch receptors because of their superificial location.
    B. They are consistently so minute as to be visible only with a microscope.
    C. They consist of the coiled terminal portion of a sensory fiber in loose connection tissue surrounded by a by a capsule.
    D. A straight terminal portion of a sensory fiber is surrounded by layers of flattened cells with fluid between the layers.
    E. They respond to temperature changes in the skin and in some mucous membranes.   A B C D E

3. Group C fibers of peripheral nerves, or group IV of dorsal roots, conduct nerve impulses for

    A. position sense
    B. pain and temperature
    C. light touch and pressure
    D. the stretch reflex
    E. fine touch   A B C D E

4. Neurotendinous spindles (Golgi tendon organs) have as their most significant role:

    A. Giving awareness of the degree of flexion at a joint
    B. Responding to painful stimuli as in inflammation of a tendon or its sheath
    C. Originating a reflex that results in contraction of the associated muscle
    D. Participation in the gamma reflex loop
    E. Constant monitoring of tension on the tendon   A B C D E

5. Motor end-plates do NOT include:

    A. a sole-plate of sarcoplasm
    B. a synaptic cleft
    C. subsarcolemmal nerve endings
    D. synaptic vesicles in nerve terminals
    E. junctional folds   A B C D E

6. Which statement about the neurolemma of a nerve fiber is correct?

    A. It represents the nucleated, cytoplasmic portions of Schwann cells
    B. It is a delicate connective tissue sheath
    C. It is a sheath of myelin
    D. It is uninterrupted at nodes of Ranvier
    E. Its extensions into the myelin sheath constitute the incisures of Schmidt-Lantermann   A B C D E

SELECT THE ONE BEST ANSWER OR COMPLETION

7. The nerve cells of spinal ganglia are

    A. of uniform size
    B. multipolar
    C. devoid of capsules
    D. spherical and unipolar
    E. centrally located in the ganglia   A B C D E

8. Which of the following statements about sensory end-bulbs is correct?

    A. They are nonencapsulated sensory endings of uniform size
    B. Their role in specific modalities of sensation is poorly understood
    C. They contain the terminal ramifications of group C fibers
    D. They are probably not sensory receptors at all
    E. They are present in mucous membranes, but not else-where   A B C D E

9. Which of the following is NOT a component of a neuro-muscular spindle?

    A. Gamma motor neuron terminal
    B. Flower spray ending
    C. Annulospiral ending
    D. Merkel ending
    E. Motor end-plate   A B C D E

10. Postganglionic visceral efferent fibers are present in

    A. dorsal spinal nerve roots   D. gray communicating
    B. ventral spinal nerve roots   rami
    C. white communicating rami   E. spinal cord   A B C D E

ANSWERS, NOTES, AND EXPLANATIONS

1. C The endoneurium, perineurium, and epineurium are connective tissue sheaths of peripheral nerves. The delicate endoneurium encloses a nerve fiber; the perineurium encloses a bundle of nerve fibers; and the entire nerve is surrounded by epineurium. Axolemma is the name given the plasma membrane of an axis cylinder, and the neurolemma consists of nucleated portions of Schwann cells external to the myelin sheath.

2. D The ellipsoidal pacinian corpuscles are from 1 to 4 mm in length. They are therefore visible to the unaided eye. The straight terminal portion of a sensory fiber occupies the cylindrical core of the corpuscle. The bulk of the corpuscle consists of thin lamellae composed of flattened cells and delicate connective tissue fibers.

28

Fluid occupies the spaces between lamellae. Pacinian corpuscles respond to slight deformation and they have proprioceptive and other functions, depending on their location in the body. They do not respond to light touch or changes in temperature.

3. B Conduction for pain and temperature is along unmyelinated group C fibers and the smallest fibers of group A. Fibers of the latter group, all of which are myelinated, afford conduction for all modalities of general somatic sensation, whereas visceral afferent fibers belong to group B. In addition to the fibers for pain and temperature, group C includes postganglionic visceral efferent fibers.

4. E Neurotendinous spindles (Golgi tendon organs) respond exclusively to tension on the tendon, greater tension being required for their stimulation than for neuromuscular spindles. Stimulation of the neurotendinous spindles causes reflex inhibition of the muscle concerned, the opposite of which is true for stimulation of neuromuscular spindles.

5. C The terminal bulbous expansions of a nerve fiber in a motor end-plate are external to the sarcolemma or surface membrane of the muscle fiber and are separated from the sarcolemma by a synaptic cleft 20-50µ m wide. The nerve terminals contain synaptic vesicles from which the neurotransmitter substance acetylcholine is released. The sarcolemma has a wavy outline produced by junctional folds, where it apposes nerve terminals. An accumulation of sarcoplasm at the motor end-plate or myoneural junction constitutes the sole-plate.

6. A The myelin sheath between one node of Ranvier and the next is laid down in the form of concentric layers of the plasma membrane of a single Schwann cell. The nucleus of the Schwann cell remains external to the myelin sheath in the attenuated cytoplastic layer; thus the neurolemma consists of cytoplasmic portions of Schwann cells, with a nucleus for each internode. The delicate connective tissue sheath external to the neurolemma is called the endoneurium. The funnel-shaped clefts in the myelin sheath known as Schmidt-Lantermann incisures are created by a loosening of the plasma membranes with retention of some cytoplasm in these particular locations.

7. D Nerve cell bodies in spinal ganglia are spherical and unipolar. They are called unipolar cells because a single process arises from each cell body and divides into peripheral and central branches. These neurons are bipolar in early embryonic development, then the two processes approach one another and fuse for a short distance. On this basis the cells are sometimes said to be pseudounipolar. Spinal ganglion cells vary in size, corresponding with the variation in thickness of their processes. They are located mainly in a peripheral zone around a central core of nerve fibers. Each nerve cell body is surrounded by a capsule consisting of an inner layer of satellite cells and an outer layer of delicate connective tissue. The inner layer is continuous with the neurolemma and the outer layer blends with the endoneurium which surrounds the cell's processes.

8. B End-bulbs are encapsulated structures of varying size and shape. Group A fibers terminate within them in an irregular configuration and they are present in a variety of tissues, both superficial and deep. End-bulbs described as having a distinctive morphology have been assigned names and specific sensory functions. For example, spherical end-bulbs of Krause and elliptical end-bulbs of Ruffini have been said to function as receptors for coolness and warmth, respectively. *Further study is needed, however, in order to identify specific types of end-bulbs on a structural and functional basis.*

9. D Merkel endings (Merkel's disks) are terminal expansions of fibers comprising simple nerve endings in the skin. They are in contact with cells in the deeper layers of the epidermis and are considered to be touch receptors. Neuromuscular spindles include two types of sensory terminal - annulospiral and flower spray endings. In addition to these, the nerve terminals on the intrafusal muscle fibers include motor end-plates for gamma motor neurons.

10. D The cell bodies of preganglionic sympathetic neurons are in the intermediolateral cell column of the spinal cord (segments Tl to L2 or L3). Their axons traverse ventral spinal nerve roots and white communicating rami to reach ganglia of the sympathetic chain, where a synapse occurs with postganglionic sympathetic neurons. From these, viceral efferent fibers proceed to spinal nerves by way of gray communicating rami and then to smooth muscle in blood vessels, arrector pili muscles of hairs, and secretory cells of sweat glands. The other postganglionic fibers enter branches of the symnpathetic chain that supply thoracic and abdominal viscera.

M U L T I - C O M P L E T I O N   Q U E S T I O N S

DIRECTIONS: In each of the following questions or incomplete statements, *one or more* of the completions given is correct. At the lower right of each question, underline A if 1, 2, and 3 are correct; B if 1 and 3 are correct; C if 2 and 4 are correct; D if only 4 is correct; and E if all are correct.

---

1. Group C fibers of peripheral nerves are characterized by

    1. fast conduction   3. presence of a myelin
    2. lack of nodes of Ranvier   4. slow conduction   A B C D E

2. Receptors for touch include:

    1. Hair follicle plexuses   3. Merkel endings
    2. Meissner's corpuscles   4. Pacinian corpuscles   A B C D E

A	B	C	D	E
1,2,3	1,3	2,4	only 4	all correct

3. Which of the following characteristics apply to nerve cell bodies in spinal ganglia of spinal nerves and general sensory ganglia of cranial nerves?

   1. A single process
   2. Absence of synapses
   3. A delicate capsule
   4. Spherical shape   A B C D E

4. Nodes of Ranvier are related to

   1. intervals between Schwann cell territories
   2. endoneurial interruptions
   3. saltatory conduction
   4. a constant spacing in fibers   A B C D E

5. Correct statements about Meissner's corpuscles include:

   1. They are touch receptors located preferentially in hairy skin
   2. As with sensory end-bulbs, their function is poorly understood
   3. They are situated in deeper layers of the epidermis
   4. They are located where tactile discrimination is best developed   A B C D E

6. Simple nerve endings responding to stimuli causing pain are

   1. terminals of both myelinated and nonmyelinated fibers
   2. nociceptive
   3. nonencapsulated
   4. present in the cornea   A B C D E

7. Correct statements concerning neuromuscular spindles include:

   1. They contain two types of sensory or afferent nerve terminal
   2. They contain special muscle fibers which are oriented in parallel with the fibers of the main muscle mass
   3. The sensory endings respond to slight stretching of the muscle
   4. Being sensory receptors, they do not require a motor innervation   A B C D E

8. A cutaneous nerve includes:

   1. Preganglionic sympathetic fibers
   2. Fibers supplying exteroceptors
   3. Gamma efferent fibers
   4. Postganglionic sympathetic fibers   A B C D E

9. Motor end-plates (myoneural junctions)

   1. are located about midway along the length of a muscle fiber
   2. contain subsarcolemmal nerve endings
   3. utilize acetylcholine as a neurotransmitter substance
   4. have a bearing on the speed of conduction of a nerve impulse

                                                      A B C D E

10. Which of the following statements concerning myelin sheaths are correct?

   1. They are lacking on group C fibers because these have no relation to Schwann cells
   2. They can be stained black with osmic acid because the chemical combines with proteins
   3. They are of uniform thickness in all group A fibers
   4. Their presence has a bearing on the speed of conduction of a nerve impulse

                                                      A B C D E

ANSWERS, NOTES, AND EXPLANATIONS

1. C <u>2 and 4 are correct</u>. *There are no nodes of Ranvier in group C fibers* because they are unmyelinated. Instead of saltatory conduction, whereby the nerve impulse skips electronically from node to node, there is a continuous action potential wave along the axolemma. This accounts for the slower speed of conduction of unmyelinated, compared with myelinated fibers. Functionally, group C fibers are afferents for pain and temperature and postganglionic visceral efferents.

2. A <u>1, 2, and 3 are correct</u>. Simple endings in the epidermis, a modification of these endings in the form of <u>Merkel endings</u>, hair <u>follicle plexuses, and Meissner's corpuscles are all regarded as touch receptors</u>. Meissner's corpuscles have a particular facility with respect to discriminative touch (two-point discrimination). Pacinian corpuscles do not function as receptors for touch as distinct from pressure because of their relatively deep location.

3. E <u>All are correct</u>. The cell bodies of primary sensory neurons for general sensation are spherical and each cell body is surrounded by a capsule consisting of two layers. The inner layer of satellite cells is continuous with the neurolemma of the cell processes, whereas the outer layer is continuous with the endoneurium. Primary sensory neurons are bipolar during early stages of development. Those in the cochlear and vestibular ganglia remain bipolar, but in the case of general sensory neurons the processes approach one another and fuse for a short distance. <u>Most primary sensory neurons are therefore unipolar</u> (or pseudounipolar); the single process bifurcates into one which

proceeds to the periphery and one which enters the central nervous system. The size of the cell body varies in accordance with the diameter of its processes.

4. B <u>1 and 3 are correct.</u> The axolemma is exposed to tissue fluid at the nodes of Ranvier, which are intervals between lengths of myelin sheath laid down by adjoining Schwann cells. The speed of impulse conduction in myelinated fibers, which is saltatory (L. <u>saltare</u>, to jump) or through tissue fluid from node to node, is faster the thicker the nerve fiber because internodal lengths vary directly according to the thickness of the fibers. The endoneurial sheath continues as elsewhere at nodal sites.

5. D <u>Only 4 is correct.</u> *Meissner's corpuscles are touch receptors situated in the dermal papillae projecting into the epidermis.* They are most numerous and best developed in cutaneous areas such as the palmar surface of the hand, especially the fingers, where tactile discrimination (two-point discrimination) is most acute. Meissner's corpuscles are usually ovoid in shape; a thin capsule encloses epithelioid cells among which the terminals of large group A nerve fibers ramify.

6. E <u>All are correct.</u> Sensory endings for pain are nonencapsulated terminal branches of small (delta) myelinated fibers of group A and unmyelinated group C fibers. The feeling of pain, as well as of heat and cold, gives warning of real or potential injury to tissues. The sensations of pain and temperature are therefore said to be nociceptive (L. <u>noceo</u>, to injure + <u>capio</u>, to take; hence responsive to injurious stimuli). This type of sensory ending has a wide distribution in the body.

7. A <u>1, 2, and 3 are correct.</u> Neuromuscular spindles not only are sensory endings responding to even slight stretching of the muscle in which they are located, but are a component of the gamma reflex loop and therefore have a motor function as well. This accounts for a more complex structure than that of sensory receptors generally. Within a fusiform capsule there are several intrafusal muscle fibers running parallel with the fibers of the main muscle mass. Annulospiral and flower spray sensory endings terminate on the intrafusal muscle fibers. In addition to these, axons of gamma motor neurons terminate in motor end-plates on the intrafusal fibers.

8. C <u>2 and 4 are correct.</u> In addition to afferent nerve fibers for cutaneous sensory receptors (exteroceptors), a cutaneous nerve contains postganglionic sympathetic fibers. The latter originate in ganglia of the sympathetic chain, enter spinal nerves via gray communicating rami, and proceed by way of cutaneous branches to blood vessels, sweat glands, and arrector pili muscles of hairs. Somatic efferent fibers, both alpha and gamma motor fibers, are components of muscle branches of spinal nerves.

9. B <u>1 and 3 are correct.</u> The nerve terminals of motor end-plates or

myoneural junctions, which are usually located about midway along the length of a muscle fibers, are in apposition with the external surface of the sarcolemma or plasma membrane of the muscle fiber. Motor end-plates have typical synaptic features, including synaptic vesicles in the nerve terminals and a synaptic cleft between these and the muscle fibers. Acetylcholine is the neurotransmitter substance at these sites. The cholinergic excitation of muscle fibers is defective in myasthenia gravis, so that contraction of voluntary muscles is impaired, beginning with small muscles such as those that move the eyes and raise the eyelids.

10. D Only 4 is correct. *Only myelinated fibers have nodes of Ranvier,* which are necessary for saltatory conduction of a nerve impulse. Differences in the thickness of myelin sheaths contribute to the size range of myelinated fibers. Conduction is faster, the larger the fiber, because the internodal distance bears a direct relation to fiber size. Osmic acid combines with the lipid component of myelin and stains it black. Several group C fibers are enclosed by a single Schwann cell, however its plasma membrane does not wrap around the axis cylinders in layers and there is therefore no myelin sheath.

F I V E - C H O I C E   A S S O C I A T I O N   Q U E S T I O N S

DIRECTIONS: Each of the following groups of questions consists of a numbered list of descriptive words or phrases accompanied by a diagram with certain parts indicated by letters, or by a list of lettered headings. For each numbered word or phrase, SELECT THE LETTERED PART OR HEADING that matches it correctly. Then insert the letter in the space to the right of the appropriate number. Each lettered heading may be selected once, more than once, or not at all.

A. Group A fibers

B. White communicating ramus

C. Spinal ganglia

D. Group C fibers

E. Gray communicating ramus

1. ____ Aggregations of primary sensory neurons

2. ____ Postganglionic sympathetic fibers only

3. ____ Fibers for proprioception

4. ____ Preganglionic sympathetic and visceral afferent fibers

5. ____ Unmyelinated fibers for pain and temperature

6. ____ Derived from neural crest cells

34

ASSOCIATION QUESTIONS

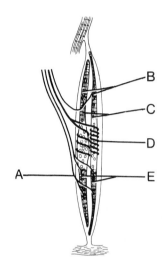

7. ____Termination of a sensory fiber called an annulospiral ending

8. ____A motor end-plate

9. ____Respond to a motor stimulus

10. ____A terminal known as a flower spray ending

11. ____An efferent or motor fiber

12. ____Nuclear bag and nuclear chain fibers

(From Barr, M.L. and Kiernan, J.A.: The Human Nervous System, 4th ed., 1983. Philadelphia, Harper & Row, Publishers Inc.)

A. Perineurium

B. Nodes of Ranvier

C. Axoplasm

D. Neurolemma

E. Axolemma

13. ___Plasma membrane of an axis cylinder

14. ____Sheath surrounding a fascicle of nerve cells

15. ____Represents nucleated, cyto-plasmic portion of Schwann cells

16. ____A special requirement for saltatory conduction

17. ____Contains cytoplasmic organelles

ASSOCIATION QUESTIONS

A. Sensory end-bulbs

B. Neurotendinous spindles

C. Myoneural junctions

D. Transducer

E. Pacinian corpuscles

18. ____A term applicable to sensory endings generally

19. ____Have an uncertain functional role

20. ____Receptors for pressure, proprioception, and vibration

21. ____Include synaptic vesicles and a snyaptic cleft

22. ____Originate impulses that inhibit motor neurons

23. ____Have a laminated structure

ANSWERS, NOTES, AND EXPLANATIONS

1. C The cell bodies of primary sensory neurons, which transmit nerve impulses from receptors to the central nervous system, are located in the spinal ganglia of spinal nerves and in the sensory ganglia of the following cranial nerves: trigeminal, facial, vestibulocochlear, glossopharyngeal, and vagus.

2. E All spinal nerves receive sympathetic fibers from the sympathetic chain lying alongside the vertebral column. The fibers are called postganglionic fibers because the cell bodies are in the ganglia of the sympathetic chain. They reach spinal nerves through gray communicating rami and are the only type of nerve fiber in these rami.

3. A Proprioceptive fibers of peripheral nerves are included in group A. They correspond to fibers of groups I and II in the numerical classification of somatic fibers in dorsal roots of spinal nerves. Afferent fibers for touch, pressure, and vibration, together with some of the fibers for pain and temperature, are likewise of the group A variety.

4. B White communicating rami connect thoracic and superior lumbar spinal nerves (T1 to L2 or L3) with the vertebral sympathetic chain. Each white ramus is located lateral to a gray ramus and includes two types of nerve fiber: visceral afferent fibers with their cell bodies in spinal ganglia, and preganglionic visceral efferent fibers. Cell bodies for the latter are situated in the intermediolateral cell column of the spinal cord, i.e., the source of the sympathetic outflow of the central nervous system. The fibers terminate on sympathetic neurons located in vertebral and prevertebral (collateral) sympathetic ganglia.

5. D Afferent fibers of group C (group IV in the classification for dorsal roots) conduct impulses for pain and temperature, as do some fibers of group A. The latter fibers are the smaller group A fibers which make up group III in the numerical system for somatic afferents in dorsal roots. As group A fibers are myelinated and permit saltatory conduction, the speed of impulse conduction is faster than for group C fibers which are unmyelinated. Impulses for pain and temperature therefore travel to the central nervous system at two speeds of conduction.

6. C Spinal ganglia (dorsal root ganglia) and sensory ganglia of cranial nerves are derived from neural crest cells, which lie along the dorsolateral borders of the embryonic neural tube. Autonomic ganglia also originate from cells of the neural crest.

7. D Annulospiral endings wind around the infrafusal muscle fibers. They are terminals of sensory fibers in the alpha range of group A, i.e., the largest myelinated nerve fibers.

8. A The motor end-plates are required because neuromuscular spindles have a motor function in the gamma reflex loop. This is in addition to the more strictly sensory function, such as providing afferent stimuli for the stretch reflex and sending proprioceptive data to higher centers, including the cerebellar and cerebral cortices.

9. C Each neuromuscular spindle contains from 2 to 10 muscle fibers which are called intrafusal fibers (within a spindle-shaped capsule) in order to distinguish them from the fibers of the main muscle mass. The infrafusal fibers are smaller than the others. Their middle zones lack cross-striations and the numerous nuclei in these zones are not in the usual subsarcolemmal location.

10. E A sensory nerve fiber terminates in the form of small expansions in contact with intrafusal muscle fibers to form a flower spray ending. This is one of two types of sensory ending in a neuromuscular spindle, the other one being an annulospiral ending.

11. B There is typically a motor end-plate on each half of an intrafusal muscle fiber. The associated nerve fiber is in the gamma range of group A, hence motor neurons for neuromuscular spindles are known as gamma motor neurons or gamma efferents.

12. C Some intrafusal muscle fibers have an expanded midregion and others do not. They are called nuclear bag and nuclear chain fibers, respectively, in part because the numerous nuclei in these regions are not in the usual subsarcolemmal position.

13. E The axolemma, or plasma membrane of the axis cylinder, is vitally concerned with nerve impulse conduction. The electrical action potential, once initiated, is self-propagated along the membrane. The event is a continuous or uninterrupted one in the case of unmyelinated fibers, whereas in myelinated fibers its occurs at the nodes of

Ranvier. There is an electronic skipping from node to node in the surrounding tissue fluid; this is called saltatory conduction.

14. A Three types of connective tissue sheath are present in peripheral nerves: epineurium, perineurium, and endoneurium which surround respectively the entire nerve, a bundle or fascicle of nerve fibers (these being destined for branches of the nerve), and an individual nerve fiber.

15. D The myelin sheath for each internodal length of a nerve fiber is formed by the plasma membrane of a Schwann cell, which is wrapped around the axis cylinder in a variable number of turns or layers. The cytoplasmic portion of the Schwann cell, together with its nucleus, is at the surface and constitutes the neurolemma of a myelinated fiber.

16. B The axolemma is bathed by tissue fluid at the nodes of Ranvier. This is required for saltatory conduction of the nerve impulse, in which the action potential skips electronically from node to node.

17. C The axoplasm (cytoplasm of the axon) contains neurofilaments, microtubules, smooth surfaced endoplasmic reticulum, and mitochondria. They are cytoplasmic organelles, as opposed to nonliving cytoplasmic inclusions.

18. D The word transducer, adopted from physics, is sometimes used for sensory endings because of the transformation of one form of energy to another. For example, energy of a mechanical nature initiates a nerve impulse, an electrical form of energy, in some sensory endings.

19. A Sensory end-bulbs are located at many sites in the body. They consist of terminal branches of nerve fibers which form an irregular pattern in a rather loose form of connective tissue surrounded by a more dense capsule. These end-bulbs vary in size and shape and specific modalities of sensory function have been ascribed to some of them. For example, spherical end-bulbs of Krause and elliptical end-bulbs of Ruffini are said to be receptors for coolness and warmth, respectively. However, there appears to be insufficient evidence for relating specific roles to specific types of end-bulbs and their functional aspects are therefore in need of further investigation.

20. E Pacinian corpuscles respond to slight pressure and their location determines the modality of sensation with which they are concerned. The correlations are as follows: subcutaneous tissue - pressure; in and near joint capsules - proprioception; adjacent to bone - vibration; in viscera and mesenteries - sensation of fullness of hollow organs and other forms of visceral sensibility.

21. C Myoneural junctions or motor end-plates are essentially synapses between nerve and muscle. Although their structure is rather more complex than that of interneuronal synapses, there are certain features in common. For example, a synaptic cleft 20 - 50 m wide intervenes

between the nerve terminal and the muscle fiber; the nerve terminals contain synaptic vesicles that release acetylcholine, the neuro-transmitter substance at myoneural junctions.

22. B Neurotendinous spindles (Golgi tendon organs) respond to tension on a tendon. The primary sensory neuron stimulates an intercalated neuron in the gray matter of the spinal cord and the intercalated neuron inhibits a motor neuron. Through this three-neuron reflex arc, relaxation of the muscle concerned is produced. Among other functions, neurotendinous spindles provide protection against damage to a muscle or a tendon resulting from excessive tension.

23. E Pacinian corpuscles consist of lamellae surrounding an elongated central core which contains the terminal portion of a sensory nerve fiber. The lamellae, separated by fluid-filled intervals, are composed of flattened cells supported by sparse collagen fibers.

FOUR

The Spinal Cord

OBJECTIVES

BE ABLE TO:

* Describe the development of the spinal cord, emphasizing the significance of the alar and basal plates.

* Discuss the positional changes of the developing spinal cord cord in relation to the vertebral column.

* Make simple sketches of the spinal cord illustrating its length, enlargements, surface markings, and the relation of the spinal cord segments and spinal nerves to the vertebral column.

* Explain the relation of the roots of the spinal nerves to the meninges and spinal ganglia.

* Describe the blood supply of the spinal cord.

* Discuss the internal structure of the spinal cord as seen in transverse sections and make simple diagrams showing the structural differences at cervical, thoracic, lumbar, and sacral levels.

* State the extent and function of the cell columns (nuclei) of gray matter.

* Discuss the stretch, gamma, and flexor reflexes with the aid of simple diagrams.

* State the origin, course, termination, and function of the major ascending and descending tracts of the spinal cord and indicate the relative positions of these tracts in a transverse section.

* Discuss briefly the main types of spinal cord lesion and interpret the basic clinical signs resulting from them.

FIVE-CHOICE COMPLETION QUESTIONS

DIRECTIONS: Each of the following questions or incomplete statements is followed by five suggested answers or completions. SELECT THE ONE BEST ANSWER OR COMPLETION in each case and underline the appropriate letter at the right.

----

1. Which statement about the adult spinal cord is <u>incorrect</u>?

   A. It is continuous with the medulla of the brain stem
   B. It lies in the vertebral canal of the vertebral column
   C. It usually ends at the inferior border of the second lumbar vertebra
   D. It narrows caudally to a slender filament
   E. It begins at the foramen magnum in the occipital bone   A B C D E

2. Which of the following spinal nerves is absent in some people?

   A. Thoracic   D. Coccygeal
   B. Cervical   E. Lumbar
   C. Sacral   A B C D E

3. Which statement about the filum terminale is <u>incorrect</u>?

   A. Attaches to the dorsum of the sacrum
   B. Has no functional significance
   C. Pierces the dura mater at the level of the second sacral vertebra
   D. Extends caudally from the conus medullaris
   E. Consists of pia mater and neuroglial elements   A B C D E

4. Select the <u>incorrect</u> statement about spinal cord levels.

   A. Cervical spinal segments are characterized by division of the dorsal white columns into two fasciculi
   B. Gray columns are maximal in the cervical and lumbosacral enlargements
   C. Sacral segments contain large amounts of white matter
   D. Cervical segments are characterized by their relatively large size and the amount of white matter
   E. Lumbar segments are characterized by their oval shape   A B C D E

41

SELECT THE ONE BEST ANSWER OR COMPLETION

5. Which statement about the nucleus dorsalis is NOT correct?

    A. A slender well-defined column of nerve cells
    B. Occupies the dorsomedial part of the dorsal horn
    C. Extends from spinal cord segments C8 through L2 or L3
    D. Largest in the twelfth thoracic and first lumbar segments
    E. It is also called Clarke's column   A B C D E

6. Identify the false statement about lamina II (substantia gelatinosa) of the spinal cord.

    A. Present in all levels
    B. Located in the apex of the dorsal gray horn
    C. Bounded externally by Lissauer's zone and lamina I of Rexed
    D. Composed chiefly of Golgi type I neurons
    E. A relay nucleus for pain and temperature data   A B C D E

7. All statements about the intermediolateral cell column are correct EXCEPT:

    A. Forms a small lateral horn of gray matter on each side
    B. Extends through the entire length of the spinal cord
    C. Is the source of preganglionic sympathetic fibers
    D. Receives stimuli from visceral afferents of dorsal roots
    E. Consists of motor-type cells that are smaller than the alpha cells of the ventral gray horn   A B C D E

8. Choose the incorrect statement.

    A. The dorsal spinocerebellar tract originates in the nucleus dorsalis
    B. The medial motor cell column extends through the whole length of the spinal cord
    C. On entering the dorsolateral tract of Lissauer, dorsal root fibers divide into short ascending and descending branches.
    D. The cuneate fasciculus conducts proprioceptive sensations from the lower limb
    E. The lateral spinothalamic tract for pain and temperature is especially important clinically   A B C D E

SELECT THE ONE BEST ANSWER OR COMPLETION

9. Which statement about the corticospinal tract is FALSE?

    A. It is also known as the pyramidal tract
    B. Fibers composing it arise mainly from the frontal lobe
    C. About 55 percent of its fibers cross at the inferior
        end of the medulla and enter the opposite side
        of the spinal cord
    D. Descends through the whole length of the spinal cord
    E. A pathway concerned with voluntary, discrete,
        skilled movements   A B C D E

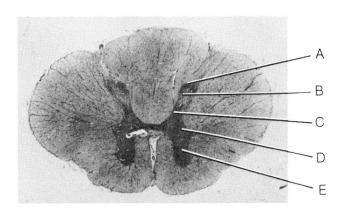

10. The nucleus proprius
    (laminae III - VI of
    Rexed) is labelled

    ____.

11. Which statement about the blood supply of the spinal
    cord is incorrect?

    A. The spinal cord is not very vulnerable to circula-
        tory impairment
    B. The blood received by the spinal arteries from the
        vertebral arteries is sufficient only for the
        cervical segments of the cord
    C. The posterior spinal artery may arise as a branch
        of the posterior inferior cerebellar artery
    D. The paired posterior spinal arteries usually arise
        from the vertebral arteries in the region of the
        medulla
    E. The spinal cord is supplied by branches of the
        vertebral arteries and multiple radicular arteries
        derived from segmental vessels of the aorta   A B C D E

43

SELECT THE ONE BEST ANSWER OR COMPLETION

12. Select the incorrect statement concerning the results of destruction or atrophy of lower motor neurons.

   A. Progressive atrophy of muscles deprived of motor fibers
   B. Diminished or absent tendon reflexes
   C. Flaccid paralysis of affected muscles
   D. No loss of somatic or visceral sensation
   E. Stroking of the sole causes upturning of the great toe   A B C D E

13. Correct statements concerning reticulospinal fibers include:

   A. Originate in the central group of reticular nuclei of the brain stem
   B. Descend in the ventral and lateral white columns
   C. Relay impulses of motor significance to lower motor neurons
   D. Terminate on both alpha and gamma motor neurons
   E. All of the above statements are correct   A B C D E

14. Which statement concerning the rubrospinal tract is FALSE?

   A. The cells bodies of fibers in this tract are in the contralateral red nucleus of the midbrain
   B. Its fibers terminate in the cervical cord and in the superior portion of the thoracic region
   C. Crosses to the opposite side of the brain stem in the medulla
   D. Runs caudally in the lateral area dorsal to the inferior olivary nucleus
   E. Is situated deeply in the tegmentum of the pons   A B C D E

ANSWERS, NOTES, AND EXPLANATIONS

1. C The spinal cord in the newborn usually terminates at the inferior border of L2 or L3 vertebrae, but in adults the spinal cord commonly ends between L1 and L2 vertebrae. The level of termination is elevated slightly by flexion of the vertebral column. In unusual cases, the inferior end of the cord may be as superior as the twelfth thoracic vertebral body or as inferior as the third lumbar vertebra.

2. D The spinal nerves are distributed as follows: cervical, 8; thoracic, 12; lumbar, 5; sacral, 5; and coccygeal, 1. The first pair of cervical nerves lacks dorsal roots in about 50 percent of persons; the coccygeal nerves are not always present.

3. A <u>The filum terminale attaches to the dorsum of the coccyx.</u> It marks the tract of regression of the caudal part of the embryonic spinal cord and lies within the cauda equina (lumbosacral nerve roots).

4. E <u>Lumbar segments are nearly circular in transverse section</u> and have massive ventral and dorsal gray horns. They also contain relatively and absolutely less white matter than cervical segments, which are characterized by their oval shape and the division of the dorsal white columns into medial and lateral fasciculi.

5. B <u>The nucleus dorsalis is located in the ventromedial part of the dorsal gray horn of the spinal cord.</u> Impulses impinging on cells in the nucleus dorsalis originate in proprioceptive endings, including neuromuscular spindles, Golgi tendon spindles, and pancian corpuscles. They receive a lesser contribution from touch and pressure receptors. Eccentric nuclei are characteristic of neurons in the nucleus.

6. D <u>Lamina II, also known as the substantia gelatinosa, consists chiefly of small Golgi type II neurons</u> with some larger neurons. This cell column should not be considered as necessarily a nucleus through which there is unaltered relay of pain and temperature data to higher centers. There may be modification of the data by other modalities of general sensation or by impulses of cortical origin.

7. B The intermediolateral cell column (nucleus) on each side of the spinal cord forms a small <u>lateral horn of gray matter from segment T1 through L2 or L3.</u> The preganglionic fibers of the sympathetic system arise from these cell columns. Similar cells in the base of the ventral gray horn in segments S2 through S4 constitute the sacral autonomic nucleus, from which the preganglionic fibers of the sacral portion of the parasympathetic system arise.

8. D <u>The gracile fasciculus and gracile nucleus deal with proprioceptive and fine touch sensations from the lower limb.</u> The cuneate fasciculus and cuneate nucleus deal with these sensations from the upper limb. As the spinal cord is ascended, axons from neurons in spinal ganglia are added to the lateral side of each fasciculus.

9. C About 85 percent of the fibers of the corticospinal tract cross at the caudal end of the medulla to the opposite side of the spinal cord through the pyramidal decussation. These crossed fibers, constituting the lateral corticospinal tract, extend throughout the cord.

10. B The nucleus proprius constitutes the entire dorsal horn of gray matter, except Lamina II (A) and the nucleus dorsalis (C). The nucleus proprius, also called the chief nucleus of the dorsal horn (laminae III - VI of Rexed), includes many internuncial neurons together with tract cells whose axons contribute to ascending fasciculi in the white matter.

11. A Radicular arteries derived from segmental vessels (i.e., ascending cervical, deep cervical, intercostal, lumbar, and sacral anterior) pass through the intervertebral foramina, divide into anterior and posterior radicular arteries, and provide the principal blood supply of thoracic, lumbar, sacral, and coccygeal segments of the cord. Hence <u>the spinal</u>

cord is vulnerable to circulatory impairment if a radicular artery is clamped. The superior thoracic and first lumbar segments are among the most vulnerable regions of the spinal cord.

12. E The sign of Babinski (upturning of the great toe and spreading of the other toes on stroking the sole) is a sign associated with an "upper motor lesion" This sign is attributed to the involvement of the cortico-spinal tract. Destruction or atrophy of lower motor neurons results in flaccid paralysis of the affected muscles, diminished or absent tendon reflexes, and progressive atrophy of muscles deprived of motor fibers.

13. E All the statements about reticulospinal fibers are correct. Among other functions, reticulospinal connections constitute an important system through which motor parts of the brain, notably the cerebral cortex and the cerebellar nuclei, are able to influence motor cells of the ventral gray horn.

14. C The rubrospinal tract arises from the red nucleus and crosses to the opposite side of the brain stem at its level of origin (midbrain). The fibers terminate on internuncial neurons or ventral horn cells superior to the midthoracic level, although conduction may continue caudally by means of spinospinalis relays. The rubrospinal and reticulospinal tracts are pathways through which the cerebral cortex and cerebellar nuclei bring their influence (via the extrapyramidal system) to bear on lower motor neurons.

M U L T I - C O M P L E T I O N   Q U E S T I O N S

DIRECTIONS: In each of the following questions or incomplete statements, one or more of the completions given is correct. At the lower right of each question, underline A if 1, 2, and 3 are correct; B if 1 and 3 are correct; C if 2 and 4 are correct; D if only 4 is correct; and E if all are correct.

----

1. Which of the following cell columns (laminae) extend throughout the spinal cord?

    1. Nucleus Dorsalis
    2. Lamina V of Rexed
    3. Intermediolateral
    4. Lamina II (substantia gelatinosa of Rolando)   A B C D E

2. The corticospinal tract

    1. is part of the pyramidal motor system
    2. originates completely from cells in the frontal lobe
    3. undergoes an incomplete decussation at the inferior end of the medulla
    4. parent cell bodies of almost all its fibers are located in the primary motor cortex   A B C D E

46

A	B	C	D	E
1,2,3	1,3,	2,4	only 4	all correct

3. <u>Correct</u> statements concerning the dorsolateral tract (of <u>Lissauer</u>) include:

    1. Fine fibers from the lateral part of the dorsal root enter the dorsal tract
    2. Lies in the interval between the apex of the dorsal horn and the surface of the spinal cord
    3. On entering this zone, dorsal root fibers divide into ascending and descending branches
    4. The branches give off collaterals that enter the dorsal horn   A B C D E

4. The longitudinal groove in the internal surface of the lateral walls of the developing spinal cord

    1. is called the sulcus limitans
    2. disappears as the mature spinal cord forms
    3. demarcates the division between the alar and basal plates
    4. marks the boundary between future motor and sensory areas   A B C D E

5. The adult spinal cord is

    1. a long cylindrical structure
    2. located in the central canal
    3. suspended in the dural sheath
    4. the same length as the vertebral column   A B C D E

6. Protection of the spinal cord is provided by the

    1. vertebral column   3. vertebral ligaments
    2. spinal meninges   4. cerebrospinal fluid   A B C D E

7. The dorsal and ventral roots

    1. join proximal to the spinal ganglion
    2. traverse the subarachnoid space
    3. form the filum terminale caudally
    4. pierce the arachnoid and dura mater   A B C D E

8. The ventral spinocerebellar tract

    1. is lateral to the spinothalamic tract
    2. first appears in the inferior lumbar region of the cord
    3. is dorsal to the site of emergence of the ventral roots
    4. is an uncrossed tract   A B C D E

A	B	C	D	E
1,2,3	1,3,	2,4	only 4	all correct

9. The spinothalamic tract is

   1. especially important clinically
   2. the main central pathway for pain, temperature, and
      light (crude) touch
   3. found in the ventrolateral column (funiculus)
   4. Formed by axons of neurons in lamina V of Rexed
      of the dorsal horn   A B C D E

10. The stretch reflex is

    1. based on a series of at least three neurons
    2. an important postural reflex
    3. protective as a response to a painful stimulus
    4. the basis of the knee-jerk test   A B C D E

11. Lesions of the spinal cord may result from

    1. trauma   3. demyelinating disorders
    3. infections   4. impairment of blood supply   A B C D E

12. The fasciculus gracilis

    1. is located in the dorsal white funiculus of the
       spinal cord
    2. contains fibers from sacral, lumbar, and
       inferior thoracic levels
    3. extends the whole length of the spinal cord
    4. transmits impulses concerned with pain and
       temperature   A B C D E

13. The nucleus dorsalis

    1. extends from C8 through L2 or L3 segments of
       the spinal cord
    2. is smallest in the twelfth thoracic and first
       lumbar segments
    3. gives origin to the dorsal spinocerebellar tract
    4. is a relay nucleus for visceral afferent impulses   A B C D E

14. Complete transection of the spinal cord between the
    cervical and lumbrosacral enlargements results in

    1. loss of all sensibility and voluntary movement
       inferior to the lesion
    2. paralysis of both legs
    3. loss of control of bladder and bowel functions
    4. a period of spinal shock lasting from eight
       weeks to a year   A B C D E

A	B	C	D	E
1,2,3	1,3,	2,4	only 4	all correct

15. Central cavitation of the spinal cord with a glial reaction
(gliosis) adjacent to the cavity, occurring in the disorder
disorder known as <u>syringomyelia</u>, usually causes

    1. upper neuron weakness
    2. yoke-like anesthesia for pain and temperature
    3. paralysis of both lower limbs (paraplegia)
    4. wasting of muscles in the upper limbs   A B C D E

16. A patient with hemisection of the upper cervical region
of the spinal cord would show which of the following
neurologic signs caudal to the lesion?

    1. Loss of position sense and the feeling of vibra-
       tion on the side of the lesion
    2. Paralysis of the body on the side of the lesion
    3. Anesthesia for pain and temperature on the
       side opposite to the lesion
    4. Little loss of touch sensation on the side of the
       lesion   A B C D E

ANSWERS, NOTES, AND EXPLANATIONS

1. C <u>2 and 4 are correct.</u> The cell columns in laminae II and V extend the
whole length of the spinal cord whereas those in the nucleus dorsalis and
the intermediolateral nucleus extend only from the level of C8 through L3
and T1 through L1 or L2 respectively. Laminae II and V are relay nuclear
areas for pain and temperature with modification of sensory input. Tract
cells for the controlateral spinothalamic tracts are located in lamina V.

2. B <u>1 and 3 are correct.</u> The sites of origin of corticospinal fibers are:
primary motor area, 30 percent; premotor and parietal cortex, 40 percent,
with the largest proportions of these coming from the first somesthetic
cortex. Although included in the corticospinal tract anatomically, many
parietal fibers are not motor but end on sensory relay neurons and
influence transmission of sensory data to the cortex.

3. E <u>All are correct.</u> Dorsal root fibers pass into the spinal cord and
enter the dorsolateral tract (of Lissauer). These fibers divide into
short ascending and descending branches. Each branch gives off numerous
collaterals. These fine caliber fibers, which are for pain and temperature, terminate mainly in laminae I, II, and V of Rexed.

4. E <u>All are correct.</u> Differential thickening of the lateral walls of the
neural tube produces a longitudinal groove, <u>the sulcus limitans</u>. This
groove is of fundamental importance because it separates the alar and
basal plates, which are later associated with afferent and efferent
functions (sensory and motor), respectively.

5. B 1 and 3 are correct. The spinal cord occupies most of the vertebral
    canal. The central canal is in the spinal cord and is derived from the
    neural canal of the neural tube. The spinal cord in adults occupies only
    the superior two-thirds of the vertebral canal (only as far as the disc
    between L1 and L2) because the vertebral column elongates more rapidly
    than the spinal cord during fetal life.

6. E All are correct. The spinal cord is suspended in the dural sheath
    by a denticulate ligament on each side, and is enclosed in three layers
    or meninges (L. membranes). The cerebrospinal fluid (CSF) in the sub-
    arachnoid space serves to support and cushion the spinal cord against
    trauma.

7. C 2 and 4 are correct. The ventral roots join the incoming sensory
    fibers immediately distal to the spinal ganglion to form the spinal
    nerve. The lumbosacral roots form the cauda equina (L. horse's tail) in
    the inferior part of the spinal canal. The cord tapers into a slender
    filament, the filum terminale, which lies in the midst of the cauda
    equina. These roots pierce the arachnoid and dura mater, at which point
    these meninges become continuous with the epineurium.

8. A 1, 2, and 3 are correct. The ventral spinocerebellar tract, unlike
    the dorsal spinocerebellar tract, is a crossed tract in the spinal cord.
    A large portion of its fibers originate in the lumbosacral enlargement,
    where the cells of origin are located in laminae V - VIII of Rexed in the
    ventral horn. The ventral and dorsal spinocerebellar tracts carry
    sensory data, predominantly proprioceptive, to the same side of the
    cerebellum.

9. E All are correct. Axons of many cells in lamina V of the dorsal horn
    give rise to the spinothalamic tract which cross the midline in the
    ventral gray and white commissures. The spinothalamic tracts are of
    considerable clinical importance. Section of the tract on one side
    (tractotomy) for relief of intractable pain results in a contralateral
    loss of pain, touch, and temperature sensations, extending superiorly to
    a level about one segment inferior to the level of the section.

10. C 2 and 4 are correct. The stretch reflex is based on a two-neuron or
    monosynaptic reflex arc. Testing for this reflex (e.g., using the knee-
    jerk test) is done in routine neurologic examinations. The reflex alters
    tension in the muscle in such a way as to maintain a constant length.

11. E All are correct. To the list of causes of lesions in the spinal cord,
    tumors should be added. Testing for impairment or loss of cutaneous
    sensation is an important part of the neurologic examination. Reflex
    contraction of muscles is also utilized in testing for the integrity of
    spinal cord segments and the spinal nerves.

12. A 1, 2, and 3 are correct. The fasciculus gracilis transmits impulses
    from proprioceptors, tactile endings, and endings that respond to
    vibration through dorsal root fibers that enter the spinal cord inferior
    to the midthoracic level. Discriminative (fine) touch sensations from
    inferior to the midthoracic level are relayed through this fasciculus to
    the nucleus gracilus, while proprioceptive impulses are relayed to the

nucleus dorsalis which in turn relays the proprioceptive impulses to nucleus of Z via collaterals from the dorsal spinocebellar tract.

13. B 1 and 3 are correct. The nucleus dorsalis (Clarke's column) is a slender, yet well-defined column of nerve cells in the ventromedial part of the dorsal horn. The column is largest in the twelfth thoracic and first lumbar segments. Impulses impinging on cells of Clarke's column originate in proprioceptive endings, including neuromuscular spindles, Golgi, tendon spindles, and pacinian corpuscles, with a lesser contribution from touch and pressor receptors.

14. A 1, 2, and 3 are correct. The initial period of spinal shock following complete transection of the cord lasts from a few days to several weeks, during which time all somatic and visceral reflex activity is abolished. On return of reflex activity, there is spasticity of muscles and exaggerated tendon reflexes.

15. C 2 and 4 are correct. Syringomyelia is characterized by central cavitation of the spinal cord, usually beginning in the cervical region. Decussating fibers for pain and temperature in the ventral gray and white commissures are interrupted early in the disease. The cavitation later spreads into the gray and white of the spinal cord. The yoke-like anesthesia for pain and temperature over the shoulder and upper limbs is one of the common signs of the disorder. Other signs are lower motor neuron weakness and wasting of the upper limb muscles owing to involvement of ventral horn cells in that area.

16. E All are correct. Hemisection of the spinal cord is unusual, but the lesion is seen most completely in knife wounds. The neurologic signs caudal to the hemisected region of the cord constitute the Brown-Sequard syndrome. The dorsal and lateral funiculi are damaged which interrupt the tracts for proprioception and tactile discrimination on the same side, inferior to the lesion. Light touch is not affected very much because of essentially bilateral conduction in the dorsal and lateral funiculi.

FIVE - CHOICE ASSOCIATION QUESTIONS

DIRECTIONS: Each of the following groups of questions consists of a numbered list of descriptive words or phrases accompanied by a diagram with certain parts indicated by letters, or by a list of lettered headings. For each numbered word or phrase, SELECT THE LETTERED PART OR HEADING that matches it correctly and insert the letter in the space to the right of the appropriate number. Each lettered heading may be selected once, more than once, or not at all.

A. Dorsolateral sulcus
B. Intermediolateral cell column
C. Ventral median fissure
D. Dorsal funiculus (column)
E. Ventrolateral sulcus

1. ____ Zone of emergence of the ventral roots

2. ____ Consists of fasciculus gracilis and fasciculus cuneatus

3. ____ Source of preganglionic sympathetic fibers

4. ____ Contains branches of the anterior spinal artery

5. ____ Bounded by the median septum and the dorsal gray horn

6. ____ Line of entrance of the dorsal roots

7. ____ Forms the lateral horn of gray matter

A. Dorsolateral tract (of Lissauer)
B. Fasciculus cuneatus
C. Ventral corticospinal tract
D. Spinal accessory nucleus
E. Medial longituidinal fasciculus (descending)

8. ____ Supplies the trapezius and sternocleidomastoid muscles

9. ____ Conducts discriminative touch sensations from the lower limb

10. ____ Also called the medial vestibulospinal tract

11. ____ Consists of dorsal root fibers

12. ____ Comprises a small portion of the pyramidal tract

13. ____ Occupies all of the dorsal funiculus in the inferior half of the cord

14. ____ Originates from the vestibular nuclei

ASSOCIATION QUESTIONS

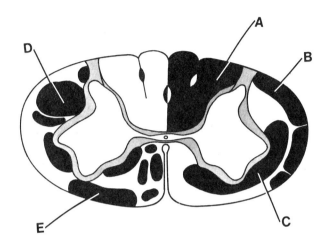

(The above photograph is modified from Barr, M.L. & Kiernan, J.A.:   The Human
Nervous System, 4th ed., 1983, Harper & Row Publishers Inc.)

15. ____Cells of origin are in the frontal and parietal lobes.

16. ____Has its origin in the nucleus dorsalis

17. ____Main central pathway for pain and temperature sensibilities

18. ____Important in the maintenance of equilibrium

19. ____Myelination not fully completed until the end of the second year

20. ____Bounded laterally by the dorsal gray horn and the dorsolateral
          tract

21. ____Also called the pyramidal tract

22. ____Spinothalamic and spinoreticular tracts

23. ____Damage to it causes a loss of discriminative touch sensations in the
          fingers

ASSOCIATION QUESTIONS

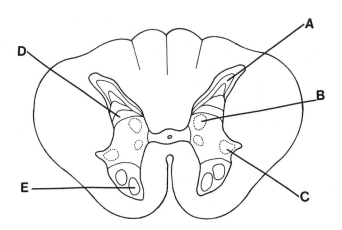

(The above photograph is modified from Barr, M.L. and Kiernan, J.A.: The Human
Nervous System, 4th ed., 1983, Harper & Row Publishers, Inc.)

24. ____Also called Clarke's column

25. ____Supplies muscles of the neck and trunk

26. ____Also known as the substantial gelatinosa (of Rolando)

27. ____Its fibers give rise to the dorsal spinocerebellar tract

28. ____Sympathetic nucleus

29. ____Gives origin to the spinothalamic tract

30. ____Its fibers conduct proprioceptive sensations to the nucleus of Z
of Brodal and Pompeiano

ANSWERS, NOTES, AND EXPLANATIONS

1. E The ventrolateral sulcus on the surface of the cord is indistinct,
but its position is clearly indicated by the zone of emergence of the

ventral roots of the spinal nerves.

2. D The dorsal funiculus of white matter in the spinal cord is bounded by the median septum and the dorsal gray horn. Superior to the mid-thoracic level, it consists of the fasciculus gracilis and fasciculus cuneatus. Caudal to the midthoracic region, the fasciculus gracilis forms the entire dorsal column.

3. B The intermediolateral cell column forms a small lateral horn on each side of the spinal cord, extending from segment T1 through L2 or L3. This column gives rise to preganglionic sympathetic fibers that emerge with axons of ventral horn cells to form the ventral roots of spinal nerves T1 to L2 or L3.

4. C The deep ventral median fissure contains connective tissue of the pia mater and branches of the anterior spinal artery.

5. D The dorsal funiculus (column) of spinal cord white matter is bounded medially by the medial septum and laterally by the dorsal gray horn superior to the midthoracic region. The faciculus gracilis and fasciculus cuneatus composing it are separated by a thin dorsal intermediate septum.

6. A The dorsolateral sulcus marks the line of (attachment) entrance of the dorsal roots of the spinal nerves. On entering the spinal cord, the dorsal root fibers divide into ascending and descending branches. They are distributed as necessary for reflex responses and transmission of sensory data to the brain. These dorsal root fibers course in the dorso-lateral tracts and fasciculus gracilis or fasciculus cuneatus.

7. B The intermediolateral cell column forms the lateral horn of gray matter in segments T1 through L2 or L3. Neurons in these columns give rise to preganglionic sympathetic fibers.

8. D Axons of neurons of the spinal accessory motor nucleus, which is located in lamina IX of the lateral region of the ventral horn in segments C1 through C5, emerge in a series of rootlets to form the spinal root of the accessory nerve. This nerve has a tortuous course through the foramen magnum and jugular foramen before it innervates the trapezius and sternocleidomastoid muscles in the neck.

9. B The fasciculus gracilis conducts discriminative touch sensations from the inferior half of the body on the same side. The large myelinated fibers of the dorsal roots, which enter the spinal cord inferior to the midthoracic level, form the fasciculus gracilis of the same side. This tract conducts discriminative touch sensations to the nucleus gracilis.

10. E The descending component of the medial longitudinal fasciculus is also called the medial vestibulospinal tract. It mainly arises from the medial vestibular nucleus and descends on the ipsilateral and contra-lateral sides of the spinal cord. The vestibulospinal tract, which arises from the lateral vestibular nucleus, is sometimes called the lateral vestibulospinal tract.

11. A The <u>dorsolateral tract (of Lissauer)</u> is made up of ascending and descending fibers from the branching of fine lateral dorsal root fibers. Fibers of this tract end in laminae I and V of Rexed as well as <u>lamina II</u> (substantial gelatinosa) within the segment of entry or in the next cranial or caudal segment of the spinal cord.

12. C The corticospinal tract, which consists of a large percentage of pyramidal cells, runs through a region of the medulla known as the pyramid; hence the alternative name of pyramidal tract. The ventral corticospinal tract comprises a small portion of the corticospinal fibers that did not cross the midline in the medulla, but descended in the ipsilateral ventral funiculus of the spinal cord.

13. A The fasciculus gracilis occupies the entire dorsal white funiculus of the spinal cord inferior to the midthoracic level. Superior to this level, the dorsal funiculus consists of a fasciculus gracilis and cuneatus. The fasciculus gracilis lies medial to the fasciculus cuneatus.

14. E The descending <u>medial longitudinal fasciculus</u> (medial vestibulospinal tract) arises from the medial vestibular nucleus in the medulla. It is involved in movements of the head required for maintaining equilibrium. It does not descend inferior to the cervical segments of the spinal cord.

15. D Parent cell bodies of about 30 percent of corticospinal fibers are located in the primary motor cortex of the frontal lobe; the remainder are other cortical areas of the frontal and parietal lobes.

16. B The dorsal (posterior) spinocerebellar tract has its origin in the nucleus dorsalis (thoracicus or Clarke's column) of the same side and begins in the superior lumbar segments. It lies along the dorsolateral periphery of the spinal cord. Most impulses carried by this tract originate in the various proprioceptive endings with an additional contribution to touch and pressure. Collaterals from this tract conduct position sense from the lower limb to the nucleus of Z of Brodal and Pompeiano, located immediately adjacent to the nucleus gracilis.

17. C The spinothalamic tract is especially important clinically. It is the main central pathway for pain, crude touch, and temperature sensibilities. However there are additional routes for pain conduction to the thalamus which are mainly through the reticular formation. The spinoreticular tract courses in the same area of the spinal cord as the spinothalmic tract.

18. E The cells of origin of the vestibulospinal (lateral) tract are in the lateral vestibular (Deiter's) nucleus of the same side. The tract extends the length of the spinal cord. The tonus of the muscle is altered according to the position of the head, and in response to head movements; thus this tract is important in the maintenance of equilibrium.

19. D Myelination of the corticospinal tracts begins in late fetal life and is not fully completed until the latter half of the second year after birth. Myelination is closely associated with the development of the functional capacity of the neurons. A sign of Babinski (upturning of the

great toe and spreading of the other toes on stroking the sole), mostly attributable to interruption of the corticospinal tract in adults, can be elicited in infants presumably because of the nonmyelinated state of the fibers at this stage. Similarly, the vestibulospinal tract is not completely myelinated at birth.

20. A In the superolateral half of the dorsal funiculus of the spinal cord, the fasiculus cuneatus is located between the fasciculus gracilis and the dorsal horn of gray matter at the dorsolateral tract. It is made up of heavily myelinated axons (fibers) entering from the dorsal roots of spinal nerves from C1 to T5. Collateral branches from the fibers of the fasciculus cuneatus end on neurons in the dorsal horn of gray matter.

21. D The corticospinal tract runs through a region of the medulla known as the pyramid, hence the alternative name of pyramidal tract. The cells of origin of this tract are in the contralateral cerebral cortex. A large percentage of these cells are called pyramidal cells (Golgi type I cells).

22. C The spinothalamic and spinoreticular tracts course together in the ventrolateral and ventral funicular area of the spinal cord. The spinothalamic tract is the main central pathway for pain, tactile and

temperature sensibilities to the center of consciousness. The spinoreticular tract conducts these sensibilities to the reticular nuclear area of the brain stem.

23. A The fasciculus cuneatus conducts ipsilateral discriminative qualities of sensation, including the ability to recognize changes readily in the positions of tactile stimuli applied to the skin of the upper limb. The fasciculus cuneatus is made up of ascending axons derived from neurons located in the dorsal root ganglia from C1 to T5. This fasciculus ends in the nucleus cuneatus.

24. B The nucleus dorsalis, often called nucleus thoracicus or Clarke's column, is a slender, well defined column of cells in the ventromedial part of the dorsal horn. The nucleus extends from C8 through L2 or L3 segments. Impulses impinging on cells in Clarke's column originate in proprioceptive endings.

25. E Lamina IX of Rexed takes the form of columns of neurons embedded in either lamina VII or VIII. Axons of neurons in lamina IX that are in the medial area of the ventral horn leave the spinal cord in the ventral roots to supply striated muscle attached to the axial skeleton, as well as intercostal and abdominal muscles. Laminae IX neurons located in the lateral enlargments of the ventral horn supply muscles of the upper and lower limbs.

26. A Lamina II of Rexed, is also known as the substantia gelatinosa (of Rolando). It is made up of densely packed neurons that have richly branched dendrites. Its axons make synaptic contact with cells in laminae I through IV. This lamina is believed to be important for the editing of sensory pain input to the spinal cord.

27. B The dorsal spinocerebellar tract has its origin in the nucleus dorsalis (thoracicus or Clarke's column) of the same side and begins in the superior lumbar segments. Its fibers ascend ipsilaterally in the dorsolateral funiculus and enter the cerebellum via the inferior cerebellar peduncle.

28. C The <u>intermediolateral cell column</u> occupies the lateral horn of the cord from segments T1 through L1 or L2. This column consists of cell bodies of preganglionic neurons of the sympathetic nervous system.

29. D <u>Lamina V (of Rexed)</u>, the widest part of the laminae of the dorsal horn, contains many large tract cells. The axons of cells in this lamina cross the midline commissural gray and white matter to ascend in the <u>contralateral spinothalamic tract</u>. This tract conducts pain, tactile, and temperature sensations from the contralateral side of the body.

30. B The nucleus dorsalis gives origin to the dorsal spinocerebellar tract. This tract passes up the ipsilateral, dorsolateral funiculus to enter the inferior cerebellar peduncle. Prior to entering the inferior cerebellar peduncle it gives off collaterals which end in the nucleus of Z. Proprioceptive sensations from the nucleus dorsalis reach the nucleus of Z via this tract.

FIVE

The Brain Stem

O B J E C T I V E S

BE ABLE TO:

* Prepare diagrams illustrating the surfaces of the brain stem.

* Give an account of the development of the brain stem and the fourth ventricle.

* List the sensory and motor pathways that pass through the brain stem.

* Draw transverse sections through rostral and caudal levels of the mid-brain, pons, and medulla to show the main anatomical features of each area.

* Identify areas of the midbrain, pons, and medulla that are derived from the alar and basal plates.

* List the important structures that would be involved in lesions of the brain stem, e.g., left side of the medulla, pons, and midbrain.

* Give a brief account of the neurological signs that would likely result from lesions affecting the various tracts and nuclear areas in the medulla, pons, or midbrain.

F I V E - C H O I C E   C O M P L E T I O N   Q U E S T I O N S

DIRECTIONS: Each of the following questions or incomplete statements is followed by five suggested answers or completions. SELECT THE ONE BEST ANSWER OR COMPLETION in each case and underline the appropriate letter at the right.

----

1. Which of the following fasciculi is located in the brain stem?

   A. Lenticular   D. Uncinate
   B. Inferior longitudinal E. Arcuate
   C. Medial longitudinal   A B C D E

SELECT THE ONE BEST ANSWER OR COMPLETION

2. Which of the following structures is located immediately deep to the floor of the fourth ventricle?

    A. Abducens nucleus
    B. Motor nucleus of facial nerve
    C. Rubrospinal tract
    D. Medial lemniscus
    E. Nucleus ambiguus   A B C D E

3. The decussation of the medial lemniscus is located in the

    A. spinal cord   D. midbrain
    B. medulla   E. diencephalon
    C. pons   A B C D E

4. The tract in the midbrain for conduction of light touch sensation from the left side of the face is located in the

    A. left tectal region   D. right cerebral
    B. right tectal region   peduncle
    C. left cerebral peduncle E. none of the above   A B C D E

5. Which of the following structures is located in the basal portion of the pons?

    A. Lateral spinothalamic tract   D. Tectospinal tract
    B. Medial lemniscus   E. Corticospinal tract
    C. Corticorubral tract   A B C D E

6. The cerebral aqueduct runs inferiorly through the

    A. telencephalon   D. metencephalon
    B. diencephalon   E. myelencephalon
    C. mesencephalon   A B C D E

7. The lateral lemniscus conducts sensory impulses for

    A. proprioception   D. all of the above
    B. touch   E. none of the above
    C. temperature   A B C D E

8. Which of the following nuclei is (are) connected with the cerebellum?

    A. Inferior olivary   D. All of the above
    B. Lateral cuneate   E. None of the above
    C. Arcuate   A B C D E

9. The decussation of the brachia conjunctiva is in the

    A. rostral midbrain   D. caudal pons
    B. caudal midbrain   E. medulla
    C. rostral pons   A B C D E

SELECT THE ONE BEST ANSWER OR COMPLETION

10. The spinal trigeminal nucleus receives general sensory sensations from

    A. cranial nerve V   D. cranial nerve X
    B. cranial nerve VII   E. all of the above
    C. cranial nerve IX   A B C D E

11. Which of the following structures is (are) found in the tectum of the midbrain?

    A. Superior colliculus
    B. Medial longitudinal fasciculus
    C. Fibers of the oculomotor nerve
    D. Ventral spinocerebellar tract
    E. All of the above   A B C D E

12. Fibers of the hypoglossal nerve in the medulla

    A. run between the pyramid and the inferior olivary nucleus
    B. decussate to the opposite side
    C. pass between the inferior cerebellar peduncle and the spinal nucleus of the cranial nerve V
    D. course between the inferior olivary nucleus and the spinal lemniscus
    E. emerge at the dorsolateral sulcus   A B C D E

13. Which of the following structures is(are) located adjacent to the midline of the medulla?

    A. Tectospinal tract   D. None of the above
    B. Medial longitudinal fasciculus E. All of the above
    C. Medial lemniscus   A B C D E

ANSWERS, NOTES, AND EXPLANATIONS

1. C The medial longitudinal fasciculus originates in the vestibular nuclear complex. The fibers making up this tract ascend and descend on the same and opposite sides of the brain stem. The other fasciculi mentioned are located in the cerebrum.

2. A The abducens nucleus is located in the floor of the fourth ventricle at the inferior end of the median eminence. Fibers from the motor nucleus of the facial nerve loop over this nucleus and form a slight swelling, called the facial colliculus. The motor nucleus of the facial nerve lies deep in the tegmentum of the pons, as does the medial lemniscus. The rubrospinal tract and the nucleus ambiguus lie deep within the tegmentum of the medulla.

3. B In the medulla, axons of neurons in the nucleus gracilis and nucleus cuneatus are known as internal arcuate fibers as they curve around the central gray matter to cross the midline in the decussation of the

medial lemniscus. In the medulla this tract is situated between the midline and the inferior olivary nucleus.

4. D. The ventral trigeminothalamic tract conducts impulses for pain, temperature, light touch (simple touch), and pressure sensations from the head area. The tract originates in the spinal nucleus of the trigeminal nerve (CN V), which is situated in the caudal end of the pons, medulla, and cephalic end of the spinal cord. Soon after emerging from the nucleus, the fibers cross obliquely to the opposite side of the brain stem, and the resulting trigeminothalamic tract terminates in the ventral posterior nucleus of the thalamus. Impulses for light touch on the left side of the face are therefore transmitted by the right trigeminothalamic tract because the constituent fibers are crossed with respect to their source and termination.

5. E The corticospinal tract descends from the middle three-fifths of the basis pedunculi into the basal portion of the pons. The tract is broken up into many small fasciculi as it passes through the basilar pons. The fasciculi begin to converge in the caudal region of the pons and form a compact tract or mass of fibers in the medullary pyramid.

6. C The cerebral aqueduct is a narrow channel extending from the third ventricle in the diencephalon, through the midbrain or mesencephalon, to the fourth ventricle.

7. E The lateral lemniscus is an auditory pathway (special sensory pathway) from the cochlear nuclei to the nucleus of the inferior colliculus. The auditory data are relayed from the inferior colliculus to the medial geniculate nucleus of the thalamus, and from it to the auditory area of the cortex.

8. D Axons of neurons in the inferior olivary, arcuate, lateral cuneate, reticular, trigeminal, and red nuclei of the brain stem project to the cerebellar cortex and nuclei via the inferior cerebellar peduncles.

9. B The superior cerebellar peduncles (brachia conjunctiva), the major efferent pathways from the cerebellum, originate from the cerebellar nuclei and pass rostrally through the midbrain to terminate in the contralateral ventral lateral nucleus of the thalamus. The peduncles "sink into" the brain stem just caudal to the inferior colliculi and undergo a prominent crossing over in the tegmentum, called the decussation of the brachia conjunctiva, between the periaqueductal gray and the inter- peduncular fossa. Having crossed the midline, the fibers terminate in the red nucleus or pass through and around it on their way to the ventral lateral nucleus of the thalamus. Fibers from this nucleus project to motor areas of the cerebral cortex.

10. E The spinal trigeminal nucleus (nucleus of the spinal tract of the trigeminal nerve) receives impulses for pain, temperature, touch, and pressure from the head region. The majority of afferent fibers to this nucleus are from CN V. However, the facial glossopharyngeal, and vagus fibers for the above sensations from the skin around the ear, the external auditory meatus, middle ear, posterior one-third of the tongue, and the walls of the pharynx terminate in the spinal trigeminal

nucleus. This nucleus projects to the contralateral ventral posterior nucleus of the thalamus by way of the trigeminothalamic tract.

11. A The tectum (L. roof) of the midbrain is made up of the corpora quadrigemina (four rounded elevations known as the superior and inferior colliculi). The colliculi indicate the extent of the midbrain on the dorsal surface. The superior colliculi are involved in the voluntary control of ocular movements and in movements of the eyes and head in response to visual and other stimuli. The other structures given as choices are located in the tegmental area of the midbrain. The tegmentum and basis pedunculi form the cerebral peduncle.

12. A Fibers from the hypoglossal nucleus, which is located primarily in the floor of the IVth ventricle between the dorsal vagal nucleus and the midline of the medulla, course ventrally through the medulla on the lateral side of the medial lemniscus. These fibers emerge along the sulcus between the pyramid and the olive. The hypoglossal nerve supplies the intrinsic muscles of the tongue and three of its extrinsic muscles (genioglossus, styloglossus, and hypoglossus).

13. E There is a vertical column of fiber tracts on each side of the midline of the medulla. This column extends dorsally from the pyramid to the hypoglossal nucleus in the floor of the IVth ventri- cle. The medial longitudinal fasciculus occupies the most dorsal part of the column; the medial lemniscus makes up its ventral two-thirds, and the tectospinal tract is between them.

M U L T I - C O M P L E T I O N   Q U E S T I O N S

DIRECTIONS: In each of the following questions or incomplete statements, one or more of the completions given is correct. At the lower right of each question, underline A if 1, 2, and 3 are correct; B if 1 and 3 are correct; C if 2 and 4 are correct; D if only 4 is correct; and E if all are correct.

---

1. The medial lemniscus originates from the

    1. dorsal cochlear nucleus
    2. nucleus gracilis
    3. ventral cochlear nucleus
    4. nucleus cuneatus   A B C D E

2. In which of the following nuclei may neurons be considered to form a final common pathway?

    1. Olivary nucleus
    2. Cochlear nucleus
    3. Cuneate nucleus
    4. Spinal accessory nucleus   A B C D E

A	B	C	D	E
1,2,3	1,3	2,4	only 4	all correct

3. The corticospinal tract crosses to the opposite side of central nervous system in the

   1. pons
   2. medulla
   3. midbrain
   4. spinal cord   A B C D E

4. The inferior brachium connects which structures?

   1. Superior colliculus
   2. Inferior colliculus
   3. Lateral geniculate body
   4. Medial geniculate body   A B C D E

5. The left middle cerebellar peduncle is made up of fibers from neurons in the:

   1. left cerebral cortex
   2. right cerebral cortex
   3. left basal pons
   4. right basal pons   A B C D E

6. Impulses for light touch sensation from the head area reach the brain stem via the

   1. trigeminal nerve
   2. facial nerve
   3. glossopharngeal nerve
   4. accessory nerve   A B C D E

7. Which of the following tracts is (are) located in the basis pedunculi of the midbrain?

   1. Corticopontine
   2. Corticospinal
   3. Corticobulbar
   4. Corticothalamic   A B C D E

8. Which of the following structures develop from the myelencephalon?

   1. Inferior olivary nucleus
   2. Hypoglossal nucleus
   3. Cuneate nucleus
   4. Facial colliculus   A B C D E

9. The ventral spinocerebellar tract is found in the

   1. spinal cord
   2. pons
   3. medulla
   4. midbrain   A B C D E

10. The junction of the spinal cord and medulla is at the

    1. upper rootlet of the second cervical nerve
    2. upper rootlet of the first cervical nerve
    3. level of the atlas
    4. level of the foramen magnum   A B C D E

11. In the medulla, the spinal lemniscus is composed of the following tract(s):

    1. spinothalamic
    2. spinoreticular
    3. spinotectal
    4. spino-olivary   A B C D E

A	B	C	D	E
1,2,3	1,3	2,4	only 4	all correct

12. Following a left hemisection through the pons, which of the following would be paralyzed?

    1. Right lateral rectus muscle
    2. Left lateral rectus muscle
    3. Muscles in the left upper limb
    4. Muscles in the right upper limb   A B C D E

13. The inferior cerebellar peduncle contains which of the following?

    1. Ventral spinocerebellar tract
    2. Dorsal spinocerebellar tract
    3. Brachium pontis
    4. Olivocerebellar fibers   A B C D E

14. In a right hemisection of the caudal pons, there would be damage to the

    1. trapezoid body
    2. spinothalamic tract
    3. medial longitudinal fasciculus
    4. spinal tract of the trigeminal nerve   A B C D E

15. Which of the following tracts originate in the midbrain?

    1. Tectospinal
    2. Central tegmental
    3. Rubrospinal
    4. Ventral trigeminothalamic   A B C D E

ANSWERS, NOTES, AND EXPLANATIONS

1. C 2 and 4 are correct. In the medulla, axons of cells from the nucleus gracilis and nucleus cuneatus (dorsal column nuclei) pursue a curved
course to the median raphe as internal arcuate fibers. After crossing the midline (the decussation of the medial lemniscus), the fibers immediately turn rostrally in the medial lemniscus. This tract traverses the brain stem and ends in the ventral posterior nucleus of the thalamus.

2. D Only 4 is correct. Axons of neurons in the cranial (nucleus ambiguus) and spinal (ventral horn C1 - C6) nuclei of the accessory nerve (CN XI) leave the medulla and spinal cord to innervate the intrinsic muscles of the larynx and muscles of the soft palate, and the trapezius and sternocleidomastoid muscles, respectively. Neurons of the central nervous system that end in striated skeletal muscles are lower motor neurons and they constitute the final common pathway (Sherrington).

65

3. C <u>2 and 4 are correct.</u> Most fibers of the corticospinal tracts begin to decussate or cross in the midline of the medulla (decussation of the pyramidal tracts). Some fibers cross more caudally (in the cephalic end of the spinal cord). Therefore the decussation of the pyramids is near the junction of the spinal cord and medulla.

4. C <u>2 and 4 are correct.</u> The inferior brachium is an elevation at the side of the midbrain, produced by fibers passing from the inferior colliculus to the medial geniculate body. The latter is a relay station in the auditory pathway. Fibers from the cochlear nuclei project to the inferior colliculus, which in turn projects to the medial geniculate body. Axons of neurons in the medial geniculate body proceed to the auditory area of cortex (anterior transverse temporal gyri).

5. D <u>Only 4 is correct.</u> The middle cerebellar peduncle (brachium pontis) consists of axons of small and medium-sized polygonal cells in the pontine nuclei located in the basal portion of the pons. Their axons cross the midline, forming the conspicuous transverse bundles of pontocerebellar fibers, and enter the cerebellum. As the ponto-cerebellar fibers approach the cerebellum, they form the large middle cerebellar peduncle.

6. A <u>1, 2, and 3 are correct.</u> Impulses concerned with general senses (pain, temperature, touch, and pressure) from the head area are conducted to the central nervous system by the trigeminal, facial, glossopharyngeal, and vagus nerves. The trigeminal nerve (CN V) provides sensory innervation for most of the head, whereas the other nerves supply the external ear, including the external acoustic meatus, the middle ear, the auditory tube, the pharynx, and the posterior one-third of the tongue. Axons of neurons from the semilunar ganglion (CN V) geniculate ganglion (CN VII), superior ganglia (CN IX and CN X), enter the brain stem and form the trigeminal spinal tract, which runs caudally in the dorsolateral area of the pons, medulla, and the cephalic end of the spinal cord. The fibers terminate in the adjacent nucleus of the trigeminal spinal tract.

7. A <u>1, 2, and 3 are correct.</u> The basis pedunculi consists of descending fibers of the pyramidal and corticopontine systems. Pyramidal fibers, most of them corticospinal, make up the middle three-fifths of this peduncle. Corticopontine fibers are divided into two large fasciculi, the frontopontine occupying the medial one-fifth and the parieto-temporopontine occupying the lateral one-fifth of the basis pedunculi. The less numerous corticobulbar fibers are located between the corticospinal and frontopontine tracts.

8. A <u>1, 2, and 3 are correct.</u> The medulla develops from the myelencephalon, one of the secondary brain vesicles. The inferior olivary nucleus, hypoglossal nucleus, and cuneate nucleus are part of the medulla. The facial colliculus, which is formed by motor fibers of the facial nerve looping over the abducens nucleus, is located in the floor of the fourth ventricle at the level of the pons.

9. E All are correct. The ventral spinocerebellar tract is a doubly crossed tract (the fibers first cross in the spinal cord) which ascends in the ventrolateral white column of the spinal cord, traverses the medulla in the periphery of the lateral area, continues through the pons and into the midbrain, and enters the cerebellum along the side of the superior cerebellar peduncle. The ventral spinocerebellar fibers again cross to the opposite side after entering the cerebellum.

10. C 2 and 4 are correct. The junction of the spinal cord and medulla is at the upper rootlet of the first cervical nerve, which is at the level of the foramen magnum. The spinal cord seems to pass imperceptibly into the medulla, insofar as surface markings are concerned. However, there is an abrupt and extensive rearrangement of the gray matter and white matter in the medulla.

11. B 1 and 3 are correct. In the medulla, the spinothalamic tract and the spinotectal tract traverse the lateral area of the medulla, dorsal to the inferior olivary nucleus. They are so close to one another that the combined tracts are called the spinal lemniscus in this location and throughout the remainder of the brain stem. The spinothalamic tract and the medial lemniscus terminate in the ventral posterior thalamic nucleus. They provide for general sensibility for the body, exclusive of the head.

12. C 2 and 4 are correct. When the pons is hemisected, all the structures on that side are damaged. The ascending sensory and descending motor tracts are interrupted and the nuclear areas are destroyed. As the left side is damaged here, the trigeminal, abducens, and facial motor nuclei are destroyed. This results in the paralysis of the muscles they supply. The left corticospinal tract crosses to the right side in the medulla (decussation of the pyramidal tract) and controls the musculature in the limbs on the right side. This tract was interrupted in the basal portion of the pons.

13. C 2 and 4 are correct. The inferior cerebellar peduncle lies on the medial aspect of the middle cerebellar peduncle, helping to form the lateral wall of the fourth ventricle. The large lateral area of the peduncle consists of olivocerebellar and dorsal spinocerebellar tract fibers, cuneocerebellar fibers from the lateral cuneate nucleus, fibers from the arcuate nucleus and the reticular formation of the medulla, and fibers from the chief sensory nucleus and the nucleus of the spinal tract of the trigeminal nerve. The medial part contains vestibular, vestibulocerebellar fibers (afferent), as well as fastigiovestibular fibers (efferent).

14. E All are correct. If the right half of the pons is damaged, all the ascending sensory and descending motor tracts are interrupted (as discussed in question 12). This involves all of the structures listed as well as other unlisted tracts.

15. A 1, 2, and 3 are correct. The tectospinal tract originates in the contralateral superior colliculus of the midbrain tectum. It courses near the midline of the pons and medulla and into the ventral column of white matter of the spinal cord. The central tegmental tract

67

originates from the red nucleus, corpus striatum, and probably other gray areas. It courses through the tegmental area of the midbrain and pons to terminate on the inferior olivary complex of the medulla. Fibers of the rubrospinal tract originate in the contralateral red nucleus of the midbrain, and terminate in laminae V, VI, and VII of Rexed in the cervical cord and the superior portion of the thoracic region of the spinal cord. The ventral trigeminothalamic tract originates in the nucleus of the spinal trigeminal tract, none of which is in the midbrain.

F I V E - C H O I C E   A S S O C I A T I O N   Q U E S T I O N S

DIRECTIONS: Each of the following groups of questions consists of a numbered list of descriptive words or phrases accompanied by a diagram with certain parts indicated by letters, or by a list of lettered headings. For each numbered word or phrase, SELECT THE LETTERED PART OR HEADING that matches it correctly and insert the letter in the space to the right of the appropriate number. Each lettered heading may be selected once, more than once, or not at all.

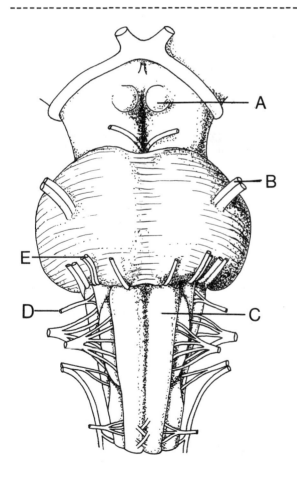

1.___Composed of corticospinal tract fibers

2.___Innervates the temporalis muscle

3.___Originates from the nucleus ambiguus

4.___Innervates the buccinator muscle

5.___Its fibers originate in the cortex of the right cerebral hemisphere

6.___Innervates the stylopharyngeus muscle

7.___Secretomotor and vasodilator to the parotid gland

(Modified from Barr, M.L. and Kiernan, J.A.; The Human Nervous System, 4th ed., 1983. Courtesy of Harper & Row, Publishers, Inc.)

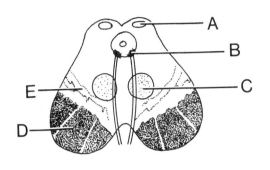

8.___Receives fibers from cerebellar nuclei

9.___Conducts impulses for proprioception from the contralateral side of the body

10.___Controls muscles in the contralateral upper limb

11.___Controls the medial rectus muscle

12.___A reflex center for eye and head movements in response to visual stimuli

13.___Originates in the ipsilateral cerebral cortex

14.___Originates from the nucleus cuneatus and nucleus gracilis

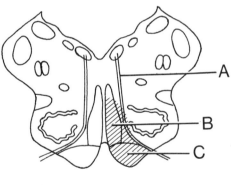

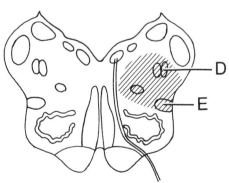

15.___Loss of proprioception on the contralateral side of the body

16.___Damage to____causes deviation of the tongue to the same side as the lesion

17.___Causes a spastic paralysis of the contralateral muscles of the upper limb

18.___Loss of pain and temperature sensations in the head area on the same side as the lesion

19.___Loss of pain and temperature sensations on the contralateral side of the body

20.___Loss of discriminative touch on the contralateral side of the body

21.___Terminates on contralateral ventral horn cells in the cervical and lumbosacral enlargements of the spinal cord

ANSWERS, NOTES, AND EXPLANATIONS

1. C The pyramid consists of descending corticospinal fibers of the pyramidal tract.

2. B The motor division of the trigeminal nerve (CN V) innervates the muscles of mastication through the mandibular division of the trigeminal nerve. In the illustration, note that the sensory division of this nerve lies caudal to the motor division.

3. D The glossopharyngeal nerve (CN IX) has sensory and motor components. The motor fibers originates in the rostral portion of the nucleus ambiguus and the sensory fibers come from the superior and inferior ganglia of the glossopharyngeal nerve.

4. E The facial nerve (CN VII) is a mixed nerve with sensory and motor components. The motor division supplies the muscles of facial expression, as well as the buccinator muscle, and includes secreto-motor fibers for the lacrimal, submandibular, and submaxillary glands. The sensory division conducts impulses for pain, temperature, touch, and pressure, from the external ear, and impulses for taste from the anterior two-thirds of the tongue.

5. C The pyramid of the medulla marks the location of corticospinal fibers of the pyramidal tract. The fibers originate in the cerebral cortex of the same side as the pyramid. At the junction of the medulla and spinal cord, about 85 percent of the fibers cross the midline in the decussation of the pyramids and form the lateral corticospinal tract. The remaining fibers form the ventral corticospinal tract.

6. D The glossopharyngeal nerve (CN IX) supplies the stylopharyngeus muscle. The motor fibers of this nerve originate in the anterior part of the nucleus ambiguus. CN IX leaves the skull via the jugular foramen in company with the Xth and XIth cranial nerves.

7. D Fibers originating in the inferior salvitory nucleus of the medulla are included in the glossopharyngeal nerve. They constitute the para-symphatic nerve supply to the parotid gland, and have secretomotor and vasodilator functions.

8. C Fibers originating in certain cerebellar nuclei (dentate, globose, and emboliform) constitute the superior cerebellar peduncle (brachium conjunctivum). They enter the midbrain where they cross to the opposite side. Some of the fibers terminate in the red nucleus, especially the large celled portion, whereas the majority of the fibers pass through and around the red nucleus en route to the ventral lateral nucleus of the thalamus.

9. E The medial lemniscus conducts impulses for proprioception, dis-criminative touch, and vibration from the opposite side of the body. This tract originates in the nucleus gracilis and nucleus cuneatus, crosses to the opposite side in the medulla, and terminates in the ventral lateral nucleus of the thalamus.

10. D The corticospinal tract is located in the <u>middle three-fifths</u> of the basis pedunculi. It descends through the pons and medulla and decussates to the opposite side (about 85 percent of its fibers) to end on ventral horn cells in the spinal cord. Voluntary control of muscles is a function of both the pyramidal (corticospinal) and extrapyramidal systems, the former conferring agility and precision, and being especially important in controlling movements of the digits.

11. B Fibers from the oculomotor nucleus innervate the extraocular muscles, with the exception of the superior oblique and the lateral rectus muscles, which are supplied by the trochlear (CN IV) and abducens (CN VI) nerves, respectively.

12. A The superior colliculus is primarily a reflex center for <u>movements of the eyes and head</u> in response to visual and other stimuli. Afferents to this area are mainly through the superior brachium. Efferents from the superior colliculus form the tectospinal tract which is distributed to ventral horn cells in the cervical region of the spinal cord, as well as to the spinal nucleus of the CN XI.

13. D Axons of pyramidal cells (for the most part) in motor areas of the cerebral cortex course through the internal capsule and into the middle three-fifths of the basis pedunculi of the midbrain as corticospinal and corticobulbar tracts. These pyramidal fibers run through the basal portion of the pons and the corticospinal fibers form the pyramid in the medulla. They then cross to the opposite side and end on ventral horn cells in the spinal cord.

14. E Axons of neurons in the nucleus cuneatus and nucleus gracilis enter the tegmental region of the medulla and cross in the midline (decussation of medial lemniscus) to form <u>the medial lemniscus</u>. This tract ascends through the brain stem and terminates in the <u>ventral posterior nucleus of the thalamus</u>. In the midbrain, the medial lemniscus is located superolateral to the substantia nigra.

15. B The right medial lemniscus is damaged so that there would be a loss of discriminative touch, vibration, and proprioceptive sensations on the left side of the body.

16. A The right hypoglossal nerve is damaged in the above lesion so there would be flaccid paralysis and eventual atrophy of the intrinsic muscles of the tongue on that side. The tongue would deviate to the paralyzed side because of the unopposed protrusor action of the unaffected left (i.e., opposite) genioglossus muscle.

17. C Damage to the corticospinal fibers at the level of the pyramid causes <u>paresis (partial paralysis) of the contralateral muscles</u> of the the upper and lower limbs. Interruption of the pyramid would likely produce contralateral hemiparesis with flaccidity. There would be good recovery in time, except for impairment of use of the digits in skilled movements. The complete upper motor neuron lesion, with spastic paralysis, is a consequence of involvement of both the pyramidal and extrapyramidal motor systems.

18. D The spinal tract and nucleus of the fifth cranial nerve (CN V) is damaged in the lesion. Impulses for pain, temperature, touch, and pressure from the head area are conducted into the brain stem by the fifth, seventh, ninth, and tenth cranial nerves. The axons of the general sensory divisions of these nerves form the spinal tract of the fifth nerve, the fibers of which synapse in the subjacent nucleus of the spinal tract. The deficit is on the same side of the head as the lesion because the sensory pathway for the thalamus eventually crosses.

19. E In the medulla the spinothalamic and spinotectal tracts form the spinal lemniscus, superolateral to the olive. The spinothalamic tract conducts pain, touch, and temperature data from the contralateral side of the body because it is a crossed pathway (in the spinal cord). This tract is damaged in this lesion, hence there is loss of pain, touch, and temperature sensations on the contralateral side of the body.

20. B The right medial lemniscus is damaged; thus there would be a loss of discriminative touch, vibration, and proprioceptive sensations on the left side of the body.

21. C Corticospinal fibers (about 85 percent) in the pyramids of the caudal end of the medulla, cross to the opposite side (decussation of the pyramids), and descend into the lateral column of white matter in the spinal cord as the lateral corticospinal tract. These fibers turn in and synapse on cells mainly in laminae IV through VII of Rexed, and a few established direct connections on lateral anterior horn cells in the cervical and lumbosacral enlargements of the spinal cord.

SIX

The Cranial Nerves

O B J E C T I V E S

BE ABLE TO:

* List the cranial nerves and indicate whether they are sensory, motor, or mixed nerves.

* Name the cranial nerves that have autonomic (parasympathetic) components.

* List the nuclei of cranial nerves which are situated in the medulla, pons, and midbrain, respectively.

* Give a brief account of the functions of each of the cranial nerves.

* Prepare simple schematic diagrams of the brain stem as viewed from the dorsal and/or median surfaces to show the location of the cranial nerve nuclei.

* Give a brief account of the cranial nerve nuclei that develop from the basal and alar plates of the embryonic brain stem.

* Make a sketch of the ventral and dorsal surfaces of the brain stem showing the sites of attachment of the cranial nerves.

* Draw transverse sections through various levels of the medulla, pons, and midbrain to show the nuclei of the cranial nerves, as well as the course of the fibers within the brain stem emanating from the motor nuclei.

* Identify the cranial nerve nuclei located in the floor of the fourth ventricle.

* State the clinical consequences of damage to the third, fourth, sixth and seventh cranial nerves.

* Identify the cranial nerves that would probably be affected by thrombosis of: (1) the posterior inferior cerebellar artery, and (2) the terminal portion of the basilar artery or the proximal portion of the posterior cerebral artery.

Note: This chapter is concerned with the cranial nerves that are attached to the brain stem, exclusive of the vestibulocochlear nerve. The olfactory, optic, and vestibulocochlear nerves are also dealt with in Chapters 15 to 18.

* List the fiber tracts that terminate in the cranial nerve nuclei which have motor components.

* Give a brief account of the symptoms that a patient would present following a unilateral lesion in the medulla, pons, or midbrain affecting the various cranial nerve nuclei.

* Describe the clinical signs and the sites of lesions with respect to Bell's palsy and Weber's syndrome.

* Classify the cranial nerves under the following functional headings: general somatic afferent, special somatic afferent, general visceral afferent, special visceral afferent, general somatic efferent, general visceral efferent, and special vsiceral efferent.

F I V E - C H O I C E   C O M P L E T I O N   Q U E S T I O N S

DIRECTIONS: Each of the following questions or incomplete statements is followed by five suggested answers or completions. SELECT THE ONE BEST ANSWER OR COMPLETION in each case and underline the appropriate letter at the right.

----

1. Sensory fibers of the fifth cranial nerve are located in the

    A. midbrain   D. spinal cord
    B. pons   E. all of the above
    C. medulla   A B C D E

2. The important cranial nerves in deglutition arise in the

    A. midbrain   D. superior cervial cord
    B. pons   E. all of the above
    C. medulla   A B C D E

3. Pain and temperature sensations from the head area reach the brain stem by way of

    A. cranial nerve III   D. cranial nerve VI
    B. cranial nerve IV   E. cranial nerve XII
    C. cranial nerve V   A B C D E

4. Postganglionic parasymnpathetic fibers that control the sphincter pupillae muscles of the eyes arise from the

    A. otic ganglion   D. ciliary ganglion
    B. submandibular ganglion E. superior cervical
    C. celiac ganglion   ganglion   A B C D E

5. The superior part of the nucleus of the right facial nerve contains cell bodies of lower motor neurons for muscles in

    A. the upper right face   D. the lower left face
    B. the upper left face   E. both right and left
    C. the lower right face   upper face regions A B C D E

74

6. Preganglionic fibers ending in the ciliary ganglion originate in the

   A. thalamus
   B. midbrain
   C. pons
   D. medulla
   E. thoracic spinal cord

   A B C D E

7. Axons of neurons of the left fourth cranial nerve emerge from the

   A. ventral surface of the left side of the midbrain
   B. ventral surface of the right side of the midbrain
   C. dorsal surface of the left side of the midbrain
   D. dorsal surface of the right side of the midbrain
   E. interpeduncular fossa

   A B C D E

8. The nucleus ambiguus develops from the

   A. telencephalon
   B. diencephalon
   C. mesencephalon
   D. metencephalon
   E. myelencephalon

   A B C D E

9. The following nuclei are located in the tegmental gray matter of the pons:

   A. Red
   B. Trochlear
   C. Oculomotor
   D. Abducens
   E. None of the above

   A B C D E

10. Which statement is NOT correct for the dorsal vagal nucleus?

   A. Located in the medulla
   B. Controls the muscles of the stomach
   C. Is stimulated by the anterior and median hypothalamic nuclei
   D. Axons from this nucleus exit through the jugular foramen
   E. Controls the muscles of the pharynx

   A B C D E

11. The glossopharyngeal nerve is composed of

   A. general visceral efferents
   B. special visceral efferents
   C. general somatic afferents
   D. special visceral afferents
   E. all of the above

   A B C D E

12. Damage to the left abducens nucleus causes

   A. adduction of the left eye
   B. abduction of the left eye
   C. adduction of the right eye
   D. abduction of the right eye
   E. elevation of the right eye

   A B C D E

13. The cell bodies of the preganglionic parasympathetic
    fibers to the heart are located in the

    A. Edingar-Westphal nucleus   D. inferior salivatory
    B. dorsal vagal nucleus   nucleus
    C. nucleus solitarius   E. none of the above   A B C D E

14. The vagus nerve does not supply the

    A. cricothyroid muscle   D. middle pharyngeal
    B. stylopharyngeus muscle   constrictor muscle
    C. muscles of the stomach   E. muscles of the duodenum   A B C D E

ANSWERS, NOTES, AND EXPLANATIONS

1. E The sensory fibers of the trigeminal nerve enter the lateral portion
    of the pons (junction of the basal portion of pons and the beginning of
    the middle cerebellar peduncle), and descend in the tegmental portion
    of the pons and medulla into the cephalic end of the spinal cord. This
    forms the spinal root of the fifth cranial nerve. These fibers synapse
    on neurons in the spinal tract of the fifth cranial nerve which lies
    immediately adjacent to these fibers. Pain, touch (discriminative and
    light), pressure, and temperature sensations are conducted in this part
    of the trigeminal nerve. Fibers for discriminative touch terminate
    solely in the chief sensory nucleus.   The fibers that conduct
    sensations for proprioception enter the pons at the same position as
    the above fibers, but ascend into the tegmental area of the midbrain as
    the mesencephalic portion of the fifth cranial nerve. These fibers are
    an exception to the general rule in that they consist of primary
    sensory neurons.

2. C In deglutition (swallowing), muscles of the pharynx, soft palate,
    and tongue come into action. These muscles are supplied by the glosso-
    opharyngeal, vagus, accessory, and hypoglossal nerves.   The nucleus
    ambiguus and the hypoglossal nucleus, containing their cells of origin,
    are located in the central gray (tegmental) area of the medulla.

3. C Impulses concerning pain and temperature sensations are conducted
    into the brain stem by the sensory divisions of the trigeminal, facial,
    glossopharyngeal, and vagus nerves.   The fifth cranial nerve conducts
    these sensations from most of the anterior part of the head, with the
    exception of the posterior one-third of the tongue, the pharynx, the
    middle and external ears, and the skin posterior to the ear. These
    areas are supplied by the glossopharngeal, vagus, and facial nerves,
    respectively.

4. D The sphincter pupillae muscles of the eyes are controlled by the
    parasymphatic and symphathetic nervous system.   Parasympathetic
    preganglionic fibers originate in the Edingar-Westphal nucleus of the

76

oculomotor nerve and pass with the motor fibers of that nerve into the orbit to synapse on neurons in the ciliary ganglion. Postganglionic fibers from this ganglion pass to the sphincter pupillae muscle of the eye. It produces pupillary constriction.

5. A The right facial nerve controls all the muscles of facial expression on the right side of the face. Axons of neurons from the superior part of the facial nucleus innervate the muscles of the forehead. Axons of neurons from the inferior half of the facial nucleus control the inferior muscles of facial expression (muscles around the mouth and nose).

6. B The Edingar-Westphal, or parasympathetic nucleus of the third cranial nerve, is at the rostral end of the oculomotor nucleus which is located in the periaqueductal gray matter of the midbrain at the level of the superior colliculus. Axons from this parasympathetic nucleus accompany motor fibers of the nerve through the tegmentum of the mid-brain, and emerge at the interpeduncular fossa. The nerve traverses the wall of cavernous sinus and enters the orbit through the superior orbital fissure. The preganglionic fibers synapse on neurons in the ciliary ganglion and postganglionic fibers course to the ciliary and sphincter pupillae muscles.

7. D The trochlear nuclei are located ventral to the aqueduct in the periaqueductal gray matter at the level of the inferior colliculi of the midbrain. The trochlear nerve fibers have an unusual course in that they wind around the periaqueductal gray matter with a caudal slope, decussate, and emerge from the dorsum of the midbrain posterior to the inferior colliculi.

8. E The nucleus ambiguus is situated in the central gray (tegmental) area of the medulla, dorsal to the inferior olivary nucleus. In the developing embryo, the medulla develops from the myelencephalon and its nuclei differentiate from its basal plates.

9. D In the tegmental gray matter of the pons (i.e., the dorsal pons), several nuclear areas are recognized. Some of them are as follows: the motor nuclei of the fifth, sixth, and seventh cranial nerves, the chief sensory nucleus, the superior portion of the spinal nucleus of the fifth cranial nerve, and the superior nucleus of the vestibular nuclear complex.

10. E The dorsal vagal nucleus is the parasympathetic nucleus of the vagus nerve (CN X). It supplies the smooth muscle and gland tissue of the gastrointestinal tract, as far as the descending colon, and the smooth muscle and gland cells of the respiratory system. The pharynx, the superior part of the esophagus, and the heart contain striated muscle which is supplied from the nucleus ambiguus via the vagus nerve.

11. E The glossopharyngeal nerve contains sensory and motor fibers. It is intimately related to the vagus nerve, the two having common intramedullary nuclei of origin, sites of termination, and similar functional components. The nerve contains: (1) a few general somatic

77

afferent fibers from the skin, posterior to the ear; (2) general visceral afferent fibers from the posterior one-third of the tongue, tonsil, pharynx, and auditory tube; (3) special visceral afferent fibers from the taste buds in the posterior one-third of the tongue; (4) general visceral efferents to the parotid gland; and (5) special visceral efferents to the stylopharyngeus muscle.

12. A The abducens nerve supplies the lateral rectus muscle of the eye. When this muscle contracts, along with the superior and inferior oblique muscles, there is horizontal deviation (abduction) away from the median plane. When the abducens nerve is paralyzed, the affected eye looks medially (adduction) because the normally functioning medial rectus muscle is unopposed.

13. E The dorsal vagal nucleus is the parasympathetic nucleus of the tenth cranial nerve. It supplies smooth muscle and gland tissue of the respiratory system and gastrointestinal tract as far as the beginning of the descending colon. The heart is supplied from the nucleus ambiguus via the vagus nerve.

14. B The vagus nerve supplies all the muscles listed except the stylopharyngeus muscle, which is the only muscle supplied by the glossopharyngeal nerve. The neurons concerned are in the rostral tip of the nucleus ambiguus; other cells in the nucleus supply the remaining muscles of the pharynx through the vagus nerve.

M U L T I - C O M P L E T I O N   Q U E S T I O N S

DIRECTIONS: In each of the following questions or incomplete statements, one or more of the completions given is correct. At the lower right of each question, underline A if 1, 2, and 3 are correct; B if 1 and 3 are correct; C if 2 and 4 are correct; D if only 4 is correct; and E if all are correct.

----

1. In the floor of the fourth ventricle the vestibular nuclei are located in the

    1. medial portion of the caudal pons
    2. lateral portion of the caudal pons
    3. medial portion of the medulla
    4. lateral portion of the medulla   A B C D E

2. Damage to the left hypoglossal nerve causes

    1. deviation of the tongue to the left side
    2. deviation of the tongue to the right side
    3. atrophy of tongue muscle on the left side
    4. atrophy of tongue muscles on the right side   A B C D E

78

A	B	C	D	E
1,2,3	1,3	2,4	only 4	all correct

3. A lesion of the right oculomotor nerve causes

    1. dilatation of the right pupil
    2. constriction of the right pupil
    3. lateral rotation of the right eye
    4. medial rotation of the right eye   A B C D E

4. The following cranial nerve nuclei lie immediately deep
   to the floor of the IVTH ventricle:

    1. Vestibular   3. Abducens
    2. Hypoglossal   4. Dorsal vagal   A B C D E

5. With respect to the nerve supply of the posterior one-
   third of the tongue, the

    1. facial nerve is for the sensation of taste
    2. vagus nerve is for taste sensation
    3. lingual nerve is for the sensation of pain
    4. glossopharyngeal nerve is for the sensation of pain   A B C D E

6. With a hemisection of the left side of the midbrain there
   would be

    1. spastic paralysis on the right side of the body
    2. spastic paralysis on the left side of the body
    3. loss of proprioception on the right side of the body
    4. loss of proprioception on the left side of the body   A B C D E

7. The facial nerve is concerned with

    1. taste sensation from the anterior two-thirds of the
       tongue
    2. pain and temperature sensations from the skin of the
       external ear
    3. innervation of the facial muscles
    4. innervation of the parotid gland   A B C D E

8. The following cranial nerve nuclei are situated in the pons:

    1. Trochlear
    2. Motor nucleus of trigeminal
    3. Dorsal vagal
    4. Motor nucleus of the facial   A B C D E

9. A large tumor in the right side of the IVth ventricle
   would destroy the

    1. abducens nucleus   3. vestibular nuclei
    2. facial nerve   4. nucleus ambiguus   A B C D E

A	B	C	D	E
1,2,3	1,3	2,4	only 4	all correct

10. The trigeminal spinal nucleus (nucleus of the spinal tract of the Vth cranial nerve) is concerned with

    1. pressure
    2. touch
    3. pain and temperature sensations
    4. proprioception   A B C D E

11. Fibers of the medial longitudinal fasciculus synapse in the following nuclei:

    1. Abducens   3. Trochlear
    2. Oculomotor   4. Facial   A B C D E

12. The accessory nerve controls the following muscles:

    1. Palatal   3. Trapezius
    2. Criothyroid   4. Platysma   A B C D E

13. Correct statements include:

    1. The oculomotor nerve supplies the superior rectus muscle
    2. The trigeminal nerve supplies the buccinator muscle
    3. The glossopharyngeal nerve supplies the stylopharyngeus muscle
    4. The abducens nerve supplies the medial rectus muscle   A B C D E

14. The dorsal vagus nucleus

    1. receives afferents from the anterior hypothalamic nuclei
    2. is partially located in the floor of the fourth ventricle
    3. controls the muscles of the jejunum
    4. controls the muscles of the pharynx   A B C D E

ANSWERS, NOTES, AND EXPLANATIONS

1. C 2 and 4 are correct. The sulcus limitans divides each half of the floor of the fourth ventricle into medial and lateral areas. The lateral area is called the vestibular area because the vestibular nuclear complex, consisting of superior, medial, lateral and inferior nuclei, lies immediately deep to it. The superior nucleus is in the pons and the remaining nuclei are in the medulla.

2. B 1 and 3 are correct. When the left hypoglossal nucleus or nerve is damaged, a flaccid paralysis and eventual atrophy of the muscles ensue on left side of the tongue. The tongue deviates to the paralyzed side on protrusion because of the unopposed protrusor action of the normal genioglossus muscle on the right side.

3. B 1 and 3 are correct. Interruption of the oculomotor nerve results in paralysis of the following muscles on the same side: superior, medial, and inferior recti, inferior oblique, and striated fibers of the levator palpebrae superioris. Parasympathetic fibers supplying the ciliary and sphincter pupillae muscles via the ciliary ganglion are likewise interrupted. The patient has an external strabismus (lateral squint) with respect to the affected eye because of the unopposed action of the lateral rectus muscle. The eye cannot be directed medially or vertically; there is drooping of the upper eyelid (ptosis), and the pupil is dilated.

4. E All are correct. The abducens, dorsal vagal, and hypoglossal nuclei lie beneath the medial area of the floor of the IVth ventricle, whereas the vestibular nuclear complex and part of the dorsal cochlear nucleus are beneath the lateral area.

5. D Only 4 is correct. Impulses for the general sensations of pain, temperature, touch, and pressure are conducted from the posterior one-third of the tongue to the brain stem by the glossopharyngeal nerve, as are impulses for the special sensation of taste. Impulses for general sensations reach the nucleus of the spinal tract of the trigeminal nerve, whereas those for taste reach the nucleus solitarius.

6. B 1 and 3 are correct. When the left side of the midbrain is damaged, all descending motor (pyramidal and extrapyramidal) tracts and ascending sensory tracts, as well as nuclear areas of gray matter, are affected in that area. The corticospinal, corticorubrospinal, and corticore- ticulospinal tracts control voluntary movements of the muscles in the upper and lower limbs on the contralateral side. This occurs because the tract decussates in the medulla and descends into the spinal cord to end on anterior horn cells in the cervical and lumbosacral enlargements. The paralysis is of a spastic type because it is the upper motor neuron that is affected. The medial lemniscus conducts proprioceptive, dis- criminative touch, and vibration sensations from the contralateral side of the body because the tract crosses to the contralateral side in the medulla.

7. A 1, 2, and 3 are correct. The facial nerve is a mixed nerve; it has general and special sensory components, as well as somatomotor and secretomotor components. Pain, temperature, touch, and pressure sensations from the skin of the external ear, a small area posterior to the external ear, the wall of the auditory canal, and the external surface of the tympanic membrane are conducted into the brain stem via this nerve. This nerve also conducts taste sensation from the anterior two-thirds of the tongue into the central nervous system. The facial nerve also supplies the muscles of facial expression and the buccinator muscle. The parasympathetic portion of the nerve stimulates secretion and causes vasodilation of the submaxillary, sublingual, and lacrimal glands.

8. C 2 and 4 are correct. In the tegmental area of the pons the following cranial nerve nuclei may be found: the motor nucleus, the chief sensory nucleus, the beginning portion of the spinal nucleus, and the beginning portion of the mesencephalic nucleus of the fifth cranial

nerve; the abducens nucleus, the motor nucleus of the seventh cranial nerve, the parasympathetic nucleus of the seventh cranial nerve (superior salivatory and lacrimal nucleus), and the rostral end of the vestibular area (superior vestibular nucleus).

9. A 1, 2, and 3 are correct. A tumor in the fourth ventricle could grow into the floor of the ventricle and damage or destroy structures in that area, such as the: abducens nucleus, medial longitudinal fasciculus (in the median eminence), vestibular nuclei, dorsal cochlear nucleus, dorsal vagal nucleus, hypoglossal nucleus, and fibers of the facial nerve as they curve over the abducens nucleus in the facial colliculus.

10. A 1, 2, and 3 are correct. The trigeminal spinal nucleus extends from the chief sensory nucleus to the caudal limit of the medulla. The nucleus is divided into three regions of subnuclei: the pars caudalis, pars interpolaris, and pars rostralis. The pars caudalis receives fibers for pain, touch, pressure, and temperature, those for pain and temperature predominating. The pars interpolaris and pars rostralis receive fibers mainly for touch (light or crude) and pressure sensibilities.

11. A 1, 2, and 3 are correct. Fibers from all of the vestibular nuclei form the medial longitudinal fasciculus which extends rostrally and caudally adjacent to the midline. The fasciculus is dorsal to the tectospinal tract. The fibers are both crossed and uncrossed but predominantly the latter. The ascending fibers terminate in the trochlear, oculomotor, and abducens nuclei. These connections have the important function of coordinating movements of the eyes and head. The medial longitudinal fasciculus also contains association fibers connecting nuclei of these cranial nerves. The descending portion of the fasciculus terminates in the ventral gray horn throughout the cervical cord, and alters the tonus of neck muscles in response to vestibular stimulation.

12. B 1 and 3 are correct. The accessory nerve, a motor nerve, has cranial and spinal portions. The cranial portion is distributed to muscles of the soft palate, except the tensor veli palatini, and the muscles of the larynx, except the cricothyroid. The fibers of this portion of the nerve originate in the nucleus ambiguus. The spinal portion supplies the trapezius and sternocleidomastoid muscles. Its nucleus is a column of cells in the lateral part of the anterior horn of the superior four or five cervical segments of the spinal cord.

13. B 1 and 3 are correct. The buccinator muscle is not a muscle of mastication, but it aids in mastication. Neither is it a muscle of facial expression, even though it develops from the same branchial arch (second) and is innervated by the same nerve (facial). The abducens nerve supplies only one muscle, the lateral rectus muscle of the eye.

14. A 1, 2, and 3 are correct. The muscles of the pharynx are supplied by the pharyngeal plexus which is made up of terminal branches of the glossopharyngeal and vagus nerves. The glossopharyngeal nerve supplies the stylopharyngeus muscle and the vagus nerve supplies the remaining

pharyngeal muscles. The motor nucleus for these nerves is the nucleus ambiguus. A few neurons in the rostral tip of the nucleus constitute the motor portion of the glossopharyngeal nerve and neurons more caudally situated give rise to the motor fibers of the vagus nerve.

FIVE-CHOICE ASSOCIATION QUESTIONS

DIRECTIONS: Each of the following groups of questions consists of a numbered list of descriptive words or phrases accompanied by a diagram with certain parts indicated by letters, or by a list of lettered headings. For each numbered word or phrase, SELECT THE LETTERED PART OR HEADING that matches it correctly and insert the letter in the space to the right of the appropriate number. Each lettered heading may be selected once, more than once, or not at all.

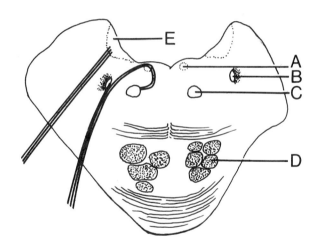

1. ____Supplies the muscles of facial expression

2. ____These fibers form the pyramids in the medulla

3. ____Controls the lateral rectus muscles

4. ____Receives fibers for light touch

5. ____Receives sensations originating the semicircular ducts

6. ____Fibers from this area form the medial longitudinal fasciculus

7. ____Axons from this nucleus form the ventral trigeminothalamic tract

83

ASSOCIATION QUESTIONS

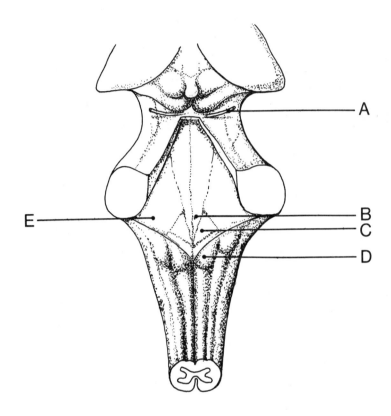

8. ____Fibers from it innervate muscles that move the tongue

9. ____Receives impulses for discriminative touch from the same side of the body

10. ____Supplies the superior oblique muscle of the eye

11. ____Innervates the muscles of the stomach

12. ____Fibers from what nucleus project to the contralateral ventral posterior nucleus of the thalamus

13. ____Fibers arising deep to this area form the medial longitudinal fasciculus

14. ____Influences the mucosal glands of the duodenum

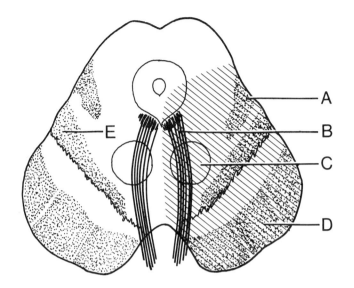

The brain stem has
been damaged in the
cross hatched area
indicated in this
diagram.

15. ____ Damage to the red nucleus
16. ____ Droooping of the eyelid on the same side as the lesion
17. ____ Loss of proprioceptive sensation on the contralateral side of the body
18. ____ Loss of pain and temperature sensations on the contralateral side of
         the body
19. ____ Spastic paralysis of the muscles of the upper limb on the contra-
         lateral side of the body
20. ____ Loss of discriminative touch on the contralateral side of the body
21. ____ Dilation of the pupil

ANSWERS, NOTES, AND EXPLANATIONS

1. C The motor nucleus of the facial nerve supplies the muscles of facial
       expression and the buccinator muscle. Fibers from the nucleus curve
       over the abducens nucleus, deep to the floor of the fourth ventricle,
       then course inferiorly and laterally to emerge well laterally at the
       caudal border of the pons.

2. D Corticospinal fibers traversing the basal portion of the pons enter
       the pons from the basis pedunculi of the midbrain and leave it to form
       the pyramids in the medulla.

3. A Fibers from the abducens nucleus supply the lateral rectus muscle.

4. B The trigeminal spinal tract, composed of sensory fibers from the fifth, seventh, ninth and tenth cranial nerves, conducts impulses for pain and temperature and touch and pressure sensations into the subjacent nucleus of the spinal trigeminal tract. The sensory data are relayed to the ventral posterior nucleus of the thalamus by the ventral trigeminothalamic tract.

5. E Axons of cells in the vestibular ganglion form the vestibular nerve, which enters the brain stem posterior to the middle cerebellar peduncle (brachium pontis) and terminates on neurons in the vestibular nuclei. The superior vestibular nucleus is located in the caudal region of the pons, whereas the other vestibular nuclei are in the medulla.

6. E Fibers from the vestibular nuclei for the medial longitudinal fasciculus (also see the explanation given for question 6).

7. B Axons of neurons in the nucleus of the spinal tract of the fifth cranial nerve form the ventral trigeminothalamic tract, which crosses to the opposite side. The tract ascends through the pons and midbrain to terminate on the ventral posterior nucleus of the thalamus. The ventral trigeminothalamic tract conducts impulses for pain, temperature, touch, and pressure to the thalamus.

8. B Fibers from the hypoglossal nucleus course through the medulla to emerge along the ventrolateral sulcus. The hypoglossal nerve passes through the anterior condyloid canal in the floor of the posterior cranial fossa and then runs anteriorly to innervate the muscles of the tongue.

9. D The fasciculus gracilis occupies the medial portion of the dorsal white column, and its fibers that function for discriminative touch terminate in the nucleus gracilis. This nucleus is located in an elevation at the rostral end of the fasciculus gracilis known as the gracile tubercle. The caudal fasciculus gracilis is concerned with proprioception, discriminative touch, and vibration, whereas the rostral fasciculus gracilis is concerned only with discriminative touch on the same side of the body.

10. A The trochlear nerve supplies the superior oblique muscle of the eye. Its fibers originate in the contralateral trochlear nucleus. It is the only cranial nerve to emerge on the dorsal aspect of the brain stem.

11. C The dorsal vagal nucleus supplies the muscles of the inferior part of the esophagus, stomach, small intestine, cecum, and colon as far as the descending limb. It also supplies the mucosal glands and associated glands of that part of the gastrointestinal tract and smooth muscles of the respiratory system.

12. D Fibers from the nucleus gracilis, and the nucleus cuneatus, pursue a curved course to the median raphe as internal arcuate fibers, cross the midline in the decussation of the medial lemniscus, and turn rostrally as the medial lemniscus. After traversing the pons and midbrain, the the tract ends in the ventral posterior nucleus of the thalamus.

13. E Fibers from the vestibular nuclei, some crossed and some uncrossed, ascend in the medial longituidinal fasciculus and terminate in the abducens, trochlear, and oculomotor nuclei. Fibers from the medial vestibular nuclei run caudally in the descending portion of the medial longitudinal fasciculus and terminate on ventral horn cells in the spinal cord.

14. C The dorsal vagal nucleus influences the mucosal glands of the duodenum (also see the explanation above for question 11).

15. C This extensive lesion in the midbrain damages the red nucleus (and the surrounding dentothalamic fibers), as well as other tegmental nuclear areas. As the red nucleus has important connections with the cerebellum, a motor sign such as an intention tremor on the side of the body opposite to the lesion is likely to follow destruction of the nucleus.

16. B The oculomotor nerve is damaged, resulting in paralysis of the "extraocular muscles", with the exception of the superior oblique and lateral rectus muscles. The constrictor muscle of the pupil and the ciliary muscle are also paralyzed. The consequences of such a lesion are external strabismus, inability to move the eye medially or vertically, and closure of the eye owing to drooping of the upper lid (ptsosis). Dilation of the pupil occurs because of the unopposed action of the dilator pupillae muscle of the iris, which has a sympathetic innervation.

17. E The fibers of the medial lemniscus are interrupted and they conduct proprioception, discriminative touch, and vibration from the contralateral side of the body. This results from crossing of the constituent fibers at the level of the medulla.

18. A The spinal lemniscus, which is made up of the spinothalamic and spinotectal tracts, is damaged in the lesion. The spinothalamic tract conducts impulses for pain, touch, and temperature from the contralateral side of the body because the constituent fibers cross the midline in the spinal cord.

19. D Damage to the corticospinal fibers in the basis pedunculi of the midbrain causes voluntary motor paresis, but flaccidity of the affected muscles on the contralateral side in the upper and lower limbs. This is explained by the fact that the pyramidal tract (corticospinal tract) crosses to the opposite side (decussation of the pyramidal tract) in the caudal end of the medulla and the rostral end of the spinal cord. The paralysis is of a spastic nature because it is an upper motor neuron that is damaged. The extrapyramidal motor system is important in the usual form of "upper motor neuron lesion", in which both the pyramidal and extrapyramidal systems are involved.

20. E Same explanation as given for question 17.

21. B Same explanation as given for question 16.

SEVEN

The Cerebellum

OBJECTIVES

BE ABLE TO:

* Give a brief account of the development of the cerebellum.

* Name the three major regions of the cerebellum that can be recognized in the horizontal plane.

* Define the following terms: vermis, flocculonodular lobe, corpus cerebelli, anterior lobe, and posterior lobe.

* State the connections of the inferior, middle, and superior cerebellar peduncles.

* Discuss the blood supply to the cerebellum.

* Make sketches of the superior and inferior surfaces of the cerebellum, showing their main anatomical features.

* State the basis for recognizing an archicerebellum, paleocerebellum, neocerebellum and discuss briefly their functions.

* Describe and illustrate the different types of neuron in the cerebellar cortex.

* Make a simple sketch to show the relative position and size of the cerebellar nuclei.

* Make a simple sketch to illustrate the cytoarchitecture of the cerebellar cortex.

* Discuss the function and connections of the cerebellar nuclei.

* Describe the cerebellar peduncles and identify the afferent efferent fibers in each one.

* Describe the signs of cerebellar dysfunction in the archicere- and cerebellar neocerebellar syndromes.

DIRECTIONS: Each of the following questions or incomplete statements is followed by five suggested answers or completions. SELECT THE ONE BEST ANSWER OR COMPLETION in each case and underline the appropriate letter at the right.

----

1. Which statement concerning the human cerebellum is <u>incorrect</u>?

    A. Has a cortex of gray matter
    B. Contains a medullary center of white matter
    C. Has three pairs of central nuclei
    D. Three pairs of peduncles connect it to the brain stem
    E. Consists of a vermis and two cerebellar hemispheres   A B C D E

2. Which of the following is a <u>correct</u> statement?

    A. The primary fissure is the first fissure to appear during fetal development
    B. The posterolateral fissure is the second fissure to appear during embryonic development
    C. The corpus cerebelli does not include the flocculonodular lobe
    D. The ventral (anterior) spinocerebellar tract is a component of the restiform body
    E. The roof of the fourth ventricle is formed by the superior medullary velum and the brachium pontis   A B C D E

3. Which nucleus is NOT embedded deep in the medullary center of the cerebellum?

    A. Fastigial   D. Dentate
    B. Amygdaloid   E. Emboliform
    C. Globose   A B C D E

4. Which of the following fiber systems is in the juxtarestiform body?

    A. Dorsal spinocerebellar   D. All of the above
    B. Cuneocerebellar   E. None of the above
    C. Olivocerebellar   A B C D E

5. There are _____ layers of cells in the cortex of a cerebellar folium

    A. three   D. six
    B. four   E. seven
    C. five   A B C D E

SELECT THE ONE BEST ANSWER OR COMPLETION

6. Which type of nerve cell is NOT present in the cerebellar cortex?

    A. Pyramidal   D. Purkinje
    B. Granule   E. Stellate
    C. Basket   A B C D E

7. Efferents from the cerebellar nuclei may terminate on the

    A. red nucleus   C. vestibular nuclei
    B. ventral lateral   D. none of the above
        thalamic nucleus   E. all of the above   A B C D E

8. The cerebellum develops from the

    A. alar plate of the myelencephalon
    B. basal plate of the myelencephalon
    C. alar plate of the metencephalon
    D. basal plate of the metencephalon
    E. basal and alar plates of the mesencephalon   A B C D E

9. Which of the following statements is incorrect?

    A. The superior vermis is clearly separated from the cere-
        bellar hemispheres
    B. The flocculus is attached to the nodule of the vermis
    C. The anterior lobe is separated from the posterior lobe
        of the primary fissure
    D. The flocculonodular lobe is the oldest component of the
        cerebellum
    E. The nodule is the rostral portion of the inferior
        vermis   A B C D E

10. Which of the following structures is considered to be part
    of the archicerebellum?

    A. Tonsil   D. Nodule
    B. Lingula   E. Pyramis
    C. Biventral lobe   A B C D E

11. Which statment concerning the cerebellum is incorrect?

    A. The vestibulocerebellum is the oldest division
    B. The paleocerebellum influences muscle tonus
    C. The neocerebellum is the largest part of the human
        cerebellum
    D. The archicerebellum is concerned with synergy of mus-
        cles composing a functional group
    E. The pontocerebellum influences the musculature of the
        same side of the body   A B C D E

ANSWERS, NOTES, AND EXPLANATIONS

1. C   There are four pairs of central nuclei embedded deep within the medullary center of the cerebellum. From a medial to lateral direction they are the fastigial, globose, emboliform, and dentate nuclei. The fastigial nucleus is the oldest phylogenetically and the dentate nucleus is the newest.

2. C   The corpus cerebelli consists of the anterior and posterior lobes. The posterolateral fissure is the first fissure to appear during development, followed by the primary fissure. The ventral (anterior) spinocerebellar tract enters the cerebellum through the superior peduncle, in which it runs along the side of the superior cerebellar peduncle en route to the vermal and paravermal cortex of the paleocerebellum. The roof of the fourth ventricle is formed by the superior medullary velum and the superior cerebellar peduncles.

3. B   The amygdaloid nucleus, one of the cerebral nuclei, is situated in the temporal lobe between the tip of the inferior horn of the lateral ventricle and the basal surface of the lentiform nucleus. Its functions are concerned with the olfactory and limbic systems of the brain. All the other nuclei named are cerebellar nuclei that are embedded deep within the medullary center.

4. E   The fibers named enter the cerebellum through the lateral area of the inferior cerebellar peduncle, together with fibers from the arcuate nuclei and the reticular formation in the medulla, and trigeminocerebellar fibers originating in the chief nucleus and the nucleus of the spinal tract of the trigeminal nerve. The medial area of the inferior peduncle contains both afferent and efferent fibers with respect to the cerebellum. The afferent fibers are from the vestibular nerve and nuclei. The efferent fibers proceed from the flocculonodular lobe, the fastigial nuclei, and to a lesser extent the globose and emboliform nuclei, to the vestibular nuclei and reticular formation of the brain stem.

5. A   Three layers of cells are recognizable in histological sections of the cerebellar cortex. From the surface to the white matter of a folium, they are: the molecular layer, the layer of Purkinje cells, and the granule cell layer.

6. A   Pyramidal cells are present in the cerebral rather than the cerebellar cortex. Purkinje, granule, stellate, basket, and Golgi cells comprise the neurons of the cerebellar cortex. The molecular layer contains scattered stellate and basket cells; the Purkinje cell layer consists of the perikarya of these cells in a single layer, and the granule cell layer consists of closely packed granule cells and occasional Golgi cells in the outer part of the layer.

7. E   Axons from the dentate, emboliform, and globose nuclei leave the cerebellum via the superior cerebellar peduncle and terminate in the ventral lateral nucleus of the thalamus, the red nucleus, or the reticular formation. Axons from the fastigial nucleus leave the cerebellum via the inferior cerebellar peduncle and terminate in the vestibular nuclear complex and the reticular formation.

8. C The cerebelum develops from symmetrical thickenings of dorsal parts of the alar plates of the metencephalon. Initially the cerebellar swellings project as small bulges into the fourth ventricle. Eventually the swellings enlarge and fuse in the midline to overgrow the rostral half of the fourth ventricle and overlap the pons and medulla.

9. A The superior vermis is not demarcated from the hemispheres. Instead, the thin transverse folia of the superior vermis continue uninterrupted into the hemispheres. However, the inferior vermis lies in a deep depression and is well delinated from the rest of the cerebellum.

10. D The archicerebellum or vestibulocerebellum is the smallest of the three functional divisions of the cerebellum and the oldest phylogenetically. It corresponds to the flocculonodular lobe, consisting of the flocculi connected by peduncles to the nodule of the inferior vermis, and the uvula of the inferior vermis immediately posterior to the nodule.

11. D. The archicerebellum or vestibulocerebellum functions in maintaining equilibrium. It projects to the brain stem and influences the lower motor neurons through the vestibulospinal tract, the medial longitudinal fasciculus, and reticulospinal fibers.

MULTI-COMPLETION QUESTIONS

DIRECTIONS: In each of the following questions or incomplete statements, one or more of the completions given is correct. At the lower right of each question, underline A if 1, 2, and 3 are correct; B if 1 and 3 are correct; C if 2 and 4 are correct; D if only 4 is correct; and E if all are correct.

---

1. Nuclei found in the medullary center of the cerebellum include;

    1. Caudate   3. Olivary
    2. Globose   4. Emboliform   A B C D E

2. The corpus cerebelli is made up of the

    1. anterior lobe   3. posterior lobe
    2. superior vermis 4. flocculonodular lobe   A B C D E

3. The cerebellum functions in

    1. maintenance of equilibrium
    2. coordination of muscle action
    3. synergy of muscle action
    4. pain and temperature sensitivity   A B C D E

	A	B	C	D	E
	1,2,3	1,3,	2,4	only 4	all correct

4. The cerebellar peduncles include:

1. Brachium pontis
2. Basis pedunculi
3. Brachium conjunctivum
4. Superior brachium

A B C D E

5. The layers evident in histological sections of the cerebellar cortex include:

1. Molecular
2. Pyramidal
3. Granular
4. Fusiform

A B C D E

6. Afferent fibers to the cerebellar cortex include:

1. Mossy
2. Spinocerebellar
3. Climbing
4. Pontocerebellar

A B C D E

7. On a functional basis, the cerebellum consists of a

1. vestibulocerebellum
2. spinocerebellum
3. pontocerebellum
4. cerebrocerebellum

A B C D E

8. Purkinje cells

1. are examples of golgi type I neurons
2. exhibit profuse dendritic branching
3. are of the order of 15 million in the cerebellum
4. terminate in central cerebellar nuclei

A B C D E

9. The cerebellum receives fibers from the

1. nuclei pontis
2. vestibular nuclei
3. nucleus dorsalis or Clarke's column of the spinal cord
4. inferior olivary nucleus

A B C D E

10. Efferent fibers from the cerebellar nuclei leave the cerebellum via the

1. brachium conjunctivum
2. restiform body
3. juxtarestiform body
4. brachium pontis

A B C D E

11. Input to cerebellar nuclei may be received from

1. Purkinje cells
2. pontocerebellar fibers
3. vestibular nuclei
4. spinocerebellar fibers

A B C D E

12. Signs characteristic of the neocerebellar syndrome include:

1. Ataxic movements
2. Dysmetria
3. Intention tremor
4. Synergy of movements

A B C D E

A	B	C	D	E
1,2,3	1,3,	2,4	only 4	all correct

13. Symptoms of the archicerebellar syndrome include:

    1. Unsteadiness on the feet   3. Sways from side to side
    2. Walks on a narrow base   4. Ataxia   A B C D E

ANSWERS, NOTES, AND EXPLANATIONS

1. C 2 and 4 are correct. The cerebellum has four pairs of central nuc-
    lei embedded deep with its medullary center. From a medial to a later-
    al direction, they are the fastigial, globose, emboliform, and dentate
    nuclei. Phylogenetically, these nuclei develop in the same order.

2. A 1, 2, and 3 are correct. The main mass of the cerebellum, i.e., all
    but the flocculonodular lobe, is called the corpus cerebelli. It
    consists of anterior and posterior lobes, of which the vermis is a part.

3. A 1, 2, and 3 are correct. The cerebellum is a motor part of the brain,
    functioning in the maintenance of equilibrium and coordination of muscle
    action in both stereotyped and nonstereotyped movements. The cerebellum
    makes a special contribution to the synergy of muscles composing a
    functional group. In spite of an abundant input from sensory receptors,
    the cerebellum does not contribute to sensory awareness, this being a
    function of the thalamus and cerebral cortex.

4. B 1 and 3 are correct. There are three cerebellar peduncles: (1) the
    superior cerebellar peduncle; (2) the middle peduncle; and (3) the infer-
    ior peduncle. The middle cerebellar peduncle contains only afferent fibers
    whereas the superior and inferior peduncles contain both afferent and ef-
    ferent fibers. The basis pedunculi of the midbrain consists of cortico-
    pontine, corticospinal, and corticobulbar fibers and the superior brachium
    consists of afferent fibers to the superior colliculus of the midbrain.

5. B 1 and 3 are correct. Three layers are evident in the cortex of the
    cerebellum. From the surface to the white matter, these are the molecular
    layer, the layer of Purkinje cells, and the granule cell layer. The
    pyramidal and fusiform cell layers are in the cerebellar cortex.

6. E All are correct. Mossy and climbing fibers are terms used to describe
    afferent fibers to the cerebellar cortex. The terminals of mossy fibers
    make synaptic contact with the claw-like endings of the short dendrites
    of granule cells. Climbing fibers, most of which come from the
    inferior olivary complex, wind among the dendritic branches of Purkinje
    cells and make synaptic contact with them. They are thought to
    originate from the nuclei pontis and reticular formation, in addition
    to the inferior olivary complex. Spinocerebellar, pontocerebellar, and
    the other afferents account for the mossy fibers.

7. A 1, 2, and 3 are correct. The functional divisions of the cerebellum
    are based primarily on the destination of afferent fiber bundles, but they
    also depend on phylogenetic development. The vestibulocerebellum or

archicerebellum, represented by the flocculonodular lobe, is the oldest division and is concerned with the maintenance of equilibrium. The spinocerebellum or paleocerebellum in the vermal and paravermal regions influences muscle tonus and synergy of muscles during stereotyped movements such as postural changes and locomotion. The pontocerebellum or neocerebellum, comprising most of the cerebellar hemispheres, ensures the synergy and delicate adjustments of muscle tonus that are necessary for accuracy of nonstereotyped movements.

8. E All are correct. There are about 15 million Purkinje cells in the cortex of the cerebellum. Classified as Golgi type I neurons, they have a flask-shaped cell body that tapers into one or two apical dendrites. Their axons traverse the granule cell layer, acquire myelin sheaths, and then pass through the medullary center to terminate in central cerebellar nuclei.

9. E All are correct. Axons from diverse regions of the brain stem and spinal cord make connections with neurons in the cerebellar cortex and nuclei. With respect to the afferent fibers named, those from the nuclei pontis compose the middle cerebellar peduncle; fibers from vestibular nuclei traverse the medial area of the inferior cerebellar peduncle and the dorsal spinocerebellar tract (originating in Clarke's column); olivocerebellar, cuneocerebellar, and medullary reticular fibers traverse the inferior peduncle.

10. B 1 and 3 are correct. Efferent fibers from the dentate, emboliform, and globose nuclei leave the cerebellum via the superior cerebellar peduncles, cross to the opposite side, and terminate mainly in the ventral lateral thalamic nucleus and the red nucleus. Fibers from the fastigial nucleus proceed to ipsilateral vestibular and reticular nuclei through the medial area of the inferior peduncle. The inferior peduncle and the middle cerebellar peduncle (brachium pontis) are composed of afferent fibers.

11. E All are correct. The input to cerebellar nuclei is: (1) intrinsic, from the Purkinje cells of the cortex, and (2) extrinsic, from neurons in the brain stem and spinal cord. The fibers from outside the cerebellum are excitatory and those from Purkinje cells are inhibitory. The fluctuating output from the cerebellar nuclei is determined by the delicate balance between excitation and inhibition at any given moment.

12. A 1, 2, and 3 are correct. When there is a destructive lesion of the corpus cerebelli or its major afferent or efferent pathways, characteristic signs are produced which are referred to as the neocerebellar syndrome. These signs are: (1) ataxia - movements are intermittent or jerky; (2) dysmetria - disturbance of power to control the range of movement; (3) asynergy or decomposition of movements - disturbance of the proper association in the contraction of muscles which assures that the components of a movement follow in proper sequence and at the proper moment, so that it is executed accurately; (4) hypotonia of muscles which tend to tire easily; (5) intention tremor occurring at the end of a particular movement; (6) nystagmus - an involuntary oscillation of the eye which may occur if the lesion encroaches on the vermis.

13. B 1 and 3 are correct. The archicerebellar syndrome results from a lesion such as a tumor which may be a medulloblastoma, causing destruction

of the flocculonodular lobe. The patient is unsteady on his/her feet, walks on a wide base, and sways from side to side. The signs are limited at first to a disturbance of equilibrium. Additional signs of cerebellar dysfunction occur when the lesion spreads to other parts of the cerebellum.

F I V E - C H O I C E   A S S O C I A T I O N   Q U E S T I O N S

DIRECTIONS: Each of the following groups of questions consists of a numbered list of descriptive words or phrases accompanied by a diagram with certain parts indicated by letters, or by a list of lettered headings. For each numbered word or phrase, SELECT THE LETTERED PART OR HEADING that matches it correctly and insert the letter in the space to the right of the appropriate number. Each lettered heading may be selected once, more than once, or not at all.

----

1. ____ Pass from medullary center to synapse with Purkinje cells

A. Purkinje cells

2. ____ Have short dendrites with claw-like endings

B. Granule cells

3. ____ Originate in the inferior olivary complex

C. Basket cells

4. ____ Have a special relation to granule cells

D. Climbing fibers

5. ____ Are Golgi type I neurons

E. Mossy fibers

6. ____ Its axon bifurcates and runs parallel with the folium

C. Basket cells

7. ____ Located in the molecular layer near Purkinje cell bodies

8. ____ Pontocerebellar fibers

A. Archicerebellum

9. ____ Includes the superior vermis and inferior vermis

B. Paleocerebellum

10. ____ Ataxic movements

C. Neocerebellum

11. ____ Consists of the flocculonodular lobe

D. Archicerebellar syndrome

12. ____ Intention tremor

E. Neocerebellar syndrome

13. ____ Disturbance of equilibrium

14. ____ Dysmetria

96

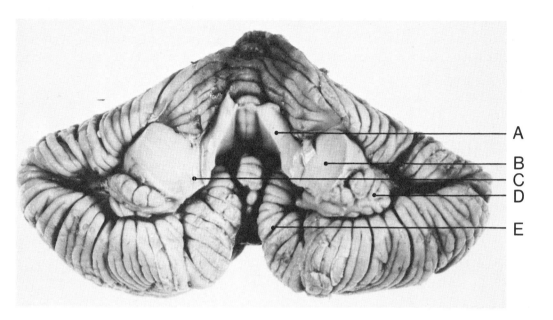

(From Barr, M.L. and Kiernan, J.A., The Human Nervous System, 4th ed., 1983. Courtesy of Harper & Row Publishers, Inc.)

15. ____ Continues to the ventral lateral thalamic nucleus
16. ____ Terminates in neocerebellar cortex
17. ____ Originates in the dentate nucleus
18. ____ Receives special sensory data from the vestibular nuclei
19. ____ Is part of the posterior lobe
20. ____ Takes origin from contralateral pontine neurons
21. ____ One of its components is the dorsal spinocerebellar tract

ANSWERS, NOTES, AND EXPLANATIONS

1. D Climbing fibers enter the cortex from the medullary center, traverse the grandule cell layer, and wind among the dendritic branches of Purkinje cells in the molecular layer, like a vine growing on a tree. Each climbing fiber makes synaptic contact with the smooth surface of the larger branches of a Purkinje cell dendrite.

2. B Granule cells contain a spherical nucleus and their scanty cytoplasm lacks clumps of Nissl substance. Their short dendrites have claw-like endings which make synaptic contact with mossy fibers. The axon of a granule cell enters the molecular layer where it bifurcates and runs parallel with the folium.

3. D Although the source of climbing fibers has been controversial for
    many years, they are now believed to originate in the inferior olivary
    complex of the medulla.

4. E Mossy fibers terminate in synaptic relation with dendrites of granule
    cells. While in the white matter of the cerebellum, mossy fibers divide
    into several branches which enter the granular layer and subdivide into
    terminal branches. Along the terminal portion of the fiber and its end,
    there are swellings known as "rosettes" with which the dendrites of
    several granule cells make synaptic contact.

5. A Purkinje cells, which are examples of Golgi type I neurons, form a
    single layer throughout the extensive cerebellar cortex. Their cell
    bodies are flask-shaped, tapering into one or two apical dendrites. The
    dendritic branching is more profuse than in any other type of nerve cell,
    occurring in a plane at right angles to the folium. The axon arises from
    the base of the cell body, gives off one or more collateral branches, and
    then traverses the white matter to synapse on neurons in the central
    cerebellar nuclei.

6. B Axons of granule cells located in the deepest layer of the cortex enter
    the superficial molecular layer, where they bifurcate and run parallel
    with the folia. Each axon traverses the dendritic trees of some 450
    Purkinje cells, with which it makes synaptic contacts. These axons may
    also synapse with dendrites of stellate, basket, and Golgi cells in the
    molecular layer.

7. C Basket cells are scattered in the molecular layer near the bodies of
    Purkinje cells. The dendrites of the basket cell branch in the trans-
    verse plane of the folium, making contact with many granule cell axons.
    The axon of a basket cell is directed transversely to a folium, and col-
    lateral branches end as basket-like arrangements, each synapsing with the
    cell body of a Purkinje cell. One basket cell may synapse with as many as
    250 Purkinje cells.

8. C The neocerebellum (pontocerebellum) is the largest functional
    division of the cerebellum in humans. Pontocerebellar fibers cross the
    midline in the basal pons as large bundles, then traverse the middle
    cerebellar peduncles and medullar center. They are distributed to the
    neocerebellar cortex, which covers most of the surface of the
    cerebrallar hemispheres.

9. B The paleocerebellum (spinocerebellum) consists of the superior
    vermis, most of the inferior vermis, and the paravermal zones on the
    superior and inferior surfaces of the hemispheres. It receives sensory
    data (proprio- ception, touch, and pressure) from the spinal cord and
    brain stem via the inferior cerebellar peduncle. The dorsal
    spinocerebellar tract is an example of a tract that conducts sensory
    data to the paleocerebellum (spinocerebellum).

10. E In the neocerebellar syndrome, several signs in varying degrees of
    severity are demonstrated. Movements tend to be ataxic (intermittent
    or jerky). There may be dysmetria (past-pointing with the finger) or
    adiodochokinesia (poor performance in rapidly alternating movements
    such as flexion and extension of the fingers). When the lesion causing

the syndrome is unilateral, as is usually the case, the signs of motor dysfunction are on the same side of the body as the lesion.

11. A   The archicerebellum (vestibulocerebellum) consists of the flocculonodular lobe, together with a small region of the inferior vermis known as the uvula, immediately adjacent to the nodule. The archicerebellum is concerned with adjustment of muscle tonus in response to vestibular stimuli and hence functions in maintaining equilibrium.

12. E   The signs of the neocerebellar syndrome include dysmetria, ataxia, asynergy, hypotonia of muscles, and sometimes nystagmus, in addition to an intention tremor. The tremor is characteristically terminal, occurring at the end of a particular movement. It can readily be distinguished from the involuntary movements occurring in the various motor disturbances coming under the heading of dyskinesias.

13. D   In the archicerebellar syndrome, characterized by a disturbance of equilibrium, the patient is unsteady on his/her feet, walks on a wide base, and sways from side to side. The disorder results from involvement of the flocculonodular lobe by a tumor or by interference with its blood supply.

14. E   The signs of the neocerebellar syndrome include dysmetria, a disturbance of the power to control the range of movement in muscular action. For example, when reaching out with the finger to touch an object, the finger overshoots the mark or deviates from it (past-pointing). Refer to the answers to question 17 and 19 for other signs of this syndrome.

15. A   The superior cerebellar peduncle, consists mainly of efferent fibers from the dentate, emboliform, and globose nuclei. The brachia enter the midbrain posterior to the inferior colliculi, cross the midline in the decussation of the superior cerebellar peduncles and continue anteriorly to the ventral lateral nuclei of the thalamus. Fibers of this peduncle also terminate in the red nucleus and reticular formation.

16. B   The middle cerebellar peduncle is composed of afferent fibers from the nuclei pontis of the opposite side of the pons. They are distributed to the nucleocerebellar (pontocerebellar) cortex, which covers most of the cerebellar hemispheres.

17. A   The superior cerebellar peduncle consists of fibers from the dentate, emboliform, and globose nuclei. They enter the midbrain immediately behind the inferior colliculi, cross the midline, and continue forward through and around the red nucleus to the ventral lateral nucleus of the thalamus. Fibers from the three central nuclei named above also terminate in the red nucleus of the midbrain, and a few fibers from the globose and emboliform nuclei end in the reticular formation of the brain stem.

18. D   The archicerebellum or vestibulocerebellum, which consists almost entirely of the flocculonodular lobe, receives fibers from the vestibular nuclear complex and fewer fibers directly from the ventibular nerve. This input is vital to the function of the archi-

cerebellum (vestibulocerebellum) in the maintenance of equilibrium.

19. E Because of their appearance, the paired swellings on the inferior surface are called the tonsils of the cerebellum. They are in the rostral part of the inferior surface of the posterior lobe, one on each side of the midline depression known as the vallecula. When the cerebellum is forced inferiorly because of some form of intracranial pathology, the tonsils may press against the medulla or herniate into the foramen magnum.

20. B The middle cerebellar peduncle (brachium pontis) is composed entirely of pontocerebellar fibers; they are axons of the small and medium-sized polygonal cells which make up the pontine nuclei in the basal pons. These fibers cross the midline in the pons, forming conspicuous transverse bundles, enter the middle cerebellar peduncles, and are distributed to the neocerebellar (pontocerebellar) cortex of the hemispheres.

21. C The inferior cerebellar peduncle lies medial to the middle cerebellar peduncle on turning dorsally to enter the cerebellum, where is forms part of the lateral wall of the fourth ventricle. The dorsal and ventral spinocerebellar tracts enter the cerebellum through the inferior and superior peduncles, respectively.

EIGHT

The Diencephalon

BE ABLE TO:

* Indicate in a median section of a brain, the junction of the midbrain and diencephalon and the boundary between the diencephalon and telencephalon.

* Describe the gross features of the diencephalon.

* List the four major divisions of the diencephalon.

* State the embryological origin of the diencephalon.

T H A L A M U S

BE ABLE TO:

* Make simple drawings of lateral and dorsal views of the thalamus showing its gross structure and major subdivisions.

* Define the following terms: stratum zonale, external medullary lamina, internal medullary lamina, hypothalamic sulcus, massa intermedia, pulvinar, medial and lateral geniculate bodies, and anterior tubercle of the thalamus.

* Identify the boundaries of the thalamus.

* Write brief notes on the functions and connections with other parts of the brain of the three main subdivisions of the thalamus (anterior, lateral, and medial nuclei).

* Discuss the thalamic syndrome.

S U B T H A L A M U S

BE ABLE TO:

* State the sensory fasciculi in the subthalamic region.

* Name the midbrain nuclei that extend into the subthalamus.

* Discuss the effects of a lesion in the subthalamic nucleus.

* Write brief notes on the following: zona incerta, subthalamic fasciculus, ansa lenticularis, and supramamillary commissure.

E P I T H A L A M U S

BE ABLE TO:

* List the components of the epithalamus.

* Describe the location and main connections of the habenular nuclei.

* Give the location of most of the cells of origin of the stria medullaris thalami, and describe the course and destination of these afferent fibers.

* Outline the pathway through which primitive aspects of brain function (basic emotional drives and sense of smell) influence the viscera.

* Describe the pineal body, including its location.

* State the probable functions of the pineal body in man and the effects of tumors in it.

H Y P O T H A L A M U S

BE ABLE TO:

* Make a simple diagram showing the location of the hypothalamus and its relationship to the fornix, thalamus, optic chiasma, and hypophysis cerebri (pituitary gland).

* List the three hypothalamic nuclei contained in the medial zone and state their general function.

* Discuss the neurosecretory activity of cells in the supraoptic and paraventricular nuclei and the relations of their secretions to the hypophysis cerebri.

* List the four main sources of afferent hypothalamic pathways.

* Name the two principal efferent pathways from the hypothalamus to the brain stem.

* Name the system through which the hypothalamus chiefly effects its responses.

* Discuss the effects of stimulating (1) the anterior hypothalamus, and (2) the posterior and lateral parts of the hypothalamus in experimental animals, and explain the significance of these responses in maintaining homeostasis in man.

DIENCEPHALON

FIVE-CHOICE COMPLETION QUESTIONS

DIRECTIONS: Each of the following questions or incomplete statements is followed by five suggested answers or completions. SELECT THE ONE BEST ANSWER OR COMPLETION in each case and underline the appropriate letter at the right.

----

1. The only external features of the diencephalon exposed to view are on the_____surface.

    A. Dorsal   D. Medial
    B. Ventral   E. Caudal
    C. Lateral   A B C D E

2. The diencephalon is divided into symmetrical halves by the

    A. massa intermedia   D. third ventricle
    B. hyothalamic sulcus E. midline nucleus
    C. Stria medullaris   A B C D E

3. Which of the following is the largest component of the diencephalon?

    A. Epithalamus   D. Hypothalamus
    B. Thalamus   E. Subthalamus
    C. Metathalamus   A B C D E

4. The diencephalon is derived from the embryonic

    A. prosencephalon   D. telencephalon
    B. mesencephalon   E. metencephalon
    C. rhombencephalon   A B C D E

5. A line traversing the _____ and the optic chiasma represents the boundary between the diencephalon and telencephalon.

    A. optic tract   D. posterior commissure
    B. anterior commissure E. interventricular
    C. mamillary body   foramen   A B C D E

6. A plane that includes the posterior commissure and the caudal margins of the_____represents the junction between the diencephalon and the midbrain.

    A. median eminence   D. geniculate bodies
    B. mamillary bodies   E. tuber cinereum
    C. optic chiasma   A B C D E

SELECT THE ONE BEST ANSWER OR COMPLETION

7. The dorsal surface of the diencephalon is partly concealed by the

    A. hippocampus   D. fornix
    B. stria medullaris thalami   E. internal capsule
    C. tuber cinereum   A B C D E

8. The lateral surface of the diencephalon is bounded by the

    A. tela choroidea   D. lamina terminalis
    B. third ventricle   E. optic tract
    C. internal capsule   A B C D E

9. Classically, the diencephalon is divided into four major parts. Which of the following is not one of these parts?

    A. Epithalamus   D. Metathalamus
    B. Hypothalamus   E. Thalamus
    C. Subthalamus   A B C D E

ANSWER, NOTES, AND EXPLANATIONS

1. B The only external features of the diencephalon visible on an undissected brain are on the ventral (basal) surface. These features are: the mamillary bodies, the hypophysial stalk (infundibular stem), and the tuber cinereum.

2. D The diencephalon is divided into symmetrical halves by the slit-like third ventricle, a derivative of the cavity of the embryonic prosencephalon. Commonly a bridge of gray matter in the third ventricle, the interthalamic adhesion (massa intermedia), joins the medial surfaces of the thalami.

3. B The thalamus comprises four-fifths of the diencephalon. The metathalamus is the most caudal and inferior part of the thalamus and is composed of the medial and lateral geniculate bodies. The large pulvinar overhangs the metathalamus.

4. A The diencephalon is derived from the prosencephalon, the rostral primary brain vesicle. During the fifth week, the prosencephalon divides into the telencephalon and the diencephalon. The telencephalon gives rise to the cerebral hemispheres and the diencephalon becomes the mature diencephalon (thalamus, epithalamus, subthalamus, and hypothalamus).

5. E A plane which passes from the interventricular foramen through the optic chiasma demarcates the boundary between the diencephalon and the telencephalon.

6. B The caudal limit of the diencephalon is represented by a line passing through the posterior commissure immediately caudal to the mamillary bodies.

7. D Dorsally the diencephalon is partly covered by the body of the fornix and the choroid plexus, which are contained in the central parts of the lateral ventricles. Immediately dorsal to the ventricles is the corpus callosum. This dorsal covering developed as the cerebral hemnispheres grew over the diencephalon during the formation of the mature brain.

8. C Laterally the diencephalon is bounded by the posterior limb of the internal capsule. The ventral (basal) exposed surface of the diencephalon is bounded on each side by the optic tract.

9. D The metathalamus, consisting of the medial and lateral geniculate bodies, is located caudally and inferiorly to the thalamus. It is part of the thalamus, one of the four divisions of the diencephalon.

M U L T I - C O M P L E T I O N   Q U E S T I O N S

DIRECTIONS: In each of the following questions or incomplete statements, one or more of the completions given is correct. At the lower right of each question, underline A if 1, 2, and 3 are correct; B if 1 and 3 are correct; C if 2 and 4 are correct; D if only 4 is correct; and E if all are correct.

----

1. The diencephalon

    1. is part of the cerebrum
    2. forms the central core of the telencephalon
    3. is almost entirely surrounded by the cerebral hemispheres
    4. is exposed to view only at its basal surface   A B C D E

2. The basal surface of the diencephalon is bounded anteriorly
    by the

    1. medial eminence   3. lamina terminalis
    2. optic tracts   4. optic chiasma   A B C D E

3. The boundary between the diencephalon and the telencephalon
    is represented by a line traversing the

    1. interventricular foramen   3. optic chiasma
    2. posterior commissure   4. mamillary body   A B C D E

4. Parts of the diencephalon include the

    1. hypothalamus   3. dorsal thalamus
    2. subthalamus   4. epithalamus   A B C D E

A	B	C	D	E
1,2,3	1,3	2,4	only 4	all correct

5. The diencephalon is the region of the brain that

    1. surrounds the third ventricle
    2. forms almost all of the walls of the third ventricle
    3. lies between the cerebral hemispheres
    4. contains relay nuclei on pathways to the cerebral
        cortex   A B C D E

6. The junction of the midbrain and the diencephalon is represented by a line passing immediately caudal to the
   mamillary body and through the

    1. anterior commissure   3. fornix
    2. interventricular foramen 4. posterior commissure A B C D E

7. Fibers of the stria medullaris thalami

    1. form a bundle of nerve fibers that arise in the
        medial olfactory area
    2. originate in the amygdaloid nuclei
    3. run along the dorsomedial border of the thalamus
    4. pass across the medial side of the tail of the
        caudate nucleus   A B C D E

8. Attachments to the roof of the diencephalon include the

    1. fornix   3. septum pellucidum
    2. tela choroidea   4. pineal body   A B C D E

ANSWERS, NOTES, AND EXPLANATIONS

1. E All are correct. The diencephalon and telencephalon, derived from
    the prosencephalon, constitute the cerebrum, of which the diencephalon
    forms the central core and the telencephalon the cerebral hemisphere.
    Being almost completely surrounded by the hemispheres, only the basal
    surface of the diencephalon is exposed to view.

2. D Only 4 is correct. The basal surface of the diencephalon that is
    exposed to view is a diamond-shaped area containing hypothalamic
    structures. This important area is bounded anteriorly by the optic
    chiasma. The optic tracts are on each side of this area and the median
    eminence is part of the basal surface of the diencephalon.

3. B 1 and 3 are correct. A plane which passes from the interventricular
    foramen immediately caudal to the optic chiasma represents the junction
    between the diencephalon and the telencephalon.

4. E All are correct. The diencephalon consists of four parts, each of
    which is represented bilaterally and differs in structure and function.
    The thalamus is the largest part, making up four-fifths of the dien-
    cephalon.

5. E All are correct. The cavity of the embryonic diencephalon forms most of the third ventricle in the mature brain. Consequently the walls of the third ventricle develop from walls of the embryonic diencephalon. The small anterior part develops from the telencephalon.

6. D Only 4 is correct. The caudal limit of the diencephalon, or of the midbrain diencephalic junction, is represented by a plane which includes the posterior commissure and the caudal margins of the mamillary bodies.

7. B 1 and 3 are correct. The stria medullaris thalami is a bundle of nerve fibers that forms an elevation along the junction of the medial and dorsal surfaces of the thalamus. Most of the cells of origin of the stria medullaris are in the medial olfactory area. This bundle should not be confused with the stria terminalis which originates in the amygdaloid nucleus; however some of its fibers turn caudally into the stria medullaris thalami.

8. C 2 and 4 are correct. The pineal body (epiphysis) develops as a midline diverticulum of the caudal part of the diencephalic roof. The tela choroidea is vascular connective tissue which forms the core of the choroid plexus in the diencephalic roof of the third ventricle, and is continuous with the vascular core of the choronoid plexuses of the lateral ventricles.

F I V E - C H O I C E   A S S O C I A T I O N   Q U E S T I O N S

DIRECTIONS: Each of the following groups of questions consists of a numbered list of descriptive words or phrases accompanied by a diagram with certain parts indicated by letters, or by a list of lettered headings. For each numbered word or phrase, SELECT THE LETTERED PART OR HEADING that matches it correctly and insert the letter in the space to the right of the appropriate number. Each lettered heading may be selected once, more than once, or not at all.

    A. Internal capsule   D. Third ventricle
    B. Diencephalon   E. Neurohypophysis
    C. Fornix

1.____Largely conceals the dorsal surface of the diencephalon

2.____Divides the diencephalon into halves

3.____A lateral boundary of the diencephalon

4.____Derived from the floor of the diencephalon

5.____Forms the walls of the third ventricle

6.____Arches over the diencephalon

ASSOCIATION QUESTIONS

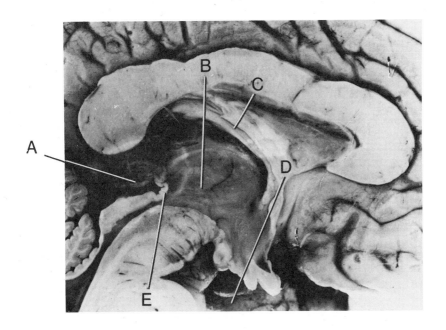

(From Barr, M.L., and Kiernan, J.A.: The Human Nervous System, 4th ed., 1983. Courtesy of Harper & Row, Publishers, Inc.)

7._____Part of the epithalamus

8._____Line indicating the caudal limit of the diencephalon

9._____Conceals the dorsal surface of the thalamus

10._____Largest part of the diencephalon

11._____An endocrine organ

12._____Line indicating the cranial limit of the diencephalon

ANSWERS, NOTES, AND EXPLANATIONS

1. C The fornix partly conceals the dorsal surface of the diencephalon. This is a robust bundle of fibers that originates in the hippocampus of the temporal lobe, curves over the thalamus, and ends mainly in the mamillary body.

2. D The diencephalon is divided into symmetrical halves by the slit-like third ventricle. This diencephalic part of the ventricular system is connected to the lateral ventricles by the interventricular foramina, and to the fourth ventricle via the cerebral aqueduct of the midbrain.

108

3.　A　The diencephalon is bounded laterally by the posterior limb of the internal capsule. The lenticothalamic portion of this important structure is between the lentiform nucleus and the thalamus.

4.　E　The neurohypophysis (neural portion of the pituitary gland) develops from the neurohypophysial bud which develops as a ventral diverticulum of the floor of the diencephalon during the eighth week of development.

5.　B　The rather extensive lateral walls of the third ventricle are formed by the diencephalon. This is understandable because the third ventricle develops almost entirely from the cavity of the embryonic diencephalon. The rostral portion of the third ventricle is derived from the cavity of the telencephalon, as are the lateral ventricles.

6.　C　The fornix (L. arch) is the efferent tract of the hippocampus that arches over the thalamus, the largest part of the diencephalon, on its way to the mamillary body of the hypothalamus.

7.　A　the pineal body and structures concerned with affective and olfactory reflex responses are part of the epithalamus. Note that this endo- crine gland is attached to the diencephalon by the pineal stalk, into which the third ventricle extends as the pineal recess.

8.　E　A line passing through the posterior commissure, immediately caudal to the mamillary body, as in this photograph of the central region of the brain in midsagittal section, demarcates the junction between the diencephalon and the midbrain.

9.　C　The fornix partly conceals the dorsal surface of the thalamus. This robust bundle of fibers originates in the hippocampus of the temporal lobe, curves over the thalamus, and ends mainly in the mamillary body.

10.　B　The thalamus is the largest part of the diencephalon; it makes up four-fifths of it. The thalamus is a mass of gray matter that is subdivided into several nuclei on the basis of their fiber connections and sequence of phylogenetic development.

11.　A　The cone-shaped pineal body is an endocrine gland that is closely related to the nervous sytem. Clinical observations of long standing suggest it has an antigonadotropic function because a pineal tumor developing around the age of puberty may alter the age of onset of pubertal changes.

12.　D　A line traversing the interventricular foramen and the optic chiasma, as in this photograph of a median section of the central region of the brain, demarcates the boundary between the diencephalon and telencephalon.

THALAMUS

FIVE-CHOICE COMPLETION QUESTIONS

DIRECTIONS: Each of the following questions or incomplete statements is
followed by five suggested answers or completions. SELECT THE ONE BEST
ANSWER OR COMPLETION in each case and underline the appropriate letter at
the right.

----

1. The internal medullary lamina divides the thalamus into ____
    gray masses.

    A. two   D. five
    B. three   E. six
    C. four   A B C D E

2. The ventral tier of the lateral nuclear mass of the thalamus
    includes the

    A. genicular nuclei   D. ventral anterior
    B. ventral posterior nuclei   nuclei
    C. ventral lateral nuclei E. all of the above   A B C D E

3. The dorsal tier of the lateral nuclear mass of the thalamus
    consists of the

    A. pulvinar   D. geniculate nuclei
    B. lateral posterior nucleus   E. all of the above
    C. lateral dorsal nucleus   A B C D E

4. Thalamic nuclei receive special sensory input for all of the
    following except

    A. general senses   D. vision
    B. taste   E. hearing
    C. smell   A B C D E

5. Which of the following thalamic nuclei is included in the
    limbic system of the brain?

    A. Anterior   D. Lateral posterior
    B. Ventral anterior   E. Ventral dorsal
    C. Ventral posterior   A B C D E

6. Which of the following nuclei produces a distinct swell-
    ing on the thalamus?

    A. Medial   D. Ventral lateral
    B. Ventral posterior   E. Ventral anterior
    C. Anterior   A B C D E

110

SELECT THE ONE BEST ANSWER OR COMPLETION

7. Which of the following thalamic nuclei has a motor function?

A. Ventral posterior
B. Lateral dorsal
C. Medial

D. Lateral posterior
E. Ventral lateral

A B C D E

8. The nucleus on the auditory pathway forming a swelling inferior to the pulvinar is the

A. medial geniculate
B. anterior
C. lateral geniculate

D. ventral posterior
E. none of the above

A B C D E

9. Which of the following is an incorrect statement concerning thalamic syndrome?

A. It is essentially a disturbance of sensory aspects of thalamic function
B. The syndrome usually results from a lesion that is vascular in origin
C. The symptons of the syndrome vary according to the location and extent of the lesion
D. The threshold for touch, pain, and temperature sensibilities is usually raised on the same side of the body as the lesion
E. The pain involved may be very disagreeable and may become intractable to analgesics

A B C D E

10. The left ventral lateral nucleus of the thalamus receives input mainly from the

A. right dentate nucleus
B. left globus pallidus
C. left dentate nucleus

D. right globus pallidus
E. substantia nigra

A B C D E

ANSWERS, NOTES, AND EXPLANATIONS

1. B The internal medullary lamina divides the thalamus into three gray masses: the lateral nuclear mass, the medial nuclear mass, and the anterior nucleus.

2. E All these nuclei are in the ventral tier of nuclei in the lateral nuclear mass of the thalamus. There are five nuclei in this tier because there are medial and lateral geniculate nuclei. Some neuroanatomists do not include the two geniculate bodies with the lateral nuclear mass, considering them instead to compose a metathalamus.

3. D The dorsal tier of lateral nuclei of the thalamus consists of the pulvinar, the lateral posterior nucleus, and the lateral dorsal nucleus. They are all situated in the dorsal part of the lateral nuclear mass and have similar connections and functions.

4. C The thalamus receives sensory input from all sensory systems except the olfactory. The main projections to the diencephalon from olfactory areas are the medial forebrain bundle to hypothalamic nuclei, and the stria medullaris thalamis to the epithalamus. The stria medullaris runs along the dorsomedial border of the thalamus, but fibers do not project into it.

5. A The anterior thalamic nucleus is included in the limbic system of the brain; thus the function of the nucleus must be in part that of the limbic system, e..g., basic emotional drives of importance to the preservation of the individual and the species.

6. C The anterior thalamic nucleus is responsible for the anterior tubercle of the thalamus which, with the fornix, bounds the interventricular foramen. The anterior end of the thalamus is narrow and the posterior end, the pulvinar, is expanded. The anterior nucleus is separated from other thalamic nuclear areas by the internal medullary lamina.

7. E The ventral lateral and ventral anterior nuclei are motor components of the thalamus and the boundary between them is arbitrary because of overlapping connections. These connections influence voluntary motor action in such a way that withdrawal or disturbance of their function contributes to the motor abnormalities coming under the general heading of dyskinesias.

8. A The medial geniculate nucleus forms a swelling, the medial geniculate body, on the posterior surface of the thalamus, inferior to the pulvinar. It is on the auditory pathway, receiving fibers via the inferior brachium from the inferior colliculus.

9. D The threshold for touch, pain, and temperature sensibilities is usually raised on the opposite side of the body, but when the threshold is reached the sensations are exaggerated, perverted, and exceptionally disagreeable.

10. A The input to the ventral lateral nucleus is mainly from the dentate nucleus of the cerebellum through the superior cerebellar peduncle. The fibers decussate in the midbrain and project to the contralateral ventral nucleus; hence, the left ventral lateral nucleus receives its input from the right dentate nucleus. Some input is received from the globus pallidus and the substantia nigra.

FIVE-CHOICE ASSOCIATION QUESTIONS

DIRECTIONS: Each of the following groups of questions consists of a numbered list of descriptive words or phrases accompanied by a diagram with certain parts indicated by letters, or by a list of lettered headings. For each numbered word or phrase, SELECT THE LETTERED PART OR HEADING that matches it correctly and insert the letter in the space to the right of the appropriate number. Each lettered heading may be selected once, more than once, or not at all.

A. Medial geniculate nucleus

B. Massa intermedia

C. Ventral lateral nucleus

D. Lateral genicular nucleus

E. Ventral posterior nucleus

1. _____ A motor component of the thalamus

2. _____ Thalamic nucleus on the auditory pathway

3. _____ Thalamic center for general senses

4. _____ Thalamic nucleus on the visual pathway

5. _____ Part of the midline nuclear complex

6. _____ Thalamic center for taste sensation

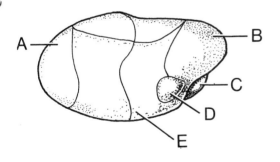

7. _____ Thalamic center for general senses

8. _____ Medial geniculate body

9. _____ Connected to association areas of the cortex

10. _____ Position of the lateral geniculate nucleus

11. _____ On the auditory pathway

12. _____ A motor component of the thalamus

(From Barr, M.L. and Kiernan, J.A.: The Human Nervous System, 4th ed., 1983. Courtesy of Harper & Row, Publishers, Inc.)

ANSWERS, NOTES, AND EXPLANATIONS

1. A The ventral lateral and ventral anterior nuclei are motor components of the thalamus that have overlapping connections. The input to the

113

ventral lateral nucleus is mainly from the dentate nucleus of the cerebellum, whereas that of the ventral anterior nucleus is from the corpus striatum (globus pallidus) and the cerebellum.

2. A The medial geniculate nucleus is on the auditory pathway. It forms a swelling, the medial geniculate body, on the posterior surface of the thalamus inferior to the pulvinar.

3. E The ventral posterior nucleus functions as a thalamic center for general senses and for the sense of taste. The contralateral medial lemniscus, the spinothalamic tract, and the trigeminothalamic tracts all terminate in this nucleus. The relay for the vestibular pathway to the cortex is also in this nucleus.

4. D The lateral geniculate nucleus is on the visual pathway to the cerebral cortex. It produces a swelling, the lateral geniculate body, beneath the pulvinar.

5. B The interthalamic adhesion (massa intermedia) forms a bridge of gray matter across the third ventricle in about 70 percent of brains. It constitutes part of the primitive midline nuclear complex. The midline nucleus is prominent in lower vertebrates, but forms a minor part of the human thalamus.

6. E The medial portion of the ventral posterior nucleus is also called the ventral posteromedial nucleus (V.P.M.). It functions as a thalamic center for taste as well as for general sensation in the head. Taste fibers are received from the gustatory nucleus in the brain stem, consisting of the rostral part of the nucleus of the solitary fasciculus. The remaining large portion (lateral) of the ventral posterior nucleus receives general sensory data from the body, exclusive of the head.

7. E The ventral posterior nucleus, as just stated, functions as a thalamic center for the general senses and the sense of taste. Fibers are received via the spinothalamic tract, the medial lemniscus, the trigeminothalamic tracts, and the gustatory and vestibular nuclei in the brain stem.

8. C The medial geniculate body is a swelling on the posterior inferomedial surface of the thalamus inferior to the pulvinar. The swelling is caused by the medial geniculate nucleus located on the auditory pathway. The nucleus receives data from the cochlear nuclei of both sides, but predominantly from the opposite side.

9. B The pulvinar, lateral posterior nucleus, and lateral dorsal nucleus are all situated in the dorsal part of the lateral nuclear mass. These three nuclei have reciprocal connections with association cortex of the parietal and occipital lobes and with the posterior part of the temporal lobe.

10. D The lateral geniculate body is a swelling on the posterior and lateral surface of the thalamus inferior to the pulvinar. It marks the position of the lateral geniculate nucleus on the visual pathway to the occipital cerebral cortex.

11. C The medial geniculate body consists of a nucleus that receives auditory fibers from the inferior colliculus. Efferents from this nucleus terminate in the auditory area (anterior transverse temporal gyri) of the temporal lobe.

12. A The ventral anterior nucleus and the ventral lateral nucleus are motor components of the thalamus that receive their input from the lentiform nucleus (globus pallidus region) through the lenticular fasciculus and the ansa lenticularis, and from the dentate nucleus of the cerebellum through the brachium conjunctivum. These two nuclei also receive connections from the substantia nigra.

S U B T H A L A M U S

        F I V E - C H O I C E   C O M P L E T I O N   Q U E S T I O N S

DIRECTIONS: Each of the following questions or incomplete statements is followed by five suggested answers or completions. SELECT THE ONE BEST ANSWER OR COMPLETION in each case and underline the appropriate letter at the right.

----

1. The subthalamus contains

    A. the medial lemmniscus, the sponthalamic tract, and the trigeminothalamic tracts
    B. fibers from the globus pallidus of the corpus striatum
    C. rostral extensions of the red nucleus and the substantia nigra
    D. fibers from the cerebellum coursing to the ventral lateral nucleus of the thalamus
    E. all of the above   A B C D E

2. Identify the incorrect statement below. Dentatothalamic fibers in the subthalamus

    A. traverse the red nucleus
    B. surround the red nucleus
    C. come from the brachium conjunctivum
    D. continue anteriorly in the field H of Forel
    E. enter the lateral dorsal nucleus of the thalamus   A B C D E

3. Which disturbance is NOT caused by a leasion in the subthalamic nucleus?

    A. Motor disturbance occurs on the opposite side of the body
    B. Involuntary movements come on suddenly
    C. Threshold for general sensations is usually limited
    D. Purposeless movements of a flailing type occur
    E. Spontaneous movements occur in the limbs   A B C D E

115

SELECT THE ONE BEST ANSWER OR COMPLETION

4. Some fibers from the globus pallidus within the subthalamus are contained in the

A. lenticular fasciculus
B. field H2 of Forel
C. ansa lenticularis
D. field H1 of Forel
E. all of the above

A B C D E

5. The major connection of the subthalamic nucleus is with the

A. globus pallidus
B. red nucleus
C. substantia nigra
D. dentate nucleus
E. ventral lateral nucleus of thalamus

A B C D E

6. Identify the <u>incorrect</u> statement about the subthalamic nucleus.

A. An extrapyramidal motor nucleus
B. Located between the internal capsule and the hypothalamus
C. Lies inferior to the lateral aspect of the thalamus
D. Sends fibers to the dentate nucleus of the cerebellum
E. Receives fibers via the subthalamic fasciculus

A B C D E

ANSWERS, NOTES, AND EXPLANATIONS

1. E The subthalamus contains all the structures mentioned. In addition, the superior cerebellar peduncle passes through the subthalamus on its way to the ventral posterior nucleus of the thalamus.

2. E The dentatothalamic fibers enter the ventral lateral nucleus of the thalamus. As their name implies, the fibers originate in the dentate nucleus of the cerebellum and pass to the thalamus via the superior cerebellar peduncle and the subthalamus. These connections influence voluntary motor action.

3. C In the thalamic syndrome the threshold for touch, pain, and temperature sensibilities is usually raised on the opposite side of the body. A lesion in the subthalamic nucleus causes a motor disturbance on the opposite side of the body called hemiballismus, in which there is a form of involuntary movement.

4. E Efferent fibers of the globus pallidus are contained in two distinct bundles, the lenticular fasciculus and the ansa lenticularis. Fibers of the lenticular fasiculus cut across the internal capsule to reach the subthalamus, where they form a band of white matter known alternatively as field H2 of Forel. The majority of fibers reverse direction in the prerubral area and enter the thalamic fasciculus or field H1 of Forel.

5. A The major connection of the subthalamic nucleus is with the globus pallidus; this consists of fibers running in both directions across the internal capsule and making up the subthalamic fasciculus.

6. D The subthalamic nucleus does not send fibers to the dentate nucleus. Dentatothalamic fibers pass through the subthalamus on their way to the ventral lateral nucleus of the thalamus, but they do not end in the subthalamic nucleus.

MULTI-COMPLETION QUESTIONS

DIRECTIONS: In each of the following questions or incomplete statements, one or more of the completions given is correct. At the lower right of each question, underline A if 1, 2, and 3 are correct; B if 1 and 3 are correct; C if 2 and 4 are correct; D if only 4 is correct; and E if all are correct.

---

1. Correct statements about the subthalamus include:

   1. In an appropriate coronal section of the diencephalon, the subthalamus can be seen medial to the internal capsule
   2. It contains an important extrapyramidal nucleus
   3. The globus pallidus provides the principal input to the subthalamus
   4. A lesion in the subthalamus, usually vascular in origin, produces hemiballismus   A B C D E

2. Which of the following nuclei, or portions of them, are included in the subthalamus?

   1. Red   3. Subthalamic
   2. Substantia nigra   4. Globus pallidus   A B C D E

3. A vascular lesion involving the subthalamic nucleus causes

   1. involuntary purposeless movements of the contralateral limbs, especially proximal parts of the arms
   2. forceful flinging movements of the contralateral limbs and sometimes involuntary contractions of muscles in the neck and face
   3. sudden, rapid, involuntary limb movements that may be choreiform or jerky
   4. loss of general sensations in the contralateral upper limb   A B C D E

4. Correct statements concerning the zona incerta include:

   1. A thin layer of gray matter between the lenticular and thalamic fasciculi
   2. A biconvex nucleus lying against the internal capsule
   3. A rostral extension of the reticular formation of the brain stem
   4. Its major connection is with the globus pallidus   A B C D E

5. The lenticular fasciculus consists of fibers which

   1. arise in the globus pallidus of the corpus striatum
   2. cut across the internal capsule to reach the subthalamus
   3. form a band of white matter known as field H2 of Forel
   4. reverse direction in the prerubral area to enter the thalamic fasciculus   A B C D E

117

A	B	C	D	E
1,2,3	1,3	2,4	only 4	all correct

6. Correct statements about the subthalamic fasciculus include:

    1. Passes through the posterior limb of the internal capsule.
    2. Consists of fibers running from the globus pallidus to the subthalamic nucleus
    3. Is a two-way array of fibers interconnecting the globus pallidus and the subthalamic nucleus
    4. Curves medially around the ventral border of the internal capsule   A B C D E

ANSWERS, NOTES, AND EXPLANATIONS

1. E All are correct. The subthalamus cannot be seen in the intact brain. To see it one must examine an appropriate coronal section of the diencephalon in which the subthalamus is medial to the internal capsule, inferior to the thalamus and lateral to the hypothalamus. Although included in the diencephalon, it is functionally part of the extrapyramidal motor system. The subthalamic nucleus is one of the extrapyramidal nuclei and is best developed in primates.

2. A 1, 2, and 3 are correct. Small portions of the substantia nigra and red nucleus extend from the midbrain into the subthalamus. The subthalamic nucleus, lying against the internal capsule, is one of the extrapyramidal nuclei. Its major connections are with the globus pallidus.

3. A 1, 2, and 3 are correct. The clinical condition caused by a lesion in the subthalamus, especially in the subthalamic nucleus, is called hemiballismus. It is characterized by violent, purposeless movements of the limbs on the contralateral side, especially the proximal parts of the arms. Although sensory fasciculi pass through the subthalamus on their way to the ventral posterior nucleus of the thalamus, they are not affected by the usual vascular type of subthalamic lesion.

4. B 1 and 3 are correct. The zona incerta is a thin lamina of gray matter in the subthalamus representing a rostral extension of the reticular formation of the brain stem. It is located between the lenticular and thalamic fasciculi, and is continuous laterally with the reticular nucleus of the thalamus.

5. E All are correct. The lenticular fasciculus is one of the fiber tracts leaving the globus pallidus of the corpus striatum. It passes through the posterior limb of the internal capsule and runs between the zona incerta and the subthalamic nucleus. Many of the fibers of the lenticular fasciculus enter the thalamic fasciculus and terminate in the ventral lateral and ventral anterior thalamic nuclei.

6. A 1, 2, and 3 are correct. The subthalamic fasciculus is the major connection between the globus pallidus and the subthalamic nucleus. It consists of fibers running in both directions across the internal capsule.

FIVE-CHOICE ASSOCIATION QUESTIONS

DIRECTIONS: Each of the following groups of questions consists of a numbered list of descriptive words or phrases accompanied by a diagram with certain parts indicated by letters, or by a list of lettered headings. For each numbered word or phrase, SELECT THE LETTERED PART OR HEADING that matches it correctly and insert the letter in the space to the right of the appropriate number. Each lettered heading may be selected once, more than once, or not at all.

----

1. ____ Lesion results in condition known as hemiballismus

A. Red nucleus

2. ____ Continuation of mesencephalic reticular formation

B. Ansa lenticularis

3. ____ Forms a sharp bend around the medial edge of the internal capsule

C. Subthalamic nucleus

D. Subthalamic fasciculus

4. ____ Interconnects the globus pallidus and the subthalamic nucleus

E. Zona incerta

5. ____ Extends from midbrain partway into the subthalamus

6. ____ Biconvex nucleus lying against the internal capsule

ANSWERS, NOTES, AND EXPLANATIONS

1. C   The subthalamic nucleus is an important site for the integration of a number of motor control centers, particularly through its connections with the globus pallidus of the corpus striatum. A lesion of one subthalamic nucleus results in the condition of hemiballismus, characterized by uncontrollable violent movements affecting the contralateral side of the body.

2. E   The mesencephalic reticular formation continues into the subthalamus, where it appears as the zona incerta between the lenticular and thalamic fasciculi.

3. B   The ansa lenticularis is a fiber tract that originates mainly in the globus pallidus and swings around the medial border of the internal capsule. Almost all its fibers terminate in the ventral lateral and ventral anterior thalamic nuclei after traversing the subthalamus.

4. D   The major connection of the subthalamic nucleus is with the globus pallidus; this consists of fibers running in both directions across the internal capsule, making up the subthalamic fasciculus.

5. A The cranial ends of two midbrain nuclei, the red nucleus and the sub-
    stantia nigra, extend into the caudal part of the subthalamus. Dentato-
    thalamic fibers of the brachium conjunctivum both surround and traverse
    the red nucleus.

6. C The subthalamic nucleus is a biconvex nucleus lying against the
    internal capsule. It is one of the extrapyramidal motor nuclei and is
    best developed in primates. Its major connection is with the globus
    pallidus. A lesion in the subthalamic nucleus causes a motor
    disturbance on the opposite side of the body known as hemiballismus.
    This condition is characterized by involuntary movements which come on
    suddenly with great force and rapidity.

E P I T H A L A M U S

F I V E - C H O I C E   C O M P L E T I O N   Q U E S T I O N S

DIRECTIONS: Each of the following questions or incomplete statements is
followed by five suggested answers or completions. SELECT THE ONE BEST
ANSWER OR COMPLETION in each case and underline the appropriate letter at
the right.

----

1. Afferents to the habenular nucleus run in the

    A. stria terminalis   D. body of the fornix
    B. fasciculus retroflexus   E. habenular commissure
    C. stria medullaris thalami   A B C D E

2. Structures which are part of a pathway in the epithalamus
    through which primitive aspects of brain function influ-
    ence the viscera include:

    A. Habenulointerpeduncular   C. Habenular nucleus
        fasciculus   D. All of the above
    B. Stria medullaris thalami   E. None of the above   A B C D E

3. Which statement about the pineal body is false?

    A. Develops from a hollow outgrowth from the caudal part of
        the roof of the diencephalon
    B. A characteristic feature of pineal bodies in children is
        the presence of corpora arenacea (brain sand)
    C. Is thought to have an endocrine secretion that has an anti-
        gonadotropic effect
    D. A pineal tumor may cause compression of the superior
        colliculus
    E. Contains neither photoreceptors nor nerve cells   A B C D E

SELECT THE ONE BEST ANSWER OR COMPLETION

4. The main destination of the habenulointerpeduncular fasciculus is the

A. amygdaloid nucleus   D. septal area
B. dorsal tegmental nucleus E. none of the above
C. habenular nucleus   A B C D E

5. Which statement about the habenular nucleus is <u>incorrect?</u>

A. Receives afferent fibers through the stria medullaris thalami
B. Many efferent fibers from it terminate in the interpeduncular nucleus
C. Forms a slight swelling in the habenular trigone
D. Site of origin of the stria terminalis
E. Gives rise to a well-defined bundle of fibers that are sometimes called the fasciculus retroflexus   A B C D E

6. Observations supporting the view that the pineal body exerts an antigonadotrophic effect include:

A. A pineal tumor in a child around the age of puberty may affect the onset of pubertal changes
B. Boys with tumors that destroyed pineal parenchyma exhibited precocious puberty
C. A child with a tumor derived from the pinealocytes shows a delay in the onset of puberty
D. Pinealectomy in young rats leads to enlargement of the reproductive organs
E. All of the above   A B C D E

ANSWERS, NOTES, AND EXPLANATIONS

1. C Afferent fibers to the habenular nucleus are received through the stria medullaris thalami, which runs along the dorsomedial border of the thalamus. The stria terminalis originates in the amygdaloid nucleus of the temporal lobe and ends mainly in the septal area and the hypothalamus. However a few of its fibers turn caudally at the anterior end of the thalamus and join the stria medullaris thalami.

2. D The stria medullaris thalami, originating mainly in the medial olfactory (septal) area on the medial surface of the frontal lobe, the habenular nucleus, and the habenulointerpeduncular fasciculus, constitute part of a pathway through which primitive aspects of brain function, e.g., basic emotional drives and the sense of smell, influence the viscera.

3. B Granules of calcium and magnesium salts normally do not appear in the pineal body until after the age of 16 years. These calcareous granules coalesce later to form larger particles, called brain sand, pineal sand, or corpora arenacea. These granules can often be used to identify the pineal body in radiographs of the skull. Identification and measure-

121

ments of the position of the pineal body in radiographs of the skull can provide useful information, especially in the diagnosis of space-occupying intracranial lesions.

4. E The habenulointerpeduncular fasciculus (tract), often called the fasciculus retroflexus, originates in the habenular nucleus and terminates in the interpeduncular nucleus in the roof of the interpeduncular fossa of the midbrain.

5. D The stria terminalis is a slender strand of fibers running along the medial side of the tail of the caudate nucleus. Originating in the amygdaloid nucleus, most of its fibers end in the septal area and the hypothalamus.

6. E All these well-documented clinical observations and the experimental evidence substantiate the belief that the pineal body is not a functionless vestigial organ, but an endocrine gland that produces a hormone that has an antigonadotropic effect. The site of action of the hormone(s) has not been established; it may be gonads, the pars distalis of the pituitary, or the hypothalamus. It appears that the pineal body has a neuroendocrine function and that it participates in the regulation of the rhythmic activity of the endocrine system.

M U L T I - C O M P L E T I O N   Q U E S T I O N S

DIRECTIONS: In each of the following questions or incomplete statements, one or more of the completions given is correct. At the lower right of each question, underline A if 1, 2, and 3 are correct; B if 1 and 3 are correct; C if 2 and 4 are correct; D if only 4 is correct; and E if all are correct.

---

1. The epithalamus includes the

    1. habenular trigone   3. stria medullaris thalami
    2. habenular nucleus   4. pineal body   A B C D E

2. Statements that correctly describe the habenular nucleus include:

    1. A nucleus on an olfactory reflex pathway
    2. Efferents from this nucleus run in the stria terminalis
    3. The main outflow pathway from this nucleus passes to the interpenduncular nucleus
    4. Part of the mesencephalic reticular formation that continues into the epithalamus   A B C D E

3. Correct statements concerning the location of the pineal body include:

    1. Lies between the habenular nuclei
    2. Partly covers the superior colliculi
    3. Attached by a stalk to the roof of the diencephalon
    4. Lies inferior to the splenium of the corpus callosum   A B C D E

	A	B	C	D	E
	1,2,3	1,3	2,4	only 4	all correct

4. Which of the following fiber bundles are included in the epithalamus?

   1. Stria medullaris thalami
   2. Stria terminalis
   3. Habenular commissure
   4. Habenulointerpenduncular fasciculus   A B C D E

5. Correct statements about the pineal body include:

   1. Contains neuroglial cells resembling astrocytes
   2. Develops as ventral bud of the floor of the diencephalon
   3. Contains a cavity that is continuous with the third ventricle
   4. Occupies the depression between the inferior colliculi   A B C D E

6. It is generally believed that the pineal body is

   1. a functionless vestigial organ in man that is of little value clinically
   2. a secretory organ, the importance of which has not been fully assessed
   3. not a useful landmark for radiologists in assessing the location of space-occupying lesions
   4. the site of formation of hormones that play a part in the regulation of peripubertal gonadal development   A B C D E

ANSWERS, NOTES, AND EXPLANATIONS

1. E All are correct. The epithalamus consists of the habenular nuclei, their connections (stria medullaris thalami and habenulointerpeduncular fasciculus), and the pineal body. The position of the habenular nucleus is indicated by a slight swelling in the habenular trigone, adjacent to the posterior end of the roof of the third ventricle.

2. B 1 and 3 are correct. The habenular nucleus is on a pathway that begins in the medial olfactory (septal) area and ends in autonomic nuclei in the brain stem. Through this pathway, primitive aspects of brain function (basic emotional drives and the sense of smell) influence the viscera.

3. E All are correct. The pineal body is a somewhat flattened, conical body lying at the posterior extremity of the roof of the third ventricle. Because it may be identified in radiographs of many persons after about 16 years of age, it is important to know its relationship to other parts of the brain. Displacement of the pineal body may result from the formation of space-occupying lesions, e.g., a tumor or a hemorrhage in the internal capsule in patients with hypertension. Because of its location, tumors of the pineal body may cause compression of the superior colliculi and the cerebral aqueduct.

4. B 1 and 3 are correct. Although a few fibers of the stria terminalis turn caudally in the region of the interventricular foramen and join the stria medullaris thalami, this slender strand of fibers is not part of the epithalamus, even though some of its fibers terminate in the habenular nucleus. The main fiber connections of the habenular nuclei are: afferent from the medial olfactory (septal) area via the stria medullaris thalami; efferents to the interpeduncular nucleus; and the habenular commissure in the dorsal wall of the stalk of the pineal body.

5. B 1 and 3 are correct. The pineal body develops as an outgrowth from the caudal part of the roof of the diencephalon. Pinealocytes or chief cells make up the bulk of the gland, whereas about 5 percent of the cells are interstitial cells which have an appearance not unlike glial cells. The pineal body is generally believed to increase in size until about the seventh year and then to regress until the age of about 14 years. After the age of 16 years, granules of calcium and magnesium salts, called brain sand, pineal sand, or corpora arenacea, appear in the gland.

6. C 2 and 4 are correct. Although the functions of the pineal body are not fully understood at present, evidence is mounting that it plays a part in the regulation of gonadal development, possibly by influencing the output of gonadotropins via the hypothalamus during the period just before puberty. There are well estabished clinical observations that suggest an antigonadotropic function because a pineal tumor developing around the age of puberty may alter the onset of secondary sexual changes.

F I V E - C H O I C E   A S S O C I A T I O N   Q U E S T I O N S

DIRECTIONS: Each of the following groups of questions consists of a numbered list of descriptive words or phrases accompanied by a diagram with certain parts indicated by letters, or by a list of lettered headings. For each numbered word or phrase, SELECT THE LETTERED PART OR HEADING that matches it correctly and insert the letter in the space to the right of the appropriate number. Each lettered heading may be selected once, more than once, or not at all.

----

	1. ____Interstitial elements
A. Neuroglial cells	2. ____Parenchymatous cells
B. Pineal recess	3. ____Hormone with a role in gonadal
C. Brain sand	development
D. Melatonin	4. ____Calcareous concretions
E. Pinealocytes	5. ____Cerebrospinal fluid
	6. ____Epithelial elements

ASSOCIATION QUESTIONS

A. Stria medullaris thalami

B. Pineal stalk

C. Fasciculus retroflexus

D. Stria terminalis

E. Habenular nucleus

7. ____Main outflow path from the nucleus

8. ____Some of its fibers join the stria medullaris thalami

9. ____Receives afferent fibers through the stria medullaris thalami

10. ____Originates in the medial olfactory area

11. ____Terminates in the interpeduncular nucleus

12. ____Attached to the posterior nucleus

ANSWERS, NOTES, AND EXPLANATIONS

1. A The neuroglial cells, which resemble astrocytes, serve as supporting elements. As these cells are situated amongst the pinealocytes, which they partially ensheath and separate, they are often called interstitial cells. Like the pinealocytes, these cells are derived from the ectodermal roof plate of the diencephalon.

2. E The pinealocytes, arranged in cords, form the parenchyma of the pineal body and constitute the main cell type. These cells produce melatonin which appears to inhibit gonadotropin secretion. The administration of pineal extracts or melatonin has been shown to delay sexual maturation in several nonprimate species.

3. D The amino acid melatonin produced by the pineal body appears to play a part in the regulation of gonadal development. Melatonin may be secreted from the gland into the blood, making it a true neuroendocrine gland, or it may be released into the pineal recess of the third ventricle.

4. C The concentrations of the pineal body, composed of calcium and magnesium granules, are called corpora arenacea, or more commonly, brain sand. These extracellular concretions begin to appear in the pineal body at about 16 years of age and increase in number with age. Their significance is unknown, but they enable one to identify the pineal body in radiographs. Measurements and identification of the position of the pineal body in radiographs of the head can provide useful information, especially in the diagnosis of space-occupying intracranial lesions.

5. B As the pineal recess is part of the third ventricle, it contains cerebrospinal fluid. Although the melatonin produced by the pinealo-

cytes may be released into the cerebrospinal fluid, it is generally believed that it is secreted into the blood in the vessels in the invest-
ing layer of pia mater.

6. E   The pinealocytes are the epithelial elements in the pineal body.
These epithelioid cells are difficult to define in routine preparations, but are easily demonstrated in silver preparations. The human
pineal body contains neither photoreceptors, as in submammalian forms,
nor nerve cells, but has some neuroglial cells in the roof of the diencephalon, from which the pineal body arose as a diverticulum.

7. C   The habenulointerpeduncular fasciculus (fasciculus retroflexus of
Meynert) is the main bundle of fibers leaving the habenular nucleus. It
terminates in the interpeduncular nucleus superior to the interpeduncular fossa of the midbrain. The habenular nucleus forms a small swelling
in the habenular trigone in the wall of the posterior part of the third
ventricle.

8. D   The cells of origin of the stria terminalis are in the amygdaloid
nucleus. As it reaches the region of the interventricular foramen, some
of the fibers of the stria terminalis turn caudally and join the stria
medullaris thalami.

9. E   The afferent fibers to the habenular nucleus are received through the
stria medullaris thalami, which is formed near the anterior pole of the
thalamus and forms the dorsomedial ridge (border) of the thalamus. Most
cells of origin of the stria medullaris are situated in the medial olfactory (septal) area, located on the medial surface of the frontal
lobe.

10. A   The stria medullaris thalami originates mainly in the medial
olfactory (septal) area. It is one of the two main projections from
this olfactory area; the other is the medial forebrain bundle. The
stria medullaris runs along the dorsomedial border of the thalamus and
ends in the habenular nucleus.

11. C   The fasciculus retroflexus, often called the habenulointerpeduncular
fasciculus, originates in the habenular nucleus and ends in the interpeduncular nucleus superior to the interpeduncular fossa of the midbrain. This tract constitutes part of a pathway through which primitive
aspects of brain function (basic emotional drives and the sense of
smell) influence the viscera.

12. B   The ventral wall of the pineal stalk is attached to the posterior
commissure and the habenular commissure traverses the dorsal wall. The
constitution and significance of the posterior commissure are imperfect-
ly understood in man. Lesions interrupting the posterior commissure are
said to reduce, but not eliminate, the consensual pupillary light
reflex.

HYPOTHALAMUS

FIVE-CHOICE COMPLETION QUESTIONS

DIRECTIONS: Each of the following questions or incomplete statements is followed by five suggested answers or completions. SELECT THE ONE BEST ANSWER OR COMPLETION in each case and underline the appropriate letter at the right.

---

1. From which of the following structures does the hypothalamus receive information?

   A. Viscera
   B. Tongue
   C. Nipples
   D. Nose
   E. All of the above

   A B C D E

2. The cells of origin of the medial forebrain bundle are chiefly in which of the following areas or structures?

   A. Septal area
   B. Intermediate olfactory area
   C. Lateral olfactory area
   D. Olfactory bulb
   E. Hippocampus

   A B C D E

3. From which of the following parts of the brain does the hypothalamus have afferent connections?

   A. Amygdaloid nucleus
   B. Septal area
   C. Hippocampus
   D. Medial thalamic nucleus
   E. All of the above

   A B C D E

4. Which of the following hypothalamic nuclei or areas of gray matter is NOT derived from the diencephalon of the embryonic forebrain?

   A. Anterior
   B. Paraventricular
   C. Ventromedial
   D. Preoptic
   E. Supraoptic

   A B C D E

5. Which statement about the dorsal longitudinal fasciculus is correct?

   A. One of two principal efferent pathways from the hypothalamus
   B. Carries impulses to parasympathetic nuclei of the brain stem
   C. Begins as paraventricular fibers beneath the ependyma of the third ventricle
   D. A major ascending pathway to the hypothalamus
   E. Carries impulses that affect lower autonomic and motor centers

   A B C D E

SELECT THE ONE BEST ANSWER OR COMPLETION

6. With which of the following does the hypothalamus have
   important efferent connections?

   A. Cerebrum   D. Spinal cord
   B. Pituitary gland   E. All of the above
   C. Brain stem   A B C D E

7. Tracts concerned with the transmission of activity in the
   hypothalamus to areas of the brain concerned with emotions
   include:

   A. Mammillotegmental tract   D. Medial forebrain
   B. Dorsal longitudinal fasciculus   bundle
   C. Mamillothalamic tract   E. All of the above   A B C D E

8. Hypothalamic function becomes manifest through

   A. autonomic nuclei in the brain stem
   B. autonomic nuclei in the spinal cord
   C. relationship with the pituitary gland
   D. all of the above
   E. none of the above   A B C D E

9. Which of the following is not a boundary of the hypothalamic region known as the tuber cinereum?

   A. Median eminence   D. Right mamillary body
   B. Optic chiasma   E. Left mamillary body
   C. Optic tract   A B C D E

10. The structure serving as a point of reference for a sagittal
    plane dividing the hypothalamus into medial and lateral zones
    is the

    A. lamina terminalis   D. tuber cinereum
    B. optic chiasma   E. median eminence
    C. fornix   A B C D E

ANSWERS, NOTES, AND EXPLANATIONS

1. E The hypothalamus receives information from all the structures men-
    tioned in subserving its role as the main integrator of the autonomic
    nervous system. Ascending visceral afferents convey data of visceral
    origin, including the senses of taste and smell. Somatic sensory in-
    formation from erotogenic zones, such as the nipples and genitalia, also
    reaches the hypothalamus.

2. A The cells of origin of the medial forebrain bundle are chiefly in the
    septal or medial olfactory area, but other fibers come from the
    intermediate and lateral olfactory areas. The medial forebrain bundle
    runs caudally in the lateral area of the hypothalamus, giving off fibers
    to hypothalamic nuclei.

3. E The hypothalamus receives information from many sources in order to serve as the main integrator of the autonomic nervous system. The central input from the viscera consists of general visceral afferents. The senses of smell and taste, which are special senses eliciting visceral resonses, come under the heading of special visceral afferents.

4. D The gray matter immediately posterior to the lamina terminalis, the preoptic area, is derived from the telencephalon, as are the lamina terminalis and the anterior commissure. The lamina terminalis is the part of the brain formed from the rostral end of the embryonic neural tube.

5. D The dorsal longitudinal fasciculus is one of the two principal efferent pathways from the hypothalamus; the other is the mamillotegmental tract. The dorsal longitudinal tract consists of descending fibers from the hypothalamus that end in nuclei giving rise to autonomic outflow from the brain stem and spinal cord, partly through relays in the reticular formation.

6. E The hypothalamus is involved in homeostatic mechanisms concerned with a person's internal welfare, and so has connections with all the structures mentioned. In addition, it has important connections with the anterior nucleus of the thalamus via the mamillothalamic tract, forming part of the limbic system.

7. C The large mamillothalamic tract (bundle of Vincq d'Azyr) connects the mamillary body with the anterior nucleus of the thalamus. This nucleus has reciprocal connections with the cortex of the cingulate gyrus. The anterior thalamic nucleus and the cingulate cortex share responsibility with other components of the limbic system for those emotions and aspects of behavior that are related to the preservation of the individual and the species.

8. D The complex role of the hypothalamus includes maintaining a constant internal body environment (homeostasis). This is accomplished in part through the autonomic outflow from the brain stem and spinal cord. Equally important are neurosecretory cells of the hypothalamus which elaborate the hormones released in the neurohypophysis and produce "releasing factors" which control the hormonal output of the adenohypophysis.

9. A The median eminence, infundibular stem, and pars nervosa of the pituitary gland together constitute the neurohypophysis. The tuber cinereum is the convex base of the hypothalamus, bordered caudally by the mamillary bodies, rostrally by the optic chiasma, and laterally by the beginning of the optic tracts. The tuber cinereum, from which the infundibular stem arises, is raised to form the median eminence.

10. C The fornix passes through the hypothalamus on its way to the mamillary body, and is located so that it serves as a point of reference for a sagittal plane dividing the hypothalamus into medial and lateral zones on each side.

MULTI-COMPLETION QUESTIONS

DIRECTIONS: In each of the following questions or incomplete statements, one or more of the completions given is correct. At the lower right of each question, underline A if 1, 2, and 3 are correct; B if 1 and 3 are correct; C if 2 and 4 are correct; D if only 4 is correct; and E if all are correct.

---

1. Correct statements about the hypothalamus include:

    1. Occupies the interval between the third ventricle and the subthalamus
    2. Extends from the lamina terminalis to the caudal border of the mamillary bodies
    3. Forms the wall of the third ventricle inferior to the hypothalamic sulcus
    4. The optic chiasma divides the hypothalamus into medial and lateral zones   A B C D E

2. Nuclei contained in the tuberal region of the hypothalamus include:

1. Ventromedial		3. Dorsomedial	
2. Posterior hypothalamic		4. Medial mamillary	A B C D E

3. The hypothalamus of man is characterized by the

    1. large size of the medial mamillary nucleus
    2. well defined lateral tuberal nucleus
    3. presence of large neurons in the posterior and lateral nuclei
    4. bulk of large neurons in the mamillary bodies   A B C D E

4. Efferent pathways from the hypothalamus to the brain include

    1. medial forebrain bundle
    2. dorsal longitudinal fasciculus
    3. stria terminalis
    4. mamillotegmental tract   A B C D E

5. Which of the following have afferent connections with the hypothalamus?

    1. Medial forebrain bundle
    2. Stria terminalis
    3. Fornix
    4. Anterior thalamic nucleus   A B C D E

A	B	C	D	E
1,2,3	1,3	2,4	only 4	all correct

6. The hypothalamus is

   1. the main integrator of the autonomic system
   2. of functional importance in proportion to its size
   3. at the crossroads between the thalamus and cerebral cortex
   4. not essential to the intimate relationship between basic emotional drives and visceral function   A B C D E

7. The neurohypophysial hormones are produced in which of the following hypothalamic nuclei?

   1. Infundibular   3. Anterior
   2. Supraoptic   4. Paraventricular   A B C D E

8. Parasympathetic responses are mostly regularly elicited by stimulation of the

   1. preoptic area   3. anterior nucleus
   2. supraoptic nucleus   4. mamillary body   A B C D E

9. Afferent fibers entering the hypothalamus that are related to basic emotional drives and the sense of smell are contained in the

   1. dorsal longitudinal fasciculus   3. lateral terminalis
   2. stria terminalis   4. medial forebrain bundle   A B C D E

10. Nuclei from which sympathetic responses are most readily elicited by electrical stimulation in experimental animals include

   1. medial hypothalamic   3. anterior hypothalamic
   2. posterior   4. lateral   A B C D E

ANSWERS, NOTES, AND EXPLANATIONS

1. A 1, 2, and 3 are correct. The fornix traverses the hypothalamus to reach the mamillary body and serves as point of reference for a sagittal plane dividing the hypothalamus into medial and lateral zones. The optic chiasma forms the rostral boundary of the tuber cinereum.

2. B 1 and 3 are correct. The tuberal region contains the ventromedial, dorsomedial and infundibular (arcuate) nuclei. The mamillary body and the posterior hypothalamic nucleus make up the mamillary region.

3. A 1, 2, and 3 are correct. Many cells of the posterior nucleus and those of the lateral nucleus of the hypothalamus are large. In man, the mamillary body consists almost entirely of a medial mamillary nucleus consisting of small neurons.

4. C **2 and 4 are correct**. There are two principal efferent pathways from the hypothalamus to the brain stem: the dorsal longitudinal fasciculus and the mamillotegmental tract. The medial forebrain bundle and the stria terminalis are afferent connections of the hypothalamus.

5. E **All are correct**. The hypothalamus receives information from many sources. In addition to the afferent connections listed, the hypothalamus receives fibers from the anterior thalamic nucleus through

   the mamillothalamic nucleus, and from the prefontal cortex. In addition, there are direct corticohypothalamic fibers.

6. E **All are correct**. Although representing only a small part of the brain, the hypothalamus is of great functional importance. Among other roles, it is essential to the intimate relationship between basic emotional drives and visceral function because it is an integral part of the limbic system of the brain.

7. C **2 and 4 are correct**. Hormones enter the blood stream from the neurohypophysis, but they are elaborated in the cells of the supraoptic and paraventricular nuclei, and reach the neurohypophysis by axoplasmic flow. The two neurohypophysial hormones are vasopressin and oxytocin. The precursors of these hormones appear in the cytoplasm of cells of the supraoptic and paraventricular nuclei as neurosecretory droplets or granules. In experimental animals, and probably in man, vasopressin (an antidiuretic hormone) is produced by the supraoptic nucleus and oxytocin by the paraventricular nucleus.

8. B **1 and 3 are correct**. Electrical stimulation of the anterior hypothalamus in experimental animals, notably the preoptic area and anterior nucleus, commonly gives parasympathetic responses, e.g., slowing of the heart rate, vasodilation, and lowering of blood pressure.

9. C **2 and 4 are correct**. The cells of origin of the medial forebrain bundle are mainly in the septal or medial olfactory areas. The medial forebrain bundle is small in the human brain compared with the brains of animals (e.g., the dog) that rely heavily on the sense of smell. The stria terminalis originates in the amygdaloid nucleus of the temporal lobe.

10. C **2 and 4 are correct**. Sympathetic responses are most regularly elicited by stimulation of the posterior and lateral hypothalamic nuclei. Typical responses are cardiac acceleration, elevation of blood pressure, cessation of peristalsis in the gastrointestinal tract, dilation of the pupils, and hyperglycemia.

DIRECTIONS: Each of the following groups of questions consists of a numbered list of descriptive words or phrases accompanied by a diagram with certain parts indicated by letters, or by a list of lettered headings. For each numbered word or phrase, SELECT THE LETTERED PART OR HEADING that matches it correctly and insert the letter in the space to the right of the appropriate number. Each lettered heading may be selected once, more than once, or not at all.

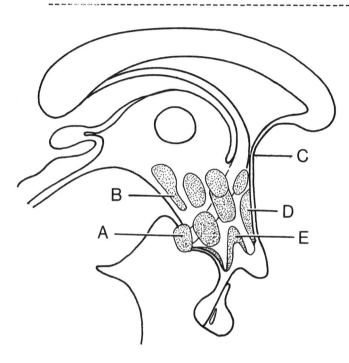

1. ____ Stimulation of it produces parasympathetic responses

2. ____ Elaborates neuro-hyposial hormones

3. ____ Contains cells of origin of mamillothalamic tract

4. ____ Represents the rostral end of the embryonic neural tube

5. ____ Serves as an osmoreceptor

6. ____ Stimulation of it produces sympathetic responses

A. Mamillary body

B. Dorsal longitudinal fasciculus

C. Medial forebrain bundle

D. Fornix

E. Medial zone of the hypothalamus

7. ____ Largest of the various fiber bundles ending in the hypothalamus

8. ____ Cells of origin are chiefly in the septal area

9. ____ Connected to the anterior thalamic nucleus

10. ____ Its fibers terminate mainly in the mamillary body

11. ____ Receives fibers from the anterior thalamic nucleus

12. ____ Principal efferent pathway from the hypothalamus

13. ____ Contains the supraoptic nucleus

14. ____ Contains afferent fibers from the hippocampus

(The above drawing is from Barr, M.L. and Kiernan, J.A.: The Human Nervous System, 4th ed., 1983. Courtesy of Harper & Row, Publishers, Inc.)

133

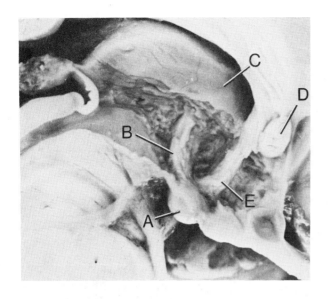

15. ____Anterior tubercle of the thalamus

16. ____Mamillary body

17. ____Connects areas of right and left temporal lobes

18. ____Fornix

19. ____Anterior commissure

20. ____Mamillothalamic tract

(From Barr, M.L. and Kiernan, J.A.: The Human Nervous System, 4th ed., 1983. Courtesy of Harper & Row, Publishers, Inc.)

ANSWERS, NOTES, AND EXPLANATIONS

1. D Stimulation of anterior parts of the hypothalamus (preoptic area (D) and anterior nucleus) in experimental animals gives parasympathetic responses, e.g., slowing of the heart.

2. E The two neurohypophysial hormones, oxytocin and vasopressin, are elaborated in cells of the supraoptic and paraventricular nuclei of the hypothalamus. The neurosecretions are carried by axoplasmic flow from the cell bodies to the axon terminals, from which they enter the blood passing through the capillary bed of the neurohypophysis.

3. A The cells of origin of the mamillothalamic tract are in the mamillary body. This large tract contains fibers running in both directions, interconnects the mamillary body with the anterior thalamic nucleus, and the latter nucleus has reciprocal connections with the cortex of the cingulate gyrus. The anterior thalamic nucleus and the cingulate cortex share with other components of the limbic system responsibility for those emotions and aspects of behavior that are related to preservation of the individual and the species.

4. C The lamina terminalis represents the rostral end of the embryonic neural tube and the site of closure of the rostral neuropore. The lamina terminalis, extending from the optic chiasma to the anterior commissure, limits the third ventricle anteriorly.

5. E The supraoptic nucleus serves as an osmoreceptor, the secretory activity of its cells being influenced by the osmolarity of the blood flowing through its highly vascular nucleus. A slight elevation of

osmotic pressure causes the cells to synthesize antidiuretic hormone (vasopressin) more rapidly, and an increased amount of the hormone enters the capillary blood of the neurohypophysis.

6. B Stimulation of the posterior (B) and lateral nuclei of the hypothalamus produces sympathetic responses, e.g, cardiac acceleration and elevation of blood pressure.

7. D The fornix, originating in the hippocampus of the temporal lobe, is the largest of the various fiber bundles ending in the hypothalamus. It arches over the thalamus and down into the hypothalamus, where the fibers terminate in several nuclei, but mainly in the mamillary body.

8. C The cells of origin of the medial forebrain bundle are chiefly in the septal or medial olfactory area. It runs caudally in the lateral area of the hypothalamus, giving off fibers to hypothalamic nuclei.

9. A The large mamillothalamic tract establishes reciprocal connections between the mamillary body and the anterior thalamic nucleus. The latter nucleus has reciprocal connections with the cortex of the cingulate gyrus.

10. D Fibers of the fornix enter the hypothalamus and terminate in several nuclei, but mainly in the mamillary body. The hypothalamus is an integral part of the limbic system of the brain and essential to the intimmate relationship between basic emotional drives and visceral function.

11. A The mamillary body receives fibers from the anterior thalamic nucleus through the mamillothalamic tract and is therefore in communication with the cingulate gyrus.

12. B The dorsal longitudinal fasciculus is one of two principal efferent pathways from the hypothalamus to the brain stem; the other is the mamillotegmental tract.

13. E Within the medial zone, the suprachiasmatic region contains nuclei. Cells in the supraoptic and paraventricular nuclei elaborate two neurohypophysial hormones: vasopressin and oxytocin.

14. D The fornix, the large fiber bundle entering the hypothalamus, originates in the hippocampus of the temporal lobe. Its fibers terminate mainly in the mamillary body.

15. C The anterior thalamic nucleus is responsible for the anterior tubercle of the thalamus, which, with the fornix, bounds the interventricular foramen. This nucleus is included in the limbic system of the brain.

16. A The mamillary bodies are swellings on the basal surface of the hypothalamus; they receive fibers from the hippocampi and the anterior thalamic nuclei.

17. D The anterior commissure, a fiber bundle connecting areas of the right and left temporal lobes, also contains some fibers connecting the ol-

factory bulbs. The anterior commissure, like the lamina terminalis, is derived from the telencephalon of the embryonic brain.

18.   E   The fornix, a Latin word meaning arch, is the efferent tract of the hippocampus. It arches over the thalamus and terminates mainly in the mamillary body of the hypothalamus.

19.   D   The anterior commissure, the lamina terminalis, and the gray areas immediately posterior to the lamina are telencephalic structures. Other hypothalamic structures are derived from the diencephalon of the embryonic forebrain.

20.   B   The mamillothalamic tract, as its name indicates, connects the mamillary body with the anterior thalamic nucleus. This large tract carries fibers to and from this region of the thalamus.

NINE

The Cerebral Hemispheres

O B J E C T I V E S

CEREBRAL CORTEX

BE ABLE TO:

* Make sketches of the dorsolateral and medial surfaces of the cerebral hemisphere to show: (1) the boundaries of the frontal, parietal, occipital and temporal lobes, and (2) the main gyri and sulci, particularly those which are landmarks for cortical areas of special function and clinical importance.

* State the basis for recognizing three main types of cortex: paleocortex, archicortex, and neocortex.

* Describe and illustrate the different types of neuron that are present in neocortex.

* Describe the basic architecture of neocortex and its principal variations.

* Make sketches showing the location of the motor and sensory areas of the cerebral cortex, and discuss the intrinsic topography, connections, and main functional properties of these areas.

* Discuss the association cortex, the language areas, and the principle of hemispheral dominance.

* Identify the neurological deficits which result from lesions in specific cortical areas.

MEDULLARY CENTER AND INTERNAL CAPSULE

BE ABLE TO:

* Describe the association fasciculi of the cerebral hemisphere.

* Describe the corpus callosum and the anterior commissure, indicating the role of the commissural system in cerebral function.

* Identify the types of cortical afferent and efferent projection fibers, based on their sites of origin and termination, which compose the corona radiata of the medullary center and the internal capsule.

* Make sketches and describe the configuration and relations of the internal capsule, and the location of its constituent groups of nerve fibers.

CORPUS STRIATUM

BE ABLE TO:

* Make sketches showing the configuration and relations of the caudate and lentiform nuclei.

* Discuss the paleostriatum and neostriatum with respect to their gross morphology, histology, and more important afferent and efferent connections.

* Describe the main syndromes (dyskinesias) which result from pathology involving the corpus striatum.

F I V E - C H O I C E   C O M P L E T I O N   Q U E S T I O N S

DIRECTIONS: Each of the following questions or incomplete statements is followed by five suggested answers or completions. SELECT THE ONE BEST ANSWER OR COMPLETION in each case and underline the appropriate letter at the right.

---

1. The movements of athetosis, one of the dyskinesias associated with pathology in the corpus striatum, are characterized by

   A. tremor at the end of a voluntary movement
   B. jerky movements involving the proximal limb musculature
   C. fine, rhythmical movement of the hands
   D. sinuous movements involving the more distal limb musculature
   E. violent, flinging movements of the limbs   A B C D E

2. Which association bundle is of special interest in connection with conduction aphasia?

   A. Cingulum
   B. Superior longitudinal fasciculus
   C. Superior occipitofrontal fasciculus
   D. Inferior longitudinal fasciculus
   E. Uncinate fasciculus   A B C D E

3. From which region are contractions of contralateral hand muscles elicited when the cortex is stimulated electrically?

   A. Paracentral lobule
   B. Inferior frontal gyrus
   C. Superior wall of the lateral fissure
   D. Inferior one-third of the precentral gyrus
   E. Midway along the precentral gyrus   A B C D E

4. The frontal lobe does NOT include

    A. the promotor area   D. the motor area
    B. orbital gyri   E. Broca's area
    C. the uncus   A B C D E

5. The correct sequence of typical neocortical layers in the
    cerebral cortex, from surface to medullary center, is:

    A. Ganglionic, inner granular, fusiform cell, outer
        granular, pyramidal cell, molecular
    B. Outer granular, pyramidal cell, inner granular,
        molecular, ganglionic, fusiform cell
    C. Molecular, outer granular, ganglionic, inner
        granular fusiform cell, pyramidal cell
    D. Molecular, outer granular, pyramidal cell, inner
        granular, ganglionic, fusiform cell
    E. Molecular, outer granular, fusiform cell, inner
        granular, ganglionic, pyramidal cell   A B C D E

6. The main projection to the general sensory cortex is
    from the

    A. ventral posterior thalamic nucleus
    B. motor and premotor cortical areas
    C. medial thalamic nucleus
    D. dorsal tier of thalamic nuclei
    E. parietal association cortex   A B C D E

7. Which correlation of terms is correct?

    A. Lentiform nucleus = putamen + caudate nucleus
    B. Neostriatum = striatum = globus pallidus + putamen
    C. Paleostriatum = caudate nucleus
    D. Neostriatum = striatum = caudate nucleus + globus
        pallidus
    E. Paleostriatum = pallidum = globus pallidus   A B C D E

8. Which statement concerning the auditory cortex is
    correct?

    A. Destruction of the area located in Heschl's convolu-
        tions causes deafness in the contralateral ear
    B. It is also known as Wernicke's area
    C. Acoustic data are received from the spiral organ of
        the same side, in addition to a major input from the
        spiral organ of the opposite side
    D. Its main afferents are fibers of the auditory radiation
        coming from the lateral geniculate nucleus of the
        thalamus
    E. Most of the auditory cortex is in the middle temporal
        gyrus   A B C D E

9. The sequential relations of certain hemispheral structures, in a medial to lateral direction, are as follows:

   A. Internal capsule, putamen, globus pallidus, extreme capsule, claustrum, external capsule, insula
   B. Internal capsule, globus pallidus, putamen, external capsule, claustrum, extreme capsule, insula
   C. Internal capsule, globus pallidus, putamen, extreme capsule, claustrum, external capsule, insula
   D. Internal capsule, globus pallidus, putamen, claustrum, external capsule, extreme capsule, insula
   E. Internal capsule, globus pallidus, external capsule, putamen, claustrum, extreme capsule, insula   A B C D E

10. Which combinations of neurological signs is likely to result from section of the corpus callosum in a right-handed person?

    A. Unimpaired intellect, poverty of language in response to sensory data reaching the right hemisphere, better performance of the left hand than the right when three-dimensional perspective is needed
    B. Loss of bimanual skills that have been well established preoperatively, in addition to an inability to transfer to the other hand skills learned postoperatively by use of one hand
    C. Impaired intelligence associated with profound aphasia
    D. Equal performance of any task by either hand and equal ability to name an object held in either hand without visual aid
    E. No significant sign of cerebral dysfunction, except for a lowering of the I.Q. score, as determined by standard tests   A B C D E

11. Which statement about the visual cortex is correct?

    A. It is relatively thick, owing to the presence of many pyramidal cells
    B. Its major input is from the medial geniculate nucleus via the geniculocalcarine tract
    C. It is thin and known as the striate area
    D. It is distributed in about equal proportions on the medial and lateral surfaces of the occipital lobe
    E. It is designated as area 18 in the Brodmann cyto-architectural map   A B C D E

12. Which area of Brodmann is NOT sensory cortex.

    A. 17   D. 43
    B. 8   C. 41
    C. 3   A B C D E

SELECT THE ONE BEST ANSWER OR COMPLETION

13. Which combination of structures include only telencephalic components of the limbic system of the brain?

    A. Hippocampus, corpus striatum, cingulate gyrus, insula
    B. Cingulate gyrus, amygdaloid nucleus, claustrum
    C. Cingulate gyrus, hippocampus, amygdaloid nucleus, dentate gyrus
    D. Hippocampus, dentate gyrus, mamillary body, amygdaloid nucleus
    E. Cingulate gyrus, anterior thalamic nucleus, amygdaloid nucleus, hippocampus   A B C D E

14. The line of Gennari

    A. is just visible to the unaided eye in Brodmann's area 4 of the cerebral cortex because of the presence of giant pyramidal cells
    B. is an especially well developed inner line of Baillarger in the visual cortex (striate area)
    C. includes many stellate cells and is therefore visible to the unaided eye in area 3 of the somesthetic cortex
    D. consists of nerve fibers running tangentially in the molecular layer of the cortex
    E. is a well developed outer line of Baillarger, consisting mainly of thalamocortical fibers, in area 17   A B C D E

15. Ablation of the arm region of the primary motor area of the left hemisphere, or destruction of this region by natural causes, results in

    A. voluntary muscle paresis of the right arm, with flaccidity of the affected muscles
    B. impairment of voluntary movements in both arms, with more pronounced motor deficit on the right side
    C. progressive atrophy of the muscles of the right arm
    D. insignificant motor deficits from the start owing to compensation by intact pyramidal and extrapyramidal neurons
    E. permanent spastic paralysis of most of the musculature of the right arm   A B C D E

16. The corpus striatum influences the motor and premotor cortical areas via

    A. the subthalamic fasciculus, ventral thalamic nuclei, and thalamocortical fibers
    B. striatocortical fibers in the internal and external capsules
    C. the lenticular fasciculus, medial thalamic nucleus, and thalamocortical fibers
    D. pallidothalamic fibers, ventral lateral and ventral anterior thalamic nuclei, and thalamocortical fibers
    E. The ansa lenticularis, intralaminar thalamic nuclei, and a thalamocortical projection   A B C D E

141

ANSWERS, NOTES, AND EXPLANATIONS

1. D Athetoid movements are slow, sinuous and aimless. They involve the distal musculature of the limb preferentially; muscles of the face, neck and tongue may be affected as well. Choreiform movements, which are likewise involuntary and purposeless, are brisk and jerky. *Both athetosis and chorea result from degenerative changes in the corpus striatum, although there may be concurrent pathology in other parts of the brain, including the cerebral cortex. A fine, rhythmic tremor is characteristic of Parkinson's disease, in which the primary pathology is in the substantia nigra.* Violent, flinging movements are typical in hemiballismus; the degenerative changes responsible for this dyskinesia are in the subthalamic nucleus. The tremor seen when there is cerebellar dysfunction occurs at the end of a voluntary movement and is called an intention tremor.

2. B The superior longitudinal fasciculus (arcuate fasiculus) runs in the frontal and parietal lobes superior to the lateral sulcus (fissure), and many of the constituent fibers curve around the posterior end of the sulcus into the temporal lobe. The cortical areas which are thereby brought into communication include Broca's motor speech area in the inferior frontal gyrus and the sensory language area, most significantly Wernicke's area in the superior temporal gyrus. Interruption of the arcuate fasciculus results in a language deficit called conduction aphasia, in which there is difficulty in repeating phrases or sentences spoken by the examiner.

3. E The primary motor area (area 4 of Brodmann) is located in the precentral gyrus and extends over the dorsomedial border of the hemisphere in the anterior part of the paracentral lobe. It is the cortical area from which motor responses are most readily elicited by electrical stimulation. The musculature of the opposite side of the body is represented in a roughly inverted sequence, and the regions controlling muscles of the head and upper limb, especially the forearm and hand, are disproportionately large. The topographical representation of the body is such that the large area controlling movements of the hand is midway along the length of the precentral gyrus. More specifically, the contralateral musculature is represented as follows, preceding superiorly from the lateral sulcus: pharynx, larynx, tongue, face, neck, hand, forearm, arm, and trunk. Most of the lower limb, as well as the anal and vesical sphincters, are represented in the anterior part of the paracentral lobule on the medial surface of the hemisphere.

4. C The parahippocampal gyrus on the basal surface of the temporal lobe hooks back on itself at its anterior end to form the uncus. The uncus is a landmark for the lateral olfactory area of cortex and the underlying amygdaloid nucleus.

5. D The molecular layer (plexiform layer) consists mainly of nerve fibers, among which are scattered a few stellate cells and horizontal cells of Cajal. The outer granular layer (layer of small pyramidal cells) contains many small pyramidal and stellate cells. The pyramidal cell layer (layer of medium-sized and large pyramidal cells) contains the cell types identified in the alternative name of the layer. The inner granular layer (layer of stellate cells) consists of closely disposed stellate cells.

142

The ganglionic layer (inner pyramidal layer) includes pyramidal cells. It derives the name "ganglionic" from the presence of giant pyramidal cells of Betz in the primary motor area (4). The fusiform cell layer (layer of poplymorphic cells) consists mainly of fusiform cells, together with cells of varying shape. Cells of Martinotti, whose axons are directed toward the surface, are present in all but the outermost layer.

6. A The ventral posterior nucleus of the thalamus is the special nucleus for the general senses and the principal source of afferents to the somesthetic area (postcentral gyrus) of the cerebral cortex. The medial portion of the nucleus receives trigeminothalamic fibers and projects to the inferior one-third of the somesthetic area. The larger, lateral portion of the ventral posterior nucleus is the terminus of the spino-thalamic tract and the medial lemniscus, and projects to the superior two-thirds of the somesthetic area. Fibers for cutaneous sensation are described as ending preferentially in the anterior strip (Brodmann's area 3) of the general sensory cortex, with those for deep sensibility terminating more posteriorly in strips corresponding to Brodmann's areas 1 and 2.

7. E The phylogenetically oldest part of the corpus striatum, i.e., the paleostriatum, is the globus pallidus or pallidum. The neostriatum, also called the striatum, became divided into the caudate nucleus and the puta-men during the fetal period because of the passage through it of pro-jection fibers of the corona radiata and internal capsule. The two components of the striatum remain in continuity through a broad band of gray matter beneath the anterior limb of the internal capsule, as well as many strands of gray matter which cut across the system of projection fibers. The corpus striatum is described, with respect to gross morphology, as consisting of the caudate nucleus and the lentiform nucleus, the latter being composed of the globus pallidus and the putamen. However, the important distinction is between the neostriatum (caudate nucleus and putamen) and the paleostriatum (globus pallidus).

8. C The inferior wall of the deep lateral sulcus is the superior surface of the superior temporal gyrus. This surface has two or more transverse temporal gyri which extend from the exposed surface to the insula, an area of cortex in the depths of the lateral sulcus. The two most anterior transverse temporal gyri, called Heschl's convolutions, are the landmark for the auditory area. This area receives the auditory radiation which originates in the medial geniculate nucleus of the thalamus and traverses the sublentiform portion of the internal capsule's posterior limb. The medial geniculate nucleus receives a significant input from the ipsila-teral spiral organ in addition to the major input from the opposite ear. Therefore, destruction of the auditory area of a hemisphere produces only slight impairment of hearing. It may be difficult to detect by routine clinical tests, although recognition of the direction from which a sound comes is said to be impaired noticeably. Wernicke's area is posterior to the auditory area. It is included in the auditory association cortex and is an important component of the sensory language area in the dominant hemisphere.

9. B The thick internal capsule is composed of projection fibers (cortical afferents and efferents) continuous with those of the corona radiata in the medullary center. The lentiform nucleus, in which the globus pallidus

is medial to the putamen, is apposed to the lateral surface of the internal capsule. The putamen is bounded laterally by the thin external capsule, which consists largely of projection fibers, including corticostriate fibers ending in the putamen and corticoreticular fibers proceeding to the reticular formation of the brain stem. Next, there is the thin sheet of gray matter known as the claustrum, the function of which is obscure. The extreme capsule is white matter associated with the overlying insula, which is composed of cortex buried in the depths of the lateral sulcus and thereby concealed from surface view.

10. A Neocortical commissural fibers constitute the corpus callosum: a relatively small number are in the anterior commissure. The role of the commissural fibers, especially those of the massive corpus callosum, in connecting comparable cortical areas of the two hemispheres has been demonstrated by commissurotomy in experimental animals, and also in man as a therapeutic measure in very severe epilepsy (status epilepticus). In addition to the desired amelioration of seizures, the following consequences of sectioning of the corpus callosum in persons with left-sided cerebral dominance were observed. Although bimanual motor activites that had become habitual could be performed, an expertise acquired by one hand subsequent to the operation was not transferable to the other hand without further training in the use of that hand. The left-sided cerebral dominance became apparent in the area of language. For example, the individual was unable to name an unseen object examined with the left hand, although he had no such difficulty when the object was examined with the right hand. In spite of being able to recognize the object, a name could not be attached to it because the right hemisphere had been rendered mute through loss of access to memory for language in the left hemisphere. However, activities that included spatial concepts were performed better by the left hand than the right, showing that the right or non-dominant hemisphere is the more proficient in functions which make use of three-dimensional perspective. Commissurotomy produced no significant changes in intellect, behavior, or emotional responses.

11. C The visual area surrounds the calcarine sulcus on the medial surface of the occipital lobe, often extending onto the occipital pole. It receives data concerning the contralateral half of the visual field by way of the geniculocalcarine tract, the cells of origin of which are in the lateral geniculate nucleus of the thalamus. The upper visual field is represented in the inferior wall of the calcarine sulcus and the lower visual field in the superior wall. A large part of the area toward the occipital pole is assigned to central or macular vision, and increasingly peripheral parts of the visual field are represented progressively more anteriorly. The visual cortex is thinner than neocortex elsewhere, being only 1.5mm in thickness. It is granular heterotypical cortex and corresponds to area 17 on the Brodmann cytoarchitectural map. The visual area is referred to as the striate area because a line of Gennari, representing a well developed outer line of Baillarger, is visible on careful inspection with the unaided eye.

12. B Brodmann's area 8 is in the middle frontal gyrus of the frontal lobe, anterior to area 6; the inferior part of area 8 is recognized as the frontal eye field for voluntary scanning movements of the eyes. The other areas listed are sensory, as follows: 17 - visual area; 3 - anterior strip of the somesthetic area; 43 - taste area; 41 - part of the auditory area.

13. C The cingulate and parahippocampal gyri are connected by an isthmus beneath the splenium of the corpus callosum to form the limbic lobe. The hippocampus, dentate gyrus, and part of the amygdaloid nucleus, together with the limbic lobe, are components of the limbic system of the brain. Of the other structures listed, the mamillary bodies are also in the limbic system, but they are in the hypothalamus of the diencephalon. (The hippocampus and dentate gyrus are sometimes added to the cingulate and parahippocampal gyri when defining the limbic lobe.)

14. E Two bands of nerve fibers seen in suitably stained sections of the neocortex are designated as lines of Baillarger. Many of the constituent fibers are branches of thalamocortical fibers that are directed tangentially to the cortical surface. The outer line is in the inner granular layer, and the inner one is in the deep portion of the ganglionic layer. In the visual area (17), the outer line of Baillarger is thicker than elsewhere. In this location, it is called the line of Gennari, which is just visible with the unaided eye as a pale line on the cut surface, and accounts for the name striate area being given the visual area.

15. A A lesion limited to the primary motor area (4), in this instance an area on the left side for muscles controlling movements of the right hand, is followed by voluntary motor paresis with decreased tonus of the affected muscles. There is considerable recovery with time, so that eventually the residual defect may be limited to individual movements of the digits. More severe impairment, i.e., paralysis of the affected muscles accompanied by spasticity, occurs when the lesion spreads beyond area 4 into the premotor area and subjacent white matter. Under these circumstances, a substantial number of extrapyramidal projections from the cortex are rendered inactive, in addition to neurons of the pyramidal system.

16. D The main efferent bundles of the globus pallidus, the efferent component of the corpus striatum, are the lenticular fasciculus, which intersects the fibers of the posterior limb of the internal capsule, and the ansa lenticularis, which curves under the posterior limb of the internal capsule. Both fasciculi enter the subthalamic region of the diencephalon, and all but a few of the constituent fibers terminate in the ventral anterior and ventral lateral nuclei of the thalamus. Axons of neurons in these nuclei project to the motor and premotor areas of the cerebral cortex; thus the sources of pyramidal and extrapyramidal motor fibers are brought under the influence of the corpus striatum.

MULTI-COMPLETION QUESTIONS

DIRECTIONS: In each of the following questions or incomplete statements, one or more of the completions given is correct. At the lower right of each question, underline A if 1, 2, and 3 are correct; B if 1 and 3 are correct; C if 2 and 4 are correct; D if only 4 is correct; and E if all are correct.

---

1. Correct statements concerning vestibular representation in the cerebral cortex include:

    1. There is evidence for the existence of a vestibular area in the parietal lobe
    2. Awareness of vestibular stimulation is the result of appropriate stimuli reaching the frontal lobe from the cerebellum
    3. There is evidence for the presence of a vestibular area in the temporal lobe
    4. The vestibular system functions solely at subcortical levels   A B C D E

2. The largest number of afferent fibers to the globus pallidus are:

    1. Corticopallidal   3. Nigropallidal
    2. Thalamopallidal   4. Striopallidal   A B C D E

3. Giant pyramidal cells are

    1. a feature of cortical area 4
    2. present in layer 5 of area 4
    3. cortical projection neurons
    4. responsible for about 3 percent of pyramidal tract fibers   A B C D E

4. Components of the corpus callosum participating in bringing the occipital lobes of the two hemispheres in communication include:

    1. Genu   3. Tapetum
    2. Forceps major   4. Splenium   A B C D E

5. Granular meterotypical cortex is

    1. characteristic of sensory or receptive areas
    2. thinner than neocortex elsewhere
    3. also known as koniocortex
    4. clearly six-layered   A B C D E

6. The corona radiata and the internal capsule include

    1. the geniculocalcarine tract
    2. the anterior thalamic radiation
    3. extrapyramidal motor fibers
    4. arcuate fibers   A B C D E

146

A	B	C	D	E
1,2,3	1,3,	2,4	only 4	all correct

7. Pathological changes in the corpus striatum are associated with

    1. Wilson's disease
    2. dystonia musculorum deformans
    3. Sydenham's and Huntington's chorea
    4. athetosis   A B C D E

8. Correct statements concerning the neocortex include:

    1. Most of it consists of the motor area and sensory areas
       in the human brain
    2. It is not possible to identify six layers in some areas
    3. The molecular layer is densely populated with small nerve
       cells
    4. It is organized functionally into minute verticals units   A B C D E

9. The visual association cortex

    1. corresponds with areas 18 and 19 in the Brodmann cyto-
       architectural map
    2. is concerned with complex aspects of vision, thereby
       supplementing area 17
    3. sends corticotectal fibers to the superior colliculus
       of the midbrain
    4. receives afferents mainly through the geniculocalcarine
       tract   A B C D E

10. Correct statements about the general sensory cortex include:

    1. It is located entirely in the postcentral gyrus on the
       dorsolateral surface of the hemisphere
    2. The opposite side of the body, although distorted as to
       proportions, is represented as inverted
    3. There is no perception of sensory stimuli from the left
       arm if the arm area of the right somesthetic cortex is
       destroyed by a lesion
    4. The principal input is from the ventral posterior nuc-
       leus of the thalamus   A B C D E

11. Thrombosis of an arterial blood vessel is most likely to result
    in motor aphasia if the area of infarction includes the

    1. superior longitudinal fasciculus of the left hemisphere
    2. inferior frontal gyrus of the right hemisphere
    3. superior temporal gyrus of the left hemisphere
    4. inferior frontal gyrus of the left hemisphere   A B C D E

12. A lesion in the temporal lobe may, depending on its precise
    location, cause

    1. a contralateral defect in the upper visual field
    2. deafness in the opposite ear
    3. sensory aphasia
    4. substantial hearing loss in both ears   A B C D E

A	B	C	D	E
1,2,3	1,3,	2,4	only 4	all correct

12. A lesion in the temporal lobe may, depending on its precise location, cause

1. a contralateral defect in the upper visual field
2. deafness in the opposite ear
3. sensory aphasia
4. substantial hearing loss in both ears   A B C D E

ANSWERS, NOTES, AND EXPLANATIONS

1. B 1 and 3 are correct. The role of the vestibular system in maintenance of equilibrium and coordination of head and eye movements is performed through reflexes involving the brain stem and spinal cord. In addition, a cortical projection contributes to motor integration at that level and to conscious spatial orientation. A vestibular area was demonstrated in the inferior part of the postcentral gyrus of the parietal lobe in experiments in which evoked potentials were elicited during stimulation of the vestibular nerve in monkeys. The possibility of a vestibular area being located rostral to the auditory area in the superior temporal gyrus is based on feelings of dizziness and vertigo that have been reported on electrical stimulation of the area during operative procedures in conscious patients. The same sensations may also appear as auras in temporal lobe epileptic seizures. The precise location of the vestibular area (or areas) is in need of further investigation.

2. D Only 4 is correct. Although there is evidence of the existence of some afferent fibers to the globus pallidus from the cerebral cortex, substantia nigra, and possibly the thalamus, these are the important sources of afferent fibers to the caudate nucleus and putamen, which together compose the striatum. The latter projects mainly to the globus pallidus and these striopallidal fibers are the predominant afferents to the pallidum. A second significant source of afferents to the globus pallidus is the subthalamic nucleus through the subthalamic fasciculus, which also includes fibers running in the reverse direction.

3. E All are correct. Layer 5 of the neocortex is called the ganglionic layer because it is the location of giant pyramidal cells, or cells of Betz, in the primary motor area. The number of Betz cells in the part of the motor area from which corticospinal fibers originate is about 35,000, the number corresponding with the 3 percent of large fibers, 10 u in diameter, in a medullary pyramid. The giant pyramidal cells therefore contribute to a small population of large, rapidly conducting fibers to the corticospinal tract, and the same principle no doubt holds for the corticobulbar tract.

4. C 2 and 4 are correct. The commissural fibers running deep to cortices of the left and right occipital lobes traverse the large posterior end, or splenium of the trunk of the corpus callosum. The resulting U-shaped configuration is called the forceps occipitalis (forceps major). A

somewhat smaller U-shaped configuration for the frontal lobes, which includes the anterior end or genu of the corpus callosum, is known as the forceps frontalis (forceps minor). The tapetum is a thin stratum of callosal fibers just superior to the temporal horn (inferior horn) of the lateral ventricle. These fibers traverse the trunk of the corpus callosum and interconnect cortices of the two temporal lobes, especially their basal surfaces.

5. A <u>1, 2, and 3 are correct</u>. The anterior strip (area 3) in the general sensory cortex, the central part of the auditory cortex (area 41), and the visual cortex (area 17) receive sensory data from the appropriate thalamic nuclei. In these areas the stellate cells, which are mainly in layer 4 elsewhere, are present in abundance in adjoining layers as well, so that there is no clear distinction between layers 2 through 5. This type of cortex is thin, in part, because of the preponderance of small neurons. Because of the large population of small cells, it is called granular cortex or koniocortex (<u>konis</u>, dust). It is said to be heterotypical because the six layers found in the remaining homotypical cortex cannot all be identified.

6. A <u>1, 2, and 3 are correct</u>. The corona radiata of the medullary center and its continuation, the internal capsule toward the base of the hemisphere, consist of projection fibers connecting the cerebral cortex with subcortical gray areas of the central nervous system. With respect to the specific projections mentioned, the geniculocalcarine tract passes from the lateral geniculate nucleus of the thalamus to the visual area; the anterior thalamic radiation provides a two-way connection between the medial thalamic nucleus and the prefrontal cortex; and extrapyramidal fibers proceed from the cortex to such motor components of the brain as the corpus striatum, red nucleus, substantia nigra, inferior olivary nucleus, and reticular formation. Arcuate fibers are short association fibers which connect the cortices of adjoining gyri by curving around the intervening sulcus in a U-shaped configuration.

7. E <u>All are correct</u>. Pathological changes in the corpus striatum occur in the dyskinesias mentioned, each of which has a characteristic type of purposeless, involuntary movement. Sydenham's chorea may be a sequel to an infectious disease, whereas Huntington's chorea is a dominant hereditary disorder. Athetosis is often part of a congenital complex of neurological signs; it occurs in a particularly disabling form in dystonia musculorum deformans. Wilson's disease, also called hepatolenticular degeneration, is caused byu a gentically determined error in copper metabolism, which causes cirrhosis of the liver as well as brain damage. Parts of the brain in addition to the corpus striatum are likely to be included in the pathological process in most of the dyskinesias.

8. C <u>2 and 4 are correct</u>. The intellectual attributes of man result from the large expanse of association cortex, which exceeds by a considerable margin the combined areas occupied by motor and sensory areas. Regions of neocortex in which six layers cannot be identifed are said to be heterotypical. The outermost molecular layer can always be identified; it consists of nerve cell processes and a few scattered stellate cells and horizontal cells of Cajal, and is an important synaptic field. The functional organization of the cortex in the form of minute vertical units that include all layers was demonstrated by making recordings from micro-

electrodes embedded in the cortex.

9. A 1, 2, and 3 are correct. The visual association cortex (areas 18 and 19) surrounds the visual cortex (area 17) and is present on the medial and lateral aspects of the occipital lobe. Area 17 receives visual data by way of the geniculocalcarine tract and is linked to areas 18 and 19 by association fibers. The association cortex permits a complex analysis of visual data, including recognition of what is seen and appreciation of its significance by relating present to past experience. Among other complex functions, the visual association cortex is thought to be involved in the recognition of color and in depth perception. Fibers proceeding from areas 18 and 19 to the superior colliculi of the midbrain tectum are part of a reflex pathway for automatic scanning movements and probably for the accommodation-convergence reaction.

10. C 2 and 4 are correct. The opposite side of the body is represented topographically in both the ventral posterior thalamic nucleus and the somesthetic area of cortex. The medial portion of the ventral posterior nucleus receives general sensory data from the head and projects to the inferior portion of the somesthetic area, and the larger, lateral portion of this nucleus receives data from the rest of the body and projects to the superior part of of the somesthetic area. The representation of parts of the body is distorted in that disproportionally large regions are assigned to body parts such as the face and hand, in which awareness of sensory stimulation is especially important. Most of the somesthetic area is in the postcentral gyrus; the area extends onto the posterior portion of the paracentral lobule on the medial surface of the hemisphere, where data are received for most of the lower limb and the anal and genital regions.

11. D Only 4 is correct. In right-handed persons, and some who are left-handed, the left hemisphere is dominant in the sense that it contains the language areas. The motor speech area occupies the triangular and opercular portions of the inferior frontal gyrus, and an infarction that includes this area causes motor aphasia. Interruption of the superior longitudinal fasciculus results in conduction aphasia. The fasciculus brings the sensory and motor language areas into communication with one another, the lack of which causes the affected person to have difficulty repeating testing phrases presented by the examiner. A lesion involving Wernicke's area in the superior temporal gyrus, again in the dominant hemisphere, is a principal cause of sensory aphasia.

12. B 1 and 3 are correct. A temporal lobe lesion which includes Meyer's loop, i.e., the part of the geniculocalcarine tract curving anteriorly in the white matter of the temporal lobe, interrupts fibers conveying data for the upper field of vision on the side opposite the lesion. A lesion that includes the sensory area for language in the dominant hemisphere, in particular Wernicke's area posterior to the auditory area in the temporal lobe, results in sensory aphasia. The auditory area receives stimuli originating in both ears, although predominantly from the one on the opposite side. A lesion that includes the auditory area causes a slight diminution of hearing in both ears, which may not be readily apparent. There is also impairment in one's ability to recognize the direction from which a sound originates.

FIVE-CHOICE ASSOCIATION QUESTIONS

DIRECTIONS: Each of the following groups of questions consists of a numbered list of descriptive words or phrases accompanied by a diagram with certain parts indicated by letters, or by a list of lettered headings. For each numbered word or phrase, SELECT THE LETTERED PART OR HEADING that matches it correctly and insert the letter in the space to the right of the appropriate number. Each lettered heading may be selected once, more than once, or not at all.

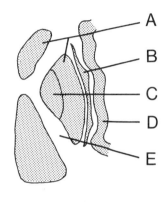

1. ____ Cortex hidden from view
2. ____ Continuous with the corona radiata
3. ____ Projects mainly to the thalamus
4. ____ Bounded by the external and extreme capsules
5. ____ The phylogenetically newer part of the corpus striatum
6. ____ Has connections with the sub-thalamic nucleus

A. Archicortex
B. Cells of Betz
C. Inner granular layer
D. Brodmann's area 4
E. Cells of Martinotti

7. ____ Agranular heterotypical cortex
8. ____ Three layered cortex
9. ____ Axons directed toward the cortical surface
10. ____ Located in layer 5 of area 4
11. ____ Consists of closely disposed stellate cells
12. ____ Primary motor cortex

A. Cingulum
B. Arcuate fasciculus
C. Anterior commissure
D. Uncinate fasciculus
E. Splenium

13. ____ Connects cortices of the temporal pole and the orbital surface of the frontal lobe
14. ____ Provides for communication between sensory and motor language areas
15. ____ Association tract for the limbic lobe
16. ____ Consists of fibers connecting cortices of the occipital lobes
17. ____ Includes fibers connecting cortices of the temporal lobes
18. ____ Connects cortices of the frontal, parietal, occipital, and temporal lobes

151

ASSOCIATION QUESTIONS

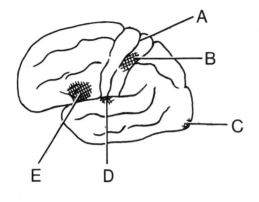

19. ____ Areas 41 and 42 in Brodmann's map
20. ____ Motor speech area
21. ____ Related to central or macular vision
22. ____ Landmark for sensorimotor strip
23. ____ General sensation in the opposite hand
24. ____ Usually present in the left rather than the right hemisphere

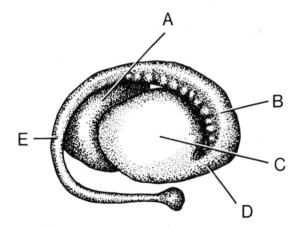

25. ____ Part of the neostriatum included in the lentiform nucleus
26. ____ Conforms to the contour of the lateral ventricle
27. ____ Largest part of the diencephalon
28. ____ Situated medial to the anterior capsule
29. ____ Continuity between the putamen and the caudate nucleus
30. ____ Conceals the globus pallidus in a lateral view

(Illustration from Barr, M.L. and Kiernan, J.A.: The Human Nervous System, 4th ed., 1983. Courtesy of Harper & Row, Publishers, inc.)

ANSWERS, NOTES, AND EXPLANATIONS

1. D The insula is an area of cortex located at the bottom of the lateral sulcus and therefore concealed from surface view.

2. E The posterior limb of the internal capsule, like the anterior limb and the genu, consists of projection fibers continuous with those composing the corona radiata of the medullary center. The fibers of the pyramidal motor system are situated in the region indicated by the pointer E, i.e., the posterior part of the lenticulothalamic portion of the posterior limb, where the corticobulbar fibers are anterior to the corticospinal fibers.

3. C The globus pallidus is the efferent component of the corpus striatum. Most of the fibers emanating from the globus pallidus form two bundles,

the lenticular fasciculus and the ansa lenticularis, and the great majority of the constituent fibers terminate in the ventral anterior and ventral lateral thalamic nuclei. Only a few fibers from the globus pallidus terminate in the brain stem; they end in a small and poorly understood nucleus in the tegmentum of the midbrain.

4.   B The claustrum, a thin sheet of gray matter the function of which is poorly understood, is coextensive with the lateral surface of the lentiform nucleus. The claustrum is bounded medially by the external capsule, which includes fibers of cortical origin passing to the putamen and the reticular formation of the brain stem. The claustrum is separated from the insula by the extreme capsule (capsula extrema), which consists of nerve fibers passing to and from the insular cortex.

5.   A The caudate nucleus and the putamen together compose a functional unit of the corpus striatum. It is known as the neostriatum because of its more recent phylogenetic origin, compared with the globus pallidus or paleostriatum.

6.   C The globus pallidus has reciprocal connections with the subthalamic nucleus through the subthalamic fasciculus, which runs across the internal capsule. The functional relationship between the subthalamic nucleus and the globus pallidus is disturbed in the dyskinesia known as hemiballismus, which is caused by some form of degenerative process involving the subthalamic nucleus.

7.   D In the primary motor area, or area 4 on the Brodmann map, layers 2 through 5 appear as a single, well developed layer, consisting of large neurons of the efferent type, mainly pyramidal cells. Area 4 therefore comes under the heading of agranular heterotypical cortex. Area 6, the premotor area, is similar histologically to area 4, the main difference being that the giant pyramidal cells of Betz are a feature of the fifth or ganglionic layer in area 4.

8.   A The cerebral cortex of submammalian vertebrates consists of three layers. This phylogenetically older cortex, compared with the six-layered neocortex of mammals, is divided in higher forms into paleocortex and archicortex. These are cortical components of the olfactory system and the limbic system, respectively.

9.   E Cells of Martinotti are present in all neocortical layers except the most superficial one. The distinguishing feature of these cells is that their axons are directed toward the cortical surface; cells of Martinotti are therefore a form of intracortical association neuron.

10. B The presence of giant pyramidal cells of Betz in layer 5 of the neocortex is responsible for the name ganglionic layer as an alternative to inner pyramidal layer, even though Betz cells are confined to the primary motor area (4).

11. C The inner granular layer, i.e., layer 4 of neocortex, consists of closely disposed stellate cells (Golgi type II cells) that receive stimuli predominantly by way of thalamocortical fibers.

12. D Brodmann's area 4 has the lowest threshold of stimulation for eliciting

muscular contractions and is therefore called the primary motor area of the cerebral cortex. About 30 percent of the fibers of the pyramidal motor system originate in area 4, 30 percent originate in area 6 of the frontal lobe and 40 percent in the parietal lobe. Many of the fibers from the parietal lobe end on sensory relay neurons and are not considered to be motor fibers.

13. D The uncinate fasciculus, an inverted U-shaped association bundle, bends around the stem of the lateral sulcus at the base of a cerebral hemisphere. It connects cortex in the region of the temporal pole with cortex of the frontal lobe, especially cortex on the inferior or orbital surface of the frontal lobe.

14. B The arcuate or superior longitudinal fasciculus is a major association bundle deep to the dorsolateral surface of the hemisphere. The longitudinal portion connects cortices of the frontal, parietal, and occipital lobes. Many fibers turn inferiorly and then anteriorly into the temporal lobe, hence the name arcuate fasciculus. The latter fibers bring the motor and sensory language areas of the dominant hemisphere into communication with one another.

15. A The cingulum is a fasciculus of nerve fibers which lies deep to the cortex of the cingulate gyrus and curves around the splenium of the corpus callosum to continue into the white matter of the parahippocampal gyrus. The constituent fibers, which are of variable lengths, are association fibers for the limbic lobe.

16. E The enlarged posterior end of the body of the corpus callosum is called the splenium of the corpus callosum. It contains fibers connecting the occipital lobes; the U-shaped configuration is called the forceps occipitalis (forceps major). The forceps frontalis (forceps minor), which includes the genu of the corpus callosum, connects cortices of the frontal lobes.

17. C The anterior commissure is a bundle of fibers which crosses the midline of the brain in the lamina terminalis, or rostral wall of the third ventricle. One component consists of fibers which connect the olfactory bulbs and the lateral olfactory areas, the landmark for the lateral olfactory area being the uncus at the anterior end of the parahippocampal gyrus of the temporal lobe. The other component consists of fibers passing between the middle and inferior temporal gyri of the two sides. The anterior commissure therefore has paleocortical and neocortical components with respect to the areas of cortex it serves.

18. B The arcuate or superior longitudinal fasciculus is a large bundle of association fibers running mainly in an anteroposterior direction in the medullary center of a cerebral hemisphere. It provides a means of communication between cortices of the frontal, parietal, occipital, and temporal lobes. The component curving anteriorly at the posterior end of the lateral sulcus and continuing into the temporal lobe is responsible for the alternative name, arcuate fasciculus.

19. D The auditory cortex corresponds with areas 41 and 42 of the Brodmann cytoarchitectural map. The landmark for the auditory area is Heschl's

convolutions, i.e., the two most anterior of the transverse temporal gyri on the superior surface of the superior temporal gyrus, which forms the floor of the lateral sulcus. Only a small portion of the auditory area extends onto the exposed surface of the superior temporal gyrus.

20. E The motor speech area, or area of Broca, occupies the triangular and opercular portions of the inferior frontal gyrus. It corresponds with Brodmann's areas 44 and 45.

21. C The visual area of cortex (the striate area or area 17) is on the medial surface of the occipital lobe, with the calcarine sulcus as the landmark. It may extend onto the occipital pole. Approximately the posterior one-third of the area receives impulses that originate in the macular region of the retina; the posterior part of the visual cortex is therefore concerned with the central field of vision.

22. A The central sulcus separates the motor area anteriorly from the general sensory area posteriorly. However, some pyramidal and extrapyramidal motor fibers originate from the sensory area and there is evidence for the termination of some sensory fibers in the motor area. Because of this overlapping, together with the functional relationship between the sensory and motor areas, the cortex surrounding the central sulcus is referred to as the sensorimotor strip.

23. B The somesthetic cortex for the opposite side of the body is situated in the postcentral gyrus of the parietal lobe, and extends onto the posterior part of the paracentral lobule on the medial surface of the hemisphere. The body parts are represented in an inverted sequence; the hand area is about midway along the postcentral gyrus. It is disproportionately large because of the importance of data originating in sensory endings in the hand.

24. E Broca's area for motor speech is in the left hemisphere in right-handed persons and in a proportion of those who are left-handed. The sensory language area in the temporoparietal region has the same hemispheral preference, and the dominant hemisphere with respect to language is therefore the left one in most individuals.

25. C Because the sketch represents a lateral view of the corpus striatum, the putamen of the lentiform nucleus presents to the surface. The putamen and the caudate nucleus compose the neostriatum or striatum, and the globus pallidus of the lentiform nucleus forms the paleostriatum or pallidum.

26. E During fetal development, part of the caudate nucleus acquires a C-shaped configuration and is called the tail of the caudate nucleus. The first part of the tail lies along the lateral border of the central part of the lateral ventricle. It then curves anteriorly into the roof of the temporal (inferior) horn and ends in the amygdaloid nucleus, with which the caudate nucleus has no functional relationship. The part of the tail of the caudate in the temporal lobe is an attenuated strand of gray matter that may be discontinuous in some human brains.

27. A The thalamus of the diencephalon, by far its largest component, is separated from the lentiform nucleus by the posterior limb of the internal

capsule.

28. B The anterior limb of the internal capsule intervenes between the head of the caudate nucleus and the lentiform nucleus. This configuration results from projection fibers growing through the neostriatum during fetal development, incompletely dividing the neostriatum into the caudate nucleus and the putamen of the lentiform nucleus.

29. D The neostriatum (striatum) is one functional unit of the corpus striatum, the other being the paleostriatum (globus pallidus or pallidum). The anatomical division of the neostriatum into the caudate nucleus and the putamen is incomplete. Their continuity is maintained by a substantial band of gray matter beneath the anterior limb of the internal capsule and by numerous strands of gray matter running across the internal capsule.

30. C The lentiform nucleus consists of the putamen and the globus pallidus, the latter being the medial component of the nucleus. The putamen extends beyond the globus pallidus in all directions except at the base of the lentiform nucleus. The smaller globus pallidus is therefore concealed by the larger putamen when the lentiform nucleus is viewed from its lateral aspect.

TEN

The Meninges and Blood Vessels

OBJECTIVES

MENINGES

BE ABLE TO:

* Describe the dura mater of the brain and spinal cord.

* Discuss the following dural folds and their attachments: (1) falx cerebri; (2) tentorium cerebelli; (3) falx cerebelli; and (4) diaphragma sellae.

* Give a brief account of the blood and nerve supply to the meninges.

* Describe the arachnoid mater of the brain and spinal cord.

* Discuss briefly the subarachnoid space and its contents.

* Make a sketch of a coronal section through the anterior part of the brain showing the meninges and their relationship to the brain.

* List the contents of the epidural space in the vertebral canal.

BLOOD VESSELS - ARTERIAL SUPPLY

BE ABLE TO:

* List and describe the branches of the internal carotid artery within the cranium.

* Name and describe the cranial branches of the vertebral artery.

* Discuss the blood supply to the spinal cord.

* Schematically illustrate the circulus arteriosus cerebri or cerebral arterial circle (circle of Willis).

* Give the clinical significance of the cerebral arterial circle and the variations in its formation.

* Give a brief account of the central arteries of the cerebrum.

* Discuss the blood supply to the lateral and medial surfaces of the cerebral hemispheres.

* Discuss the blood supply to the cerebellum.

* Identify the major arterial vessels of the brain and recognize their normal position in angiograms.

* Point out the cerebral vessels in which aneurysms most frequently develop.

* Make a sketch of a transvere section of the spinal cord to show its arterial blood supply.

BLOOD VESSELS - VENOUS DRAINAGE

BE ABLE TO:

* Describe briefly the superficial venous drainage of the cerebral hemispheres.

* Give a brief account of the deep veins of the cerebrum.

* List the veins emptying into the great cerebral vein (of Galen).

* Identify the major venous sinuses of the brain.

* Make a sketch of the cavernous sinus showing its contents.

* Discuss the venous drainage of the spinal cord.

F I V E - C H O I C E   C O M P L E T I O N   Q U E S T I O N S

DIRECTIONS: Each of the following questions or incomplete statements is followed by five suggested answers or completions. SELECT THE ONE BEST ANSWER OR COMPLETION in each case and underline the appropriate letter at the right.

----

1. The long central artery (recurrent artery of Heubner) is a branch of the ____ artery.

    A. internal carotid   D. anterior cerebral
    B. middle cerebral   E. anterior communi-
    C. anterior choroidal   cating   A B C D E

2. Which of the following are found in the subdural space?

    A. Cerebrospinal fluid   D. Cranial nerves
    B. Cerebral arteries   E. None of the above
    C. Cerebral veins   A B C D E

3. The pia mater lies immediately adjacent to the

    A. precentral gyrus   D. pyramids
    B. flocculus   E. all of the above
    C. optic tract   A B C D E

4. The superior petrosal sinus lies in the margin of the

    A. tentorium cerebelli   D. diaphragma sellae
    B. falx cerebelli   E. greater wing of the
    C. falx cerebri   sphenoid bone   A B C D E

5. The anterior meningeal artery is a branch of the _____
    artery.

    A. vertebral   D. middle meningeal
    B. ophthalmic   E. accessory meningeal
    C. occipital   A B C D E

6. The ____ artery is the largest cranial branch of the
    vertebral artery.

    A. anterior spinal   D. anterior inferior
    B. posterior spinal   cerebellar
    C. posterior inferior   E. medullary   A B C D E

7. The striate arteries (anterolateral, central, or gang-
    lionic arteries) supply the

    A. uncus   D. preoptic area of the
    B. putamen   hypothalamus
    C. pulvinar of thalamus   E. tectum of the midbrain A B C D E

8. The internal auditory artery commonly arises from the

    A. middle cerebral
    B. posterior cerebral
    C. posterior inferior cerebellar
    D. vertebral
    E. basilar   A B C D E

9. The basilar artery

    A. is formed from the junction of the two vertebral
        arteries
    B. terminates by forming left and right posterior
        cerebral arteries
    C. gives rise to the superior cerebellar artery
    D. terminates at the anterior border of the basal
        portion of the pons
    E. all of the above are correct completions   A B C D E

159

SELECT THE ONE BEST ANSWER OR COMPLETION

10. The anterior spinal artery supplies the

    A. pyramids
    B. vestibulospinal tracts
    C. anterior horn of cervical gray matter
    D. anterior corticospinal tract
    E. all of the above are correct completions   A B C D E

11. The _____ sinus occupies the free margin of the falx cerebri.

    A. occipital   D. cavernous
    B. inferior sagittal   E. superior sagittal
    C. straight   A B C D E

12. The superior sagittal sinus begins at the

    A. sigmoid sinus   D. straight sinus
    B. transverse sinus   E. foramen cecum
    C. cavernous sinus   A B C D E

13. Name the dural venous sinus that has a cranial nerve and an artery coursing through it.

    A. Superior sagittal   D. Intercavernous
    B. Cavernous   E. Sigmoid sinus
    C. Confluence of sinuses   A B C D E

14. The posterior spinal veins drain blood from the

    A. nucleus gracilis and nucleus cuneatus
    B. posterior column of white matter of the
        cervical spinal cord
    C. posterior horn of cervical gray matter
    D. tract of Lissauer
    E. all of the above are correct completions   A B C D E

ANSWERS, NOTES, AND EXPLANATIONS

1. D The long central artery (recurrent artery of Heubner) is also called the striate artery because of its contribution to the blood supply of the corpus striatum. It arises from the anterior cerebral artery just proximal to the anterior communicating artery. This large artery penetrates the anterior perforated substance along with the other anteromedial branches and supplies the ventral part of the head of the caudate nucleus, the adjacent portion of the putamen, and the anterior limb and genu of the internal capsule.

2. E None of the structures named are found in the subdural space because this is only a potential space between the dura mater and the arachnoid mater. It contains a minute quantity of serous fluid which

moistens the smooth surfaces of the opposed membranes. The structures listed are found in the subarachnoid space.

3. E The pia mater, a microscopic thin layer, closely invests the brain and spinal cord. It contains a network of fine blood vessels and dips between cerebral gyri and cerebellar folia. It follows all the contours of the central nervous system. The penetrating blood vessels to the brain and spinal cord are surrounded for a short distance by a sleeve of pia mater. Within this sleeve, the subarachnoid space extends into the perivascular spaces (Virchow-Robin spaces).

4. A The superior petrosal sinuses, small and narrow, drain the cavernous sinuses into the tranverse sinuses. The superior petrosal sinus runs posterolaterally in the attached margin of the tentorium cerebelli, which is attached to the petrous ridge of the temporal bone. The superior petrosal sinus terminates by joining the transverse sinus where the latter curves inferiorly to become continuous with the sigmoid sinus.

5. D The anterior meningeal artery is the larger branch of the middle meningeal artery which arises from the maxillary artery deep to the lateral pterygoid muscle. The middle meningeal artery passes through the foramen spinosum; it then runs anterolaterally in the groove on the anterior part of the squamous part of the temporal bone and divides into frontal and parietal branches. The anterior meningeal artery supplies the meninges in the caudal, frontal, and anterior parietal areas.

6. C The posterior inferior cerebellar artery is the largest branch of the vertebral artery. It pursues an irregular course between the lateral medulla and the inferior region of the cerebellum, as far as the pontine cerebellar angle; it then courses onto the inferior surface of the cerebellum. Branches from this clinically important artery are distributed to the posterior part of the cerebellar hemisphere, the inferior vermis, the central nuclei of the cerebellum, the choroid plexus of the fourth ventricle, and the dorsolateral region of the medulla oblongata. Occlusion of this vessel results in the lateral medullary syndrome (Wallenberg's syndrome).

7. B The anterolateral ganglionic or striate arteries arise from the proximal portion of the middle cerebral artery. The region supplied by these arteries is mostly the corpus striatum (head of the caudate nucelus, anterior limb of the internal capsule, putamen, and lateral part of the globus pallidus). The other structures listed are supplied either by other ganglionic arteries or by the anterior and posterior choroidal vessels.

8. E The internal auditory artery is usually a branch of the basilar artery, but it is not uncommon for it to originate from the anterior inferior cerebellar artery. The internal auditory artery ramifies throughout the membranous labyrinth of the internal ear, which it reaches by way of the internal auditory canal in company with the facial (VII) and auditory (VIII) cranial nerves.

9. E The basilar artery, so named from its position at the base of the brain and skull, is formed by the junction of the two vertebral arteries. It extends from the posterior to the anterior border of the basal portion of the pons. It is contained within the cisterna pontis (large subarachnoid space). It lies between the two abducens nerves near its beginning and between the two oculomotor nerves near its termination, where it forms the left and right posterior cerebrals. Its branches are as follows: anterior inferior cerebellar, pontine, internal auditory, superior cerebellar, and posterior cerebrals.

10. E The anterior spinal artery is formed by a contribution from each vertebral artery. This forms a Y-shaped configuration which runs caudally in the ventral median fissure of the caudal end of the medulla and the entire length of the spinal cord. This artery is reinforced at intervals by segmental branches from the vertebral artery, the posterior intercostal branches of the thoracic aorta, and lumbar branches of the abdominal aorta. Central branches pass into the ventral median fissure from the anterior spinal artery to supply the anterior gray matter, the base of the posterior gray column, and the adjacent white matter. All the structures listed would be supplied by these penetrating central branches.

11. B The inferior sagittal sinus is smaller than the superior sagittal sinus. It runs along the free border of the posterior one-half to two-thirds of the falx cerebri. It increases in size as it passes posteriorly and ends in the straight sinus at the point where the great cerebral vein (of Galen) joins the straight sinus. It receives several veins from the falx cerebri and a few from the medial surfaces of the hemispheres.

12. E The superior sagittal sinus, the largest sinus in the falx cerebri, occupies the attached convex margin of the falx cerebri. It commences anterior to the crista galli of the ethmoid bone, where the foramen cecum is located and where there may be a narrow communication with nasal veins. Venous lacunae lie alongside the superior sagittal sinus and open into it. The superior cerebral veins drain into this sinus or into the lateral lacunae. The superior sagittal sinus usually turns to the right at the internal occipital protuberance and continues as the right transverse sinus.

13. B A cavernous sinus is situated on each side of the body of the sphenoid bone. The cavernous sinuses receive the ophthalmic veins and the superficial middle cerebral vein. It drains into the transverse sinus through the superior and inferior petrosal sinuses. The internal carotid artery, surrounded by a plexus of sympathetic filaments, passes anteriorly through the sinus as does the abducens nerve which lies inferolateral to this artery. The oculomotor, trochlear, ophthalmic, and maxillary divisions of the trigeminal nerve are located in the lateral wall of the cavernous sinus.

14. E The posterior spinal veins, three in number, are located in the subarachnoid space of the spinal cord. They are situated in the dorsal midline, and in the left and right dorsolateral sulci. The spinal veins are drained at intervals by up to 12 posterior radicular veins. Blood is drained from the interior of the dorsal half of the entire

length of the spinal cord and the caudal end of the medulla by venules. They course from the interior of the gray and white matter and empty into the posterior spinal veins. All structures contained in the posterior aspect of the spinal cord (posterior and dorsolateral column of white matter and posterior horn of gray matter) are drained of blood through these vessels.

MULTI-COMPLETION QUESTIONS

DIRECTIONS: In each of the following questions or incomplete statements, one or more of the completions given is correct. At the lower right of each question, underline A if 1, 2, and 3 are correct; B if 1 and 3 are correct; C if 2 and 4 are correct; D if only 4 is correct; and E if all are correct.

----

1. The meningeal vessels are contained in the

    1. dura mater   3. subarachnoid space
    2. epidural space   4. inner periosteum   A B C D E

2. The spinal dura mater is separated from the wall of the
    spinal cord by

    1. adipose tissue
    2. an arterial plexus
    3. a venous plexus
    4. a spinal nerve plexus   A B C D E

3. The falx cerebri is attached to the

    1. crista galli
    2. anterior clinoid process
    3. tentorium cerebelli
    4. petrous ridge of the temporal bone   A B C D E

4. The cranial dura mater is supplied by the following nerves:

    1. Ophthalmic   3. Mandibular
    2. Maxillary   4. Vagus   A B C D E

5. The blood supply to the lateral surface of the cerebral
    hemisphere is derived from the____artery.

    1. anterior cerebral   3. middle cerebral
    2. posterior cerebral   4. anterior choroidal   A B C D E

6. The blood supply to the occipital cortex is derived from the
    ____artery.

    1. posterior choroidal   3. anterior cerebral
    2. middle cerebral   4. posterior cerebral   A B C D E

A	B	C	D	E
1,2,3	1,3,	2,4	only 4	all correct

7. The following arteries are branches of the cranial portion of the internal carotid artery:

   1. Ophthalmic
   2. Anterior choroidal
   3. Hypophysial
   4. Posterior choroidal   A B C D E

8. The anterior choroidal artery supplies the

   1. globus pallidus
   2. amygdala
   3. uncus
   4. choroid plexus in inferior horn of lateral ventricle   A B C D E

9. Within the cranium, branches of the vertebral artery include:

   1. Anterior inferior cerebellar artery
   2. Posterior inferior cerebellar artery
   3. Internal auditory (labyrinthine) artery
   4. Posterior spinal artery   A B C D E

10. The medulla is supplied by the

   1. vertebral artery
   2. anterior and posterior spinal arteries
   3. anterior inferior cerebellar artery
   4. posterior inferior cerebellar artery   A B C D E

11. The central nuclei of the cerebellum are supplied by the

   1. anterior inferior cerebellar artery
   2. posterior inferior cerebellar artery
   3. superior cerebellar artery
   4. internal auditory artery   A B C D E

12. The thalamus is supplied by the

   1. posteromedial ganglionic artery
   2. anterior choroidal artery
   3. posterior choroidal artery
   4. posterolateral ganglionic arteries   A B C D E

13. The straight sinus is formed from the

   1. superior sagittal sinus
   2. inferior sagittal sinus
   3. inferior cerebral vein
   4. great cerebral vein   A B C D E

14. The confluence of the sinuses is formed by the following sinuses:

   1. Superior sagittal
   2. Straight
   3. Occipital
   4. Transverse   A B C D E

A	B	C	D	E
1,2,3	1,3,	2,4	only 4	all correct

15. The basal vein is formed from the following veins:

    1. Deep middle cerebral   3. Anterior cerebral
    2. Superficial middle cerebral   4. Posterior cerebral   A B C D E

16. Branches from the following arteries supply the cranial meninges:

    1. Ophthalmic   3. Occipital
    2. Maxillary (internal maxillary) 4. Superficial temporal   A B C D E

ANSWERS, NOTES, AND EXPLANATIONS

1. D Only 4 is correct. The meningeal vessels are contained in the inner periosteum. They appear as if they lie between the bone and the dura mater. These vessels should be called periosteal arteries instead of meningeal arteries because they are located outside the meninges and mainly supply the overlying bone.

2. B 1 and 3 are correct. Unlike the cranial dura mater, which is firmly attached to the inner periosteum of the skull, the spinal dura mater is separated from the wall of the vertebral canal by a epidural space containing adipose tissue and a rich venous plexus.

3. B 1 and 3 are correct. The falx cerebri is attached to the crista galli of the ethoid bone anteriorly, to the midline of the cranial vault (frontal, parietal, and occipital bones) as far posteriorly as the internal occipital protuberance, and to the tentorium cerebelli. It has no attachments to the anterior clinoid process or to the petrous portion of the temporal bone.

4. E All are correct. The cranial dura has a rich sensory supply of nerves which originates mainly from the three sensory branches of the trigeminal nerve. They supply the dura in the anterior and middle cranial fossa. The dura in the area of the posterior cranial fossa is supplied by meningeal branches from the vagus nerve and by branches from the superior cranial nerves.

5. A 1, 2, and 3 are correct. The blood supply to the lateral surface of the cerebral hemisphere is derived from the anterior, middle, and posterior cerebral arteries. Branches from the middle cerebral artery supply most of the cortex; however branches, especially the calcarine and parietooccipitals from the posterior cerebral arteries, send branches around the superior border and posterior pole of the hemisphere to supply a peripheral strip on the dorsolateral surface. The posterior cerebral artery supplies all the cortex on the medial surface.

6. C 2 and 4 are correct. The blood supply to the cortex of the occipital lobe is mainly derived from the middle cerebral and posterior cere-

bral arteries. Branches from the middle cerebral artery supply most of the cortex. However branches, especially the calcarine and parieto-occipitals from the posterior cerebral arteries, send branches around the superior border and posterior pole of the hemisphere to supply a peripheral strip on the dorsolateral surface. The posterior cerebral artery supplies all the cortex on the medial surface.

7. A 1, 2, and 3 are correct. Within the cranium the internal carotid artery gives off several collateral branches before terminating to form the middle and anterior cerebral arteries. Some of these collateral branches are as follows: (1) hypophysial, originating in the cavernous sinus; (2) cavernous, arising in the cavernous sinus; (3) meningeal (a very small branch), also arising from the cavernous portion of the internal carotid artery; (4) ophthalmic, originating immediately after the internal carotid artery leaves the cavernous sinus and enters the subarachnoid space; (5) posterior communicating, arising very close to the terminal bifurcation of the internal carotid (it may also arise from the middle cerebral), and (6) anterior choroidal, arising from the distal part of the internal carotid, or like the posterior communicating, it may arise from the middle cerebral. The posterior choroidal artery is not a branch of the internal carotid; it arises from the posterior cerebral artery.

8. E All are correct. The anterior choroidal artery has a very extensive supply to many of the deep structures of the cerebrum. Some of the structures that it supplies are as follows: (1) choroidal plexus in the inferior horn of the lateral ventricle; (2) optic tract; (3) uncus; (4) amygdala; (5) hippocampus; (6) globus pallidus; (7) lateral geniculate body; (8) ventral aspect of the internal capsule; (9) thalamus; and (10) subthalamus.

9. C 2 and 4 are correct. Within the cranium, the vertebral artery has many branches; one or two of these are important clinically because involvement of them can lead to serious dysfunction of areas of the brain. The cranial branches of the vertebral artery are as follows: (1) small meningeal; (2) posterior spinal (may also arise from the posterior inferior cerebellar); (3) anterior spinal; (4) posterior inferior cerebellar; and (5) medullary. The anterior inferior cerebellar, like the internal auditory artery, is a branch of the basilar artery.

10. E All are correct. The medulla has an extensive blood supply. Branches from the vertebral arteries, as they course along each ventrolateral side of the medulla, are the main source of supply. However, the anterior inferior cerebellar artery, a branch from the basilar artery, contributes to its blood supply. Branches from the posterior inferior cerebellar artery are the most important. Other sources of blood supply to the medulla are as follows: (1) anterior spinal; (2) posterior spinal; and (3) medullary.

11. A 1, 2, and 3 are correct. The central nuclei (dentate, globose, emboliform, and fastigial) of the cerebellum are supplied by branches from the three main arteries to the cerebellum: the superior, anterior inferior, and posterior inferior cerebellar arteries. Although the internal auditory artery may arise from the anterior inferior cerebellar

artery, it does not send any branches to the cerebellum or its nuclei.

12. E All are correct. The thalamus, as well as other deep structures of the cerebrum, has a good blood supply from posterior branches of the cerebral arterial circle and internal carotid artery. Some of these branches are as follows: the posteromedial and posterolateral ganglionic (central) arteries, the anterior choroidal (from the internal carotid), and the posterior choroidal (from the posterior cerebral) arteries. Branches from the anterior part of the cerebral arterial circle contribute little or nothing to the blood supply of the thalamus.

13. C 2 and 4 are correct. The straight sinus, situated in the line of junction of the falx cerebri with the tentorium cerebelli, is formed by the union of the inferior sagittal sinus and the great cerebral vein. The straight sinus receives some of the superior cerebellar veins. The straight sinus usually continues as the left transverse sinus, whereas the superior sagittal sinus, which is not involved in the formation of the straight sinus, usually continues as the right transverse. Remember that the left and right internal cerebral veins unite to form the great cerebral vein (of Galen) under the splenium of the corpus callosum.

14. A 1, 2, and 3 are correct. The confluence of the sinuses (confluens sinuum) is usually formed by the superior longitudinal, straight, and occipital sinuses. They empty into a common pool from which the left and right transverse sinuses arise and conduct blood to the sigmoid sinus and the internal jugular vein. At the region of the internal occipital protuberance, a confluence of the sinuses is no more common than deviation of the superior sagittal sinus to one side and the straight sinus to the other side to form the transverse sinus with only a slender communication between them. The transverse sinus does not help form the confluence when present, but it conducts blood from this "common pool."

15. B 1 and 3 are correct. The basal vein begins at the anterior perforated substance by the union of: (1) a small anterior cerebral vein which accompanies the anterior cerebral artery; (2) the deep middle cerebral vein which receives tributaries from the insula and neighbouring gyri and runs in the floor of the lateral sulcus; and (3) striate veins which pass through the anterior perforated substance to join the above structures. The superficial middle cerebral vein, located in the subarachnoid space in the lateral sulcus, empties into the cavernous sinus. There are no posterior cerebral veins named as such.

16. A 1, 2, and 3 are correct. The cranial meninges have a very extensive blood supply from branches of the external carotid (maxillary and occipital) and internal carotid (directly and from the ophthalmic) arteries. Some of these named branches are as follows: (1) direct meningeal branches from the occipital artery; (2) a meningeal branch from the mastoid branch of the occipital artery; (3) middle and accessory meningeal branches from the maxillary artery; (4) direct meningeal branches from the ophthalmic artery; and (5) a recurrent meningeal branch from the lacrimal division of the ophthalmic artery.

DIRECTIONS: Each of the following groups of questions consists of a numbered list of descriptive words or phrases accompanied by a diagram with certain parts indicated by letters, or by a list of lettered headings. For each numbered word or phrase, SELECT THE LETTERED PART OR HEADING that matches it correctly and insert the letter in the space to the right of the appropriate number. Each lettered heading may be selected once, more than once, or not at all.

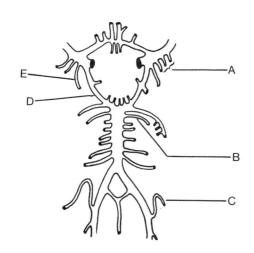

1. ____ Connects the posterior cerebral artery with the carotid artery

2. ____ Supplies the uncus and globus pallidus, as well as the choroid plexus in the temporal horn of the lateral ventricle

3. ____ Its branches are distributed to the posterior part of the cerebellar hemisphere, the inferior vermis, and the dorsolateral region of the medulla oblongata

4. ____ The oculomotor and trochlear nerves emerge between this artery and the posterior cerebral artery

5. ____ Supplies the major portion of the corpus striatum

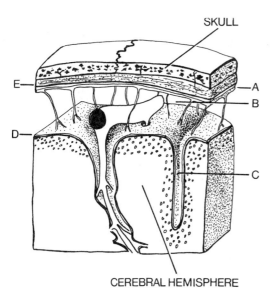

CEREBRAL HEMISPHERE

6. ____ Contains cerebrospinal fluid and cerebral blood vessels

7. ____ Provides support for the brain and is attached intimately to the inner periosteum of the skull

8. ____ Thin microscopic layer of tissue that adheres to the surface of the brain

9. ____ Cerebral sulcus

10. ____ Arachnoid

168

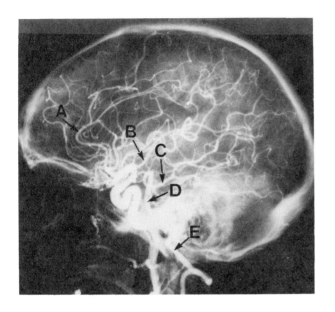

11. _____ Middle cerebral artery

12. _____ Anterior cerebral artery

13. _____ Basilar artery

14. _____ Posterior cerebral artery

15. _____ Vertebral artery

ANSWERS, NOTES, AND EXPLANATIONS

1. D The posterior communicating artery connects the posterior cerebral artery with the internal carotid artery. The anterior communicating connects the two anterior cerebrals. By means of these communicating arteries, a cerebral arterial circle is formed at the base of the brain.

2. E The anterior choroidal artery, a branch of the distal part of the internal carotid artery, or the beginning of the middle cerebral artery, passes into the choroid fissure at the medial edge of the temporal lobe and into the temporal (inferior) horn of the lateral ventricle. It supplies the choroid plexus of the temporal horn of the lateral ventricle, the uncus, amygdala, hippocampus, globus pallidus, lateral geniculate nucleus, and ventral part of the internal capsule.

3. C The posterior inferior cerebellar artery, the largest branch of the vertebral artery, has an irregular tortuous course between the medulla and cerebellum. It supplies the posterior part of the cerebellar hemisphere, the inferior vermis, the central nuclei of the cerebellum, the choroid plexus of the fourth ventricle, and the dorsolateral region of the medulla.

4. B The superior cerebellar artery arises close to the posterior cerebral artery (terminal bifurcation of the basilar artery), and runs parallel with this artery for a short distance before it ramifies over the dorsal surface of the cerebellum to supply the cortex, medullary center, and central nuclei. The third and fourth cranial nerves course between these two vessels as they run parallel to one another near the

169

anterior border of the basilar pons.

5. A The anterolateral ganglionic (central) arteries arise mainly from
    the proximal portion of the middle cerebral artery and pierce the
    anterior perforated substance. They are also known as striate arteries
    (lateral striate) because they supply the major portion of the corpus
    striatum. These vessels supply the following structures: head of the
    caudate nucleus, putamen, lateral part of the globus pallidus, much of the
    internal capsule (anterior limb, genu, and dorsal portion of posterior
    limb), external capsule, claustrum, and lateral area of hypothalamus.

6. B The subarachnoid space is located between the arachnoid and pia
    mater. These two layers may be combined under the heading of the pia-
    arachnoid; they bound the subarachnoid space filled with cerebrospinal
    fluid. The cerebral arteries and external cerebral veins, as well as
    the spinal arteries and veins, are contained in this space. Numerous
    trabeculae (connective tissue strands) passing through this space
    connect the arachnoid mater with the pia mater.

7. E The cranial dura mater is a dense, thick, compact layer of collagen-
    ous connective tissue that is firmly attached to the periosteum of the
    skull. It, along with the other meningeal layers, provides support and
    protection for the brain in addition to that afforded by the skull.

8. D The pia mater is a microscopic thin layer consisting of extremely
    thin areolar tissue and a minute plexus of blood vessels. It closely
    invests all of the brain and spinal cord. It is attached to the arach-
    noid by delicate strands known as trabeculae and the two layers are
    often referred to as the pia-arachnoid; together they constitute the
    leptomeninges (L. slender membranes).

9. C A cerebral sulcus, furrow, or groove is located between cerebral
    convolutions or gyri. It is lined with pia mater. The arachnoid does
    not dip into the sulci of the cerebral hemispheres. This subarachnoid
    extension is filled with cerebral spinal fluid and many branches of
    cerebral vessels are located in the sulci.

10. A The arachnoid is a delicate membrane enveloping the brain and spinal
    cord. It lies between the pia mater internally and the dura mater ex-
    ternally. It is separated from the dura by a potential subdural space
    containing a thin film of fluid. The external surface of the arachnoid
    is covered by a thin layer of fluid. The external surface of the
    arachnoid is covered by a thin layer of squamous epithelial cells. The
    arachnoid surrounds the cranial and spinal nerves, enclosing them in
    loose sheaths as far as their points of exit from the skull and
    vertebral canals.

11. B The middle cerebral artery is a terminal branch of the internal
    carotid artery; it courses laterally into the lateral sulcus between
    the frontal and temporal lobes. Within the lateral sulcus, it curves
    over the insula and divides into many branches which ramify over the
    lateral surface of the hemisphere.

12. A The anterior cerebral artery, the smaller terminal branch of the in-
    ternal carotid artery, is directed medially, superior to the optic

nerve to the median longitudinal fissure. The anterior cerebral artery ascends in the longitudinal fissure, bends posteriorly around the genu of the corpus callosum, and gives off branches to the medial surface of the cerebral hemispheres as far posteriorly as the parietooccipital fissure.

13. D The basilar artery is formed by the junction of the two vertebral arteries at the base of the skull. It extends from the posterior to the anterior border of the pons. It lies in a shallow median groove on the ventral surface of the pons. At the anterior border of the pons, it divides into two terminal posterior cerebral arteries.

14. C The posterior cerebral artery, a terminal branch of the basilar artery, curves around the cerebral peduncle to reach the medial surface of the hemisphere inferior to the corpus callosum. Branches of the posterior cerebral artery ramify over the inferior surface of the temporal lobe and on to the posteromedial surface to supply the occipital lobe.

15. E The vertebral artery, a branch of the subclavian artery, ascends on each side through the foramina of the transverse processes of the superior six cervical vertebrae. At the base of the skull the artery winds around the lateral mass of the atlas, pierces the atlanto-occipital membrane, and then enters the subarachnoid space at the level of the foramen magnum. The vertebral artery runs anteriorly on the ventral surface of the medulla, joining its fellow of the opposite side to form the basilar artery at the posterior border of the basal portion of the pons.

ELEVEN

The Ventricular System and Cerebrospinal Fluid

O B J E C T I V E S

BE ABLE TO:

* Discuss early development of the ventricular system.

* Describe the main features of each ventricle.

* Make a simple diagram illustrating the structures in the floor of the ventricle.

* List the contents of the lateral ventricles and the structures in the floor and roof of these ventricles.

* Describe the formation of cerebrospinal fluid and its absorption into the venous system.

* Discuss the circulation of cerebrospinal fluid.

* Discuss external, internal, and communicating hydrocephalus.

* Recognize the normal shape and position of the ventricles as seen in ventriculograms and tomograms (CT scans).

F I V E - C H O I C E   C O M P L E T I O N   Q U E S T I O N S

DIRECTIONS: Each of the following questions or incomplete statements is followed by five suggested answers or completions. SELECT THE ONE BEST ANSWER OR COMPLETION in each case and underline the appropriate letter at the right.

----

1. Which statement concerning the posterior horn of a lateral ventricle is <u>correct</u>?

    A. It is surrounded by white matter of the medullary center
    B. The calcar avis protrudes into it
    C. The bulb of the posterior horn is in its medial wall
    D. None of the above
    E. All of the above   A B C D E

SELECT THE ONE BEST ANSWER OR COMPLETION

2. The body of a lateral ventricle is adjacent to

   A. the head of the caudate nucleus   D. all of the above
   B. the hippocampus   E. none of the
   C. the fibria of the fornix   above   A B C D E

3. Which statement concerning the floor of the fourth ventricle
   is incorrect?

   A. It is divided into symmetrical halves by a median sulcus
   B. The locus ceruleus is located at the rostral end of the
      sulcus limitans
   C. It is covered by ependymal epithelium
   D. The facial colliculus is a slight swelling at the superior
      end of the median eminence
   E. The vestibular area lies deep to most of the lateral
      area of the rhomboid fossa   A B C D E

4. Which statement about the third ventricle is incorrect?

   A. The membranous roof of the third ventricle is attached
      along the striae medullares thalami
   B. Cerebrospinal fluid enters the third ventricle through
      the cerebral aqueduct of the midbrain
   C. The interventricular foramen is bounded by the fornix
      and the anterior tubercle of the thalamus
   D. The anterior wall of the third ventricle is formed by
      the lamina terminalis
   E. The posterior commissure forms a slight prominence
      superior to the entrance to the cerebral aqueduct of
      the midbrain   A B C D E

5. The roof of the inferior horn of a lateral ventricle is NOT
   related to the

   A. dentate gyrus
   B. tail of the caudate nucleus
   C. vena terminalis
   D. stria terminalis
   E. ependymal epithelium   A B C D E

6. Which statement concerning a lateral ventricle is correct?

   A. It develops from the lateral recess of the lumen of
      the diencephalon
   B. A lateral ventricle communicates with the third ven-
      tricle via the cerebral aqueduct
   C. It is lined by microglial epithelium
   D. The hippocampus is related to the inferior horn of a
      lateral ventricle
   E. The head of the caudate nucleus is adjacent to the
      posterior horn of a lateral ventricle   A B C D E

173

SELECT THE ONE BEST ANSWER OR COMPLETION

8. Which statement is <u>incorrect</u>?

 A. The average amount of cerebrospinal fluid in the ven-
    tricules and subarachnoid space is approximately 130 ml
 B. The ventricular system alone contains approximately 60-70
    ml of cerebrospinal fluid at any one time
 C. The normal pressure of cerebrospinal fluid is from 80 to
    180 mm of water when a person is recumbent
 D. The normal pressure of cerebrospinal fluid in the inferior
    spinal subarachnoid space is approximately 160-360 mm of
    water when a person is in a sitting position
 E. The specific gravity of normal cerebrospinal fluid is
    1.003 - 1.008.   A B C D E

9. Which statement about the choroid epithelium as seen in
   electron micrographs is <u>incorrect</u>?

 A. The abundant cytoplasm and numerous mitrochondria in the
    epithelial cells are indicative of an active process con-
    cerned with the formation of cerebrospinal fluid
 B. The plasma membrane at the free surface of the epithelial
    cells is greatly increased in area by irregular microvilli
 C. There is no basement membrane separating the epithelium
    from the subjacent stroma
 D. In an embryo the choroid epithelial cells bear motile cilia
 E. The membranes of adjoining cells are thrown into complicated
    folds at the base of the cells   A B C D E

ANSWERS, NOTES, AND EXPLANATIONS

1. E The occipital (posterior) horn of a lateral ventricle, which is
   variable in length, is surrounded by the medullary center of the hemisphere. There are two elevations on the medial wall of the occipital
   horn. The dorsal prominence, for which the forceps occipitalis is responsible, is referred to as the bulb of the occipital horn; the lower
   prominence, formed by the calcarine sulcus, is called the calcar avis.

2. E The head of the caudate nucleus bulges into the frontal or anterior
   horn of a lateral ventricle, whereas the first part of the tail lies
   along the lateral edge of the central part of a lateral ventricle. The
   hippocampus occupies the floor of the temporal or inferior horn of a
   lateral ventricle. Efferent fibers of the hippocampus form a ridge or
   fimbria along its medial border. The fimbria continues as the crus of
   the fornix when the hippocampus terminates beneath the splenium of the
   corpus callosum.

3. D The facial colliculus, a slight swelling at the inferior end of the
   median eminence, is formed by fibers from the motor nucleus of the
   facial nerve looping over the abducens nucleus.

4. B Cerebrospinal fluid enters the third ventricle from the lateral ventricles through the interventricular foramina. The fluid leaves the

174

third ventricle via the cerebral aqueduct of the midbrain, flows through the fourth ventricle, and enters the subarachnoid space through the median and lateral apertures of the fourth ventricle.

5. A The dentate gyrus, which has a toothed or beaded appearance, occupies the interval between the fimbria of the hippocampus and the parahippocampal gyrus, along the medial edge of the temporal lobe. The dentate gyrus is produced by a further extension of the hippocampus during the development of the brain.

6. D The hippocampus develops in the fetal brain by a process of continuing expansion of the medial edge of the temporal lobe. It does so in such a way that the gyrus comes to occupy the floor of the temporal or inferior horn of a lateral ventricle. The lateral ventricles develop from lateral recesses of the lumen of the telencephalon. They are roughly C-shaped cavities lined by ependymal epithelium. Each lateral ventricle communicates with the third ventricle through an opening known as the interventricular foramen.

7. B The floor of the central part of a lateral ventricle includes part of the dorsal surface of the thalamus. The lateral surface of the thalamus lies immediately adjacent to the posterior limb of the internal capsule.

8. B The ventricular system normally contains 15 to 40 ml of cerebrospinal fluid. When the median and lateral apertures leading from the fourth ventricle are blocked, the fluid increases in volume and pressure and the ventricles become enlarged. Blockage of the ventricular system may also occur at other sites (e.g., the cerebral aqueduct).

9. C A prominent basement membrane separates the choroid epithelium from the subjacent stroma with its vascular network. The epithelial cells bear motile cilia in the embryo and patches of ciliated epithelium persist postnatally for varying periods. The large spherical nucleus, abundant cytoplasm, and numerous mitochondria indicate that the production of cerebrospinal fluid is in part an active process requiring expenditure of energy by these cells.

M U L T I - C O M P L E T I O N   Q U E S T I O N S

DIRECTIONS: In each of the following questions or incomplete statements, one or more of the completions given is correct. At the lower right of each question, underline A if 1, 2, and 3 are correct; B if 1 and 3 are correct; C if 2 and 4 are correct; D if only 4 is correct; and E if all are correct.

---

1. Structures deep to the floor of the fourth ventricle, medial to the sulcus limitans, include:

    1. Vestibular nuclei
    2. Facial colliculus
    3. Cochlear nuclei
    4. Hypoglossal trigone   A B C D E

A	B	C	D	E
1,2,3	1,3,	2,4	only 4	all correct

2. Cerebrospinal fluid enters the subarachnoid space through the

    1. lateral apertures of the fourth ventricle
    2. foramen of Magendie
    3. median aperture of the fourth ventricle
    4. foramina of Luschka   A B C D E

3. The following structures lie anterior to the interventricular
   foramen:

    1. Anterior commissure   3. Lamina terminalis
    2. Column of the fornix   4. Thalamic tubercle   A B C D E

4. The forepart of the roof of the fourth ventricle is formed
   by the

    1. brachium conjunctivum   3. superior medullary velum
    2. brachium pontis   4. superior vermis   A B C D E

5. Which structures are included in the lateral wall of the
   fourth ventricle?

    1. Foramen of Magendie
    2. Recess leading to the foramen of Luschka
    3. Superior cerebellar peduncle
    4. Inferior cerebellar peduncle   A B C D E

6. Cerebrospinal fluid is produced mainly by the choroid
   plexus in the

    1. lateral ventricles   3. fourth ventricle
    2. third ventricle   4. central canal   A B C D E

7. Structures within the inferior horn of a lateral ventricle
   include:

    1. Anterior choroidal   3. Choroid plexus
       artery   4. Tail of caudate
    2. Dentate gyrus   nucleus   A B C D E

8. Which components of the ventricular system might become
   dilated subsequent to occlusion of the median and lateral
   apertures of the fourth ventricle?

    1. Lateral ventricle   3. Fourth ventricle
    2. Third ventricle   4. Cerebral acqueduct   A B C D E

9. Normal cerebrospinal fluid is

    1. clear   3. colorless
    2. a pale amber color   4. opaque   A B C D E

10. In the choroid plexus, capillary blood is separated from the ventricular lumen by

1. endothelium
2. a basement membrane

3. choroid epithelium
4. ependymal cells   A B C D E

ANSWERS, NOTES, AND EXPLANATIONS

1. C 2 and 4 are correct. The sulcus limitans divides each half of the floor of the fourth ventricle into a medial and a lateral area. Motor nuclei of cranial nerves are located beneath the medial area. The hypoglossal and vagal triangles indicate the position of the rostral ends of the hypoglossal nucleus and the dorsal nucleus of the vagus nerve, respectively. The facial colliculus, a slight swelling near the inferior end of the median eminence, is formed by fibers from the motor nucleus of the facial nerve looping over the abducens nucleus. The medial longitudinal fasciculus is situated beneath the medial area adjacent to the median sulcus. The vestibular nuclear complex lies beneath most of the lateral area.

2. E All are correct. The median aperture of the fourth ventricle, formerly known as the foramen of Magendie, is a deficiency of variable size in the inferior medullary velum. It provides a communication between the ventricular system and the subarachnoid space. Lateral recesses of the fourth ventricle extend around the sides of the medulla and open ventrally as the lateral apertures of the fourth ventricle, through which cerebrospinal fluid also enters the subarachnoid space. These apertures are situated at the junction of the pons, medulla, and cerebellum.

3. A 1, 2, and 3 are correct. The lamina terminalis, extending from the optic chiasma to the rostrum of the corpus callosum, represents the rostral end of the embryonal neural tube. The anterior commissure lies immediately posterior to the superior portion of the lamina terminalis. It separates it from the column of the fornix which curves ventrally anterior to the interventricular foramen. The anterior tubercle of the thalamus is the posterior boundary of this foramen.

4. B 1 and 3 are correct. The tent-shaped roof of the fourth ventricle protrudes into the cerebellum. The forepart of the roof is formed by the superior cerebellar peduncles. The V-shaped interval between the converging peduncles is bridged by the superior medullary velum, a thin sheet consisting of pia mater and ependyma with some nerve fibers between them.

5. C 2 and 4 are correct. The lateral walls of the fourth ventricle include the inferior cerebellar peduncles, which curve from the medulla into the cerebellum on the medial aspect of the middle cerebellar peduncles. The lateral recesses of the fourth ventricle extend around the sides of the medulla and open ventrally as the lateral apertures of the fourth ventricle. The superior cerebellar peduncles form most of

the anterior part of the roof of the fourth ventricle.

6. A 1, 2, and 3 are correct. The cerebrospinal fluid is produced mainly
by the choroid plexuses of the lateral, third, and fourth ventricles,
those in the lateral ventricles being the largest and most important.
From the ventricles, cerebrospinal fluid passes through the median
aperture and the foramina of the lateral recesses of the fourth
ventricle into the subarachnoid space.

7. B 1 and 3 are correct. Major branches of the anterior choroidal
artery enter the temporal or inferior horn of the lateral ventricle
through the choroidal fissure. They supply the choroid plexus situated
within the ventricle. The tail of the caudate nucleus, stria terminalis, and vena terminalis are in the roof of the temporal horn. The
floor of the temporal horn consists of the hippocampal formation, made
up of the hippocampus and dentate gyrus, and the associated alveus and
fibria of the hippocampus.

8. E All are correct. Internal hydrocephalus refers to dilation of the
ventricles. All the ventricles would be enlarged if the median and
lateral apertures of the fourth ventricle were occluded. The lateral
and third ventricles would be dilated if the obstruction were in the
cerebral aqueduct of the midbrain, whereas only one lateral ventricle
would enlarge following occlusion of an interventricular foramen.

9. B 1 and 3 are correct. Cerebrospinal fluid is clear and colorless,
with a specific gravity of 1.003 - 1.008. It contains small amounts of
protein and glucose, larger amounts of potassium and sodium chloride,
and traces of sulphate, phosphate, calcium, and uric acid. Three to
eight lymphocytes are present in each cubic millimeter of normal
cerebrospinal fluid.

10. A 1, 2, and 3 are correct. Capillary blood is separated from the ventricular lumen by endothelium, a basement membrane, and choroidal
epithelium. The junctions between capillary endothelial cells appear
to be more permeable than elsewhere, and the cells have fenestrations
or pores closed by thin diaphragms. Some components of plasma pass
through these layers with difficulty; others enter the cerebrospinal
fluid readily by diffusion, and still others reach the fluid with the
assistance of metabolic activity on the part of choroid epithelial
cells.

FIVE-CHOICE ASSOCIATION QUESTIONS

DIRECTIONS: Each of the following groups of questions consists of a numbered list of descriptive words or phrases accompanied by a diagram with certain parts indicated by letters, or by a list of lettered headings. For each numbered word or phrase, SELECT THE LETTERED PART OR HEADING that matches it correctly and insert the letter in the space to the right of the appropriate number. Each lettered heading may be selected once, more than once, or not at all.

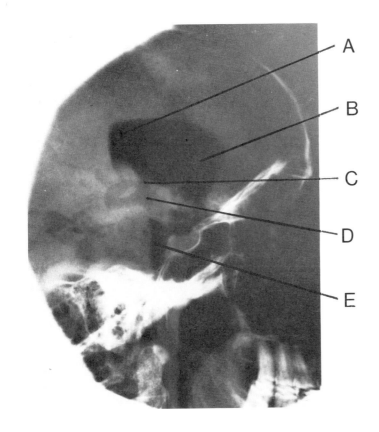

1. ____The genu of the corpus callosum forms its anterior boundary

2. ____The tail of the caudate nucleus is located in its roof

3. ____Its floor includes part of the dorsal surface of the thalamus

4. ____The anterior tubercle of the thalamus is a posterior boundary

5. ____It is bounded laterally by the medial surface of the thalamus

6. ____Appears as a triangular slit in a coronal section

179

ASSOCIATION QUESTIONS

A. Floor of fourth ventricle

B. Occipital horn of lateral ventricle

C. Median aperture

D. Central part of lateral ventricle

E. Third ventricle

7. ____Vena terminalis

8. ____Facial colliculus

9. ____Massa intermedia

10. ____Calcar avis

11. ____Opens into cisterna magna

12. ____Sulcus limitans

13. ____Lamina terminalis

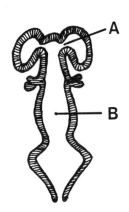

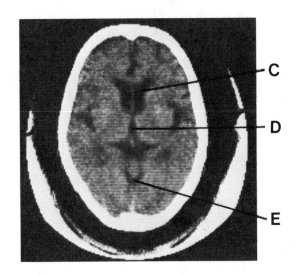

14. ____Frontal horn of laternal ventricle

15. ____Continuity between lateral and third ventricles

16. ____Opens into the subarachnoid space

17. ____Bounded medially by the septum pellucidum

18. ____Third ventricle

19. ____Courses through the midbrain

ANSWERS, NOTES, AND EXPLANATIONS

1. B The frontal horn extends anteriorly from the central part of the lateral ventricle into the frontal lobe, beginning at the level of the interventricular foramen. The corpus callosum continues as the roof and the genu of the corpus callosum limits the horn anteriorly.

2. E The temporal horn begins at the collateral trigone and extends rostrally into the median part of the temporal lobe, ending about 2.5 cm from the temporal pole. The roof and lateral wall are largely formed by the tapetum and the optic radiations. In the medial region of the roof, a small part is furnished by the tail of the caudate nucleus, which extends anteriorly as far as the amygdaloid nucleus. It is accompanied by the stria terminalis.

3. A The central part of the lateral ventricle, a relatively shallow cavity, extends from the interventricular foramen to the splenium of the corpus callosum, where it enlarges in the region of the collateral trigone at the junction of the occipital and temporal horns. Its roof is formed by the corpus callosum, and its floor by a number of structures. In a lateral to medial direction, these are: the tail of the caudate nucleus, stria terminalis and vena terminalis, dorsal surface of the thalamus, and fornix. The choroid plexus is attached along the interval between the dorsal surface of the thalamus and the fornix.

4. C The interventricular foramen is a crescentic slit, through which the third ventricle communicates with a lateral ventricle. The foramen is bounded anteriorly by the curving column of the fornix and posteriorly by the convex anterior tubercle of the thalamus. It is closed posteriorly by a reflection of ependyma between the fornix and the thalamus.

5. D Each lateral wall of the third ventricle consists of a superior portion formed by the thalamus and an inferior portion formed by the hypothalamus. The hypothalamic sulcus, which extends from the interventricular foramen to the cerebral aqueduct of the midbrain, is the line of demarcation between the two parts of the lateral wall of the third ventricle.

6. B The frontal horn of a lateral ventricle appears as a triangular slit in a coronal section. The anterior part of the corpus callosum forms the flat roof and the septum pellucidum, the vertical medial wall. The head of the caudate nucleus produces a convex bulge in the lateral wall of the frontal horn.

7. D The vena terminalis (thalamostriate vein) begins in the region of the amygdaloid nucleus and follows the curve of the tail of the caudate nucleus on its medial side. In the floor of the central part of the lateral ventricle, the vein runs anteriorly in the groove between the caudate nucleus and the dorsal surface of the thalamus. The vena terminalis joins the choroid vein in the region of the interventricular foramen to form the internal cerebral vein.

8. A The facial colliculus, a slight swelling at the inferior end of the

181

median eminence, is in the medial area of the floor of the fourth ventricle. It is formed by fibers from the motor nucleus of the facial nerve looping over the abducens nucleus.

9.   E The lateral walls of the third ventricle are often joined to each other across the cavity of the ventricle by a band of gray matter, named the massa intermedia (interthalamic connection). It is present in about 70 percent of brains. A shadow created by the massa intermedia in a pneumoencephalogram may provide a useful radiological landmark. Likewise, shadows of the anterior commissure and a calcified pineal body can be identified in many radiographs.

10. B The calcar avis is a longitudinal elevation on the medial wall ·of the occipital horn of the lateral ventricle, produced by deep penetration of the calcarine sulcus. A more dorsal prominence, for which the forceps occipitalis is responsible, is called the bulb of the occipital horn.

11. C The median aperture of the fourth ventricle provides the principal communication between the ventricular system and the subarachnoid space. It is a deficiency of variable size in the inferior medullary velum and opens into the cerebellomedullary cistern (cisterna magna).

12. A The floor of the fourth ventricle is divided into symmetrical halves by the median sulcus. The sulcus limitans divides each half into medial and lateral area. The sulcus limitans forms a groove in the wall of the embryonic neural tube, separating the basal and alar laminae.

13. E The anterior wall of the third ventricle is formed by the lamina terminalis, which represents the cephalic end of the primitive neural tube. The anterior commissure crosses the midline in the superior part of the lamina. The lamina terminalis stretches from the optic chiasma to the rostrum of the corpus callosum.

14. C The photograph is from a tomograph (C.T. scan) of a human brain. The frontal horn of the lateral ventricle is clearly seen on each side of the cerebrum. The genu of the corpus callosum limits the frontal horn anteriorly and the septum pellucidum separates the frontal horns of the two ventricles. The head of the caudate nucleus bulges into the lateral side of the frontal horn.

15. A The sketch is of the embryonic brain vesicles and the developing ventricular system. During the sixth week of development, the prosencephalon subdivides into a telencephalon and a diencephalon. The large cavities within each segment are the primordia of the lateral and third ventricles, respectively. The interventricular foramen, a large opening posterior to the lamina terminalis, provides continuity between the third ventricle and the cavity of the expanding cerebral hemisphere i.e., the primitive lateral ventricle.

16. E The ventricular system communicates with the subarachnoid space through the median aperture of the fourth ventricle and the paired lateral apertures of the fourth ventricle. The median aperture is in that part of the ventricular roof formed by the inferior medullary

velum, and the lateral apertures opening on the ventral surface of the brain are at the ends of the lateral recesses of the fourth ventricle. Through these openings, cerebrospinal fluid gains access to the sub-arachnoid space.

17. C   In the frontal lobe, the frontal horn of the lateral ventricle extends anteriorly from the level of the interventricular foramen. Its roof and rostral wall are formed by the body and genu of the corpus callosum, respectively, and is separated from the frontal horn of the opposite ventricle by the thin vertical lamina of the septum pellucidum.

18. D   The third ventricle is a narrow slit-like cavity interposed between the lateral ventricles and the more caudally placed cerebral aqueduct and fourth ventricle. It is bounded on each side by the thalamus and hypothalamus. The anterior wall of the third ventricle is composed of the lamina terminalis and the anterior commissure, and the roof is formed by a thin layer of ependyma and pia mater.

19. B   During the sixth week of development, the primary brain vesicles (prosencephalon, mesencephalon, and rhombencephalon) are converted into five secondary brain vesicles, the telencephalon, diencephalon, mesencephalon, metencephalon, and myelencephalon. The large cavities of the brain vesicles are continuous with the lumen of the central canal of the spinal cord; they are the primordia of the ventricular system. With continued brain growth, the lumen of the mesencephalon becomes narrowed to form the cerebral aqueduct of the midbrain.

PART TWO

The Systems

TWELVE

The General Sensory Systems

O B J E C T I V E S

BE ABLE TO:

* Illustrate the various peripheral receptors for the general senses.

* Discuss the concept of primary, secondary, and tertiary sensory neurons.

* Describe the somatic sensory pathways to the cerebral cortex for: (1) (1) pain and temperature; (2) light touch and pressure: and (3) discriminitive touch, proprioception, and vibration.

* Discuss the sensory deficit resulting from a lesion which interrupts a general sensory pathway at various points along its course.

F I V E - C H O I C E   C O M P L E T I O N   Q U E S T I O N S

DIRECTIONS: Each of the following questions or incomplete statements is followed by five suggested answers or completions. SELECT THE ONE BEST ANSWER OR COMPLETION in each case and underline the appropriate letter at the right.

----

1. The chief sensory nucleus of the trigeminal nerve receives fibers for

    A. proprioception   D. temperature
    B. pain   E. all of the above
    C. discriminative touch   A B C D E

2. Which sensory deficit may be expected inferior to the level of the lesion subsequent to section of the left ventral quadrant of the spinal cord?

    A. Proprioception on right side   D. Pain on left side
    B. Pain on right side   E. Touch on both sides
    C. Touch on left side   A B C D E

187

SELECT THE ONE BEST ANSWER OR COMPLETION

3. Specific thalamocortical fibers for general sensation run in the

    A. posterior limb of the internal capsule
    B. genu of the internal capsule and the corona radiata
    C. retrolenticular portion of the posterior limb of the internal capsule
    D. external capsule
    E. anterior limb of the internal capsule and the corona radiata   A B C D E

4. Which sensory ending does not function as a proprioceptor?

    A. Golgi tendon organ
    B. Meissner's corpuscle
    C. Neuromuscular spindle
    D. Nonencapsulated ending
    C. Pacinian corpuscle   A B C D E

5. With respect to cranial nerves, cutaneous sensation is fully provided by the

    A. trigeminal nerve
    B. trigeminal and facial nerves
    C. ophthalmic and mandibular divisions of the trigeminal nerve
    D. trigeminal, facial, and vagus nerves
    E. trigeminal and facial nerves   A B C D E

6. Which statement concerning the spinal lemniscus is correct?

    A. It is an uncrossed general sensory pathway in the brain stem
    B. It terminates in the medial portion of the ventral posterior nucleus of the thalamus
    C. It consists of axons of second order sensory neurons for muscle, joint, and tendon sense
    D. It is situated in the medial part of the brain stem
    E. Its fibers terminate in the lateral portion of the ventral posterior thalamic nucleus and the superior colliculus   A B C D E

7. The somesthetic cortical area consists of

    A. cortex supplied entirely by the middle cerebral artery
    B. area 6 of Brodmann
    C. cortex with afferents mainly from the dorsal tier of thalamic nuclei
    D. cortex in the postcentral gyrus and the posterior part of the paracentral lobule
    E. agranular heterotypical cortex   A B C D E

SELECT THE ONE BEST ANSWER OR COMPLETION

8. Which sensory deficit is characteristic of an infarction in the
    lateral medulla, dorsal to the inferior olivary nucleus?

    A. Proprioceptive loss on the opposite side of the body
    B. Anesthesia for pain and temperature limited to the
        opposite side of the face
    C. Lack of thermal sensitivity on the same side of the
        head and body
    D. Loss of discriminative touch ipsilaterally
    E. Anesthesia for pain and temperature on the same side of
        the face and the opposite side of the body   A B C D E

ANSWERS, NOTES, AND EXPLANATIONS

1. C Fibers for discriminative touch in the sensory root of the trigeminal
    nerve terminate in the chief or principal nucleus in the dorsal pons.
    Some fibers for light touch and pressure bifurcate on entering the pons;
    one branch ends in the chief sensory nucleus and the other descends in
    the spinal tract of the trigeminal nerve and ends in the nucleus of the
    spinal tract. Fibers for pain and temperature terminate in the nucleus
    of the trigeminal spinal tract. Proprioceptive fibers are peripheral
    branches of cells in the mesencephalic nucleus of the trigeminal nerve.

2. B Section of the ventrolateral quadrant of the spinal cord interrupts
    the spinothalamic tract for pain, touch, and temperature on the opposite
    side of the body. Conduction for proprioception is in the dorsal white
    column which is spared in the present lesion.

3. A Specific thalamocortical fibers for general sensation run from the
    ventral posterior nucleus of the thalamus to the somesthetic area in the
    parietal lobe. They traverse the posterior limb of the internal capsule,
    i.e., posterior to the genu, and continue into the corona radiata of the
    medullary center.

4. B The principal proprioceptive endings are neuromuscular spindles,
    neurotendinous spindles or Golgi tendon organs, pacinian corpuscles ad-
    jacent to joints, and nonencapsulated terminal branches of sensory fibers
    in ligaments and capsules of joints. Meissner's corpuscles, located in
    dermal papillae, are receptors for touch, especially fine or discrimina-
    tive touch.

5. D The ophthalmic, maxillary, and mandibular divisions of the trigeminal
    nerve supply large cutaneous areas. The external ear, most of the exter-
    nal acoustic meatus and tympanic membrane, and an area posterior to the
    ear are supplied by the facial and vagus nerves, the second and third
    cervical spinal nerves, and sometimes the glossopharyngeal nerve.

6. E On reaching the level of the inferior olivary nucleus in the medulla,
    the spinothalamic tract and the spinotectal tract merge to form the
    spinal lemniscus. The cell bodies for fibers of these tracts are in the
    dorsal horn of the contralateral gray matter of the spinal cord. Spino-
    tectal fibers leave the spinal lemniscus in the midbrain and terminate in

the superior colliculus, whereas the spinothalamic fibers continue to the lateral portion of the ventral posterior nucleus of the thalamus (ventral posterolateral nucleus).

7. D The general sensory or somesthetic cortex in the parietal lobe occupies the postcentral gyrus on the dorsolateral surface and the posterior part of the paracentral lobule on the medial surface. The opposite side of the body is represented as inverted, with disproportionately large regions assigned to the head and the hand. The most dorsal region for the lower limb is supplied by the anterior cerebral artery, the remainder by the middle cerebral artery. The somesthetic area corresponds to areas 3, 1, and 2 in the Brodmann cytoarchitectural map. Area 3, the anterior strip, is classified as granular heterotypical cortex and areas 1 and 2 are homotypical cortex. The somesthetic area receives specific thalamocortical afferents from the ventral posterior thalamic nucleus, one of the nuclei in the ventral tier of the thalamus.

8. E An infarction in the lateral medulla (located as described) would be produced by thrombosis of a medullary branch of the posterior inferior cerebellar artery or the vertebral artery. The resulting signs and symptoms characterize the lateral medullary or Wallenberg's syndrome. Involvement of the spinal tract of the trigeminal nerve and the nucleus of the spinal tract, together with the spinal lemniscus, produces loss of pain and temperature sensibility on the same side of the face as the lesion and the opposite side of the body. Proprioception and discriminative touch are spared because the medial lemniscus near the midline is not included in the area of the lesion. Other signs of the lateral medullary syndrome include difficulty in swallowiong and phonation because of destruction of the nucleus ambiguus. Horner's syndrome is added if the pathway from the hypothalamus to the sympathetic outflow in the spinal cord is interrupted. Signs of vestibular and cerebellar dysfunction are also added when the infarcted area extends dorsally to the vestibular nuclei and the inferior cerebellar peduncle.

M U L T I - C O M P L E T I O N   Q U E S T I O N S

DIRECTIONS: In each of the following questions or incomplete statements, one or more of the completions given is correct. At the lower right of each question, underline A if 1, 2, and 3 are correct; B if 1 and 3 are correct; C if 2 and 4 are correct; D if only 4 is correct; and E if all are correct.

----

1. The dorsolateral fasciculus in the spinal cord consists of

    1. long thickly myelinated fibers
    2. fibers for pain and temperature
    3. descending motor fibers
    4. group A and group C fibers   A B C D E

A	B	C	D	E
1,2,3	1,3,	2,4	only 4	all correct

2. Which fibers terminate in the ventral posterior nucleus of the thalamus?

   1. Trigeminothalamic tract
   2. Spinothalamic tract
   3. Medial lemniscus
   4. Fibers from the gustatory and vestibular nuclei

   A B C D E

3. The mesencephalic nucleus of the trigeminal nerve

   1. is concerned with proprioception
   2. receives afferents from cells in the trigeminal ganglion
   3. consists of primary sensory neurons
   4. is situated lateral to the red nucleus

   A B C D E

4. Modalities of general sensation conducted ipsilaterally in the spinal cord include:

   1. Vibration
   2. Two-point touch discrimination
   3. Muscle, joint, and tendon sense
   4. Coolness and warmth

   A B C D E

5. An infarction in the lateral portion of the tegmentum of the midbrain may cause a contralateral sensory deficit for

   1. touch
   2. proprioception
   3. pain
   4. temperature

   A B C D E

6. Correct statements concerning the nucleus of the spinal tract of the trigeminal nerve include:

   1. It is confined to the medulla oblongata
   2. It is so called because it sends fibers to the spinal cord
   3. Axons from the nucleus are distributed through the spinal tract of the trigeminal nerve
   4. It has properties shared with the dorsal gray horn of the spinal cord

   A B C D E

7. Contralateral sensory deficits caused by obstruction of the anterior cerebral artery include:

   1. Proprioception in the leg
   2. Anesthesia in the arm
   3. Touch in the leg
   4. Pain the leg

   A B C D E

ANSWERS, NOTES, AND EXPLANATIONS

1. C 2 and 4 are correct. Dorsal root fibers for pain and temperature are group C fibers (unmyelinated) and thinly myelinated fibers of group A.

They bifurcate on entering the spinal cord and constitute the dorsolateral fasciculus. These fibers terminate in the laminae I, II (mainly), and V of Rexed within the segment of entry or at the most in the adjacent segment.

2. E All are correct. In addition to pathways for the general senses, the ventral posterior thalamic nucleus receives fibers from the gustatory nucleus (rostral portion of the nucleus of the tractus solitarius) and the vestibular nuclei. It is therefore a thalamic relay nucleus to the cerebral cortex for taste and the vestibular system, as well as for the general senses. The ventral posterior nucleus also receives some fibers from the lateral cervical nucleus, situated in the superior two cervical segments of the spinal cord, and extending for a short distance into the medulla. This nucleus is the termination of the spinocervical tract which provides an alternative route for the various general senses.

3. B 1 and 3 are correct. The mesencephalic nucleus of the trigeminal nerve consists of a slender strand of cells in the periaqueductal gray matter of the midbrain, and beneath the rostral end of the floor of the fourth ventricle. They are the cell bodies of primary sensory neurons in an unusual location, i.e., in the central nervous system rather than a ganglion of a spinal or cranial nerve. The single process of these unipolar neurons divides into a peripheral and a central branch. The peripheral branches terminate in proprioceptive endings, including those associated with the muscles of mastication and the temporomandibular joint. The central branches synapse with neurons in the reticular formation, the axons of which join the trigeminothalamic tract or complete the afferent limb of a reflex arc by synapsing with cells in the motor nucleus of the trigeminal nerve.

4. A 1, 2, and 3 are correct. Axons of second order neurons for pain and temperature cross the midline at all levels of the spinal cord to form the spinothalamic tract. In the case of the dorsal column system for proprioception, fine touch, and vibration, the crossing takes place in the decussation of the medial lemniscus in the medulla.

5. E All are correct. The spinal lemniscus, medial lemniscus, and trigeminothalamic tract all traverse the lateral region of the tegmentum of the midbrain. An infarction or other lesion so situated would affect transmission for all modalities of general sensation to the thalamus and cerebral cortex.

6. D Only 4 is correct. The nucleus of the spinal tract of the trigeminal nerve extends throughout the medulla and as far rostrally as the chief sensory nucleus of the trigeminal nerve in the pons. The caudal half of the nucleus of the spinal tract is similar histologically to the substantia gelatinosa and subjacent gray matter of the dorsal horn in the spinal cord. Also, this portion of the nucleus of the spinal tract receives fibers for pain and temperature from the dorsolateral fasciculus. Axons from the trigeminal spinal nucleus make up a large proportion of the trigeminothalamic tract.

7. B 1 and 3 are correct. The anterior cerebral artery supplies the dorsal portion of the somesthetic area of cortex, i.e., the region assigned to the contralateral leg. A lesion so situated results in loss of sensation

192

from the leg, except that pain is still felt in a crude form, as well as extremes of temperature, as a result of neural mechanisms in the dorsal horn of the spinal gray matter. The remainder of the somesthetic area is supplied by the middle cerebral artery.

F I V E - C H O I C E   A S S O C I A T I O N   Q U E S T I O N S

DIRECTIONS: Each of the following groups of questions consists of a numbered list of descriptive words or phrases accompanied by a diagram with certain parts indicated by letters, or by a list of lettered headings. For each numbered word or phrase, SELECT THE LETTERED PART OR HEADING that matches it correctly and insert the letter in the space to the right of the appropriate number. Each lettered heading may be selected once, more than once, or not at all.

A. Nucleus cuneatus
B. Hair follicle plexus
C. Dorsolateral fasciculus
D. Terminus of second order trigeminal fibers
E. Proprioception in lower limbs

1. ____ Ventral posteromedial nucleus of thalamus
2. ____ Light touch
3. ____ Rhomberg test
4. ____ Dorsal portion of medial lemniscus in medulla
5. ____ Pain and temperature
6. ____ Fasciculus gracilis

A. Substantia gelatinosa
B. Spinothalamic tract
C. Mesencephalic nucleus of trigeminal nerve
D. Meissner's corpuscles capsule
E. Posterior limb of internal capsule

7. ____ Light touch and pressure
8. ____ Specific thalamocortical fiber
9. ____ Proprioception
10. ____ Fine touch
11. ____ Lamina II of Rexed
12. ____ Formed by second order sensory neurons

ANSWERS, NOTES, AND EXPLANATIONS

1. D The ventral posteromedial nucleus of the thalamus is the termination of the trigeminothalamic tract. It is concerned with general senses for the opposite side of the head.

2. B The nonencapsulated plexuses surrounding hair follicles are stimulated by the slightest movement of hairs and are exquisitely sensitive sensors for light and simple touch.

3. E The Rhomberg test is performed by asking the patient to stand erect

with the eyes closed; balance is normally maintained because of information reaching the central nervous system from proprioceptors in the lower limbs.

4. A Axons originating in the nucleus cuneatus enter the contralateral medial lemniscus. They are in the dorsal part of the medial lemniscus in the medulla and in the medial part in the pons and midbrain. The remainder of the medial lemniscus consists of axons originating in the contralateral nucleus gracilis, the lateral cervical nucleus, and the nucleus of Z of Brodal and Pompeiano.

5. C The dorsolateral fasciculus consists of short ascending and descending branches of dorsal root fibers for pain and temperature; they soon terminate in laminae I, II (the majority terminate here) and V of Rexed.

6. E Superior to the midthoracic level, axons of primary sensory neurons for proprioception, fine touch, and vibration reach the nucleus cuneatus in the medulla by traversing the fasciculus cuneatus in the lateral area of the dorsal white column of the spinal cord. Proprioception from the lower limb passes through the lower fasciculus gracilis to the nucleus dorsalis, thjen to the nucleus Z of Brodal and Pompeiano via collaterals from the dorsal spinocerebellar tract. From the nucleus of Z fibers enter the medial lemniscus.

7. B The spinothalamic tract conducts light touch and pressure sensations, in addition to the important pain and temperature sensations.

8. E The specific thalamocortical fibers for the general senses traverse the posterior limb of the internal capsule en route to the somesthetic area in the postcentral gyrus of the parietal lobe. Specific thalamocortical fibers for vision and hearing run in the retrolenticular and sublenticular portions of the internal capsule, respectively.

9. C The mesencephalic nucleus of the trigeminal nerve sends fibers to proprioceptors specifically. It is unusual in that it consists of cell bodies of primary sensory neurons which, with this exception, are in the spinal ganglia of spinal nerves and sensory ganglia of cranial nerves.

10. D Meissner's corpuscles, located in dermal papillae, are most numerous in hairless skin. They contribute to one's ability to appreciate that points on the skin are touched separately, even though close together (two-point discrimination).

11. A Lamina II of Rexed is also known as the substantia gelatinosa (of Rolando). It consists of densely packed neurons (gelatinosa cells) having richly branched axons and dendrites.

12. B The spinothalamic tract consists of axons of second order neurons on the pathway for pain, temperature, light touch and pressure. Small neurons often intervene between those with long processes that are designated as primary, secondary, and tertiary neurons in sensory pathways.

194

THIRTEEN

The Recticular Formation

OBJECTIVES

BE ABLE TO:

* Describe the basic nature of the reticular formation of the brain stem.

* Identify the reticular nuclei which: (a) are concerned with cerebellar function exclusively; (b) constitute the lateral or "sensory" portion of the reticular formation; and (c) constitute the medial portion of the reticular formation.

* Discuss the ascending reticular activating system under the following headings: (a) sensory input; (b) projections to the diencephalon and thence to the cerebral cortex; and (c) the role of the activating system in determining the level of consciousness and the degree of alterness and attention.

* Discuss the contribution of the reticular formation to motor and visceral activities.

* Identify certain small nuclei of the brain stem that have a functional relationship with nuclei of the reticular formation proper.

FIVE-CHOICE COMPLETION QUESTIONS

DIRECTIONS: Each of the following questions or incomplete statements is followed by five suggested answers or completions. SELECT THE ONE BEST ANSWER OR COMPLETION in each case and underline the appropriate letter at the right.

----

1. Of the following sensory systems, select the one which does NOT contribute afferents to the reticular formation.

    A. Dorsal column   D. Acoustic
    B. Spinal lemniscal   E. Visual
    C. Olfactory
                                                    A B C D E

SELECT THE ONE BEST ANSWER OR COMPLETION

2. The reticular formation participates in motor functions by means of

   A. its projection to the
      corpus striatum
   B. a projection to area 4 of
      the cerebral cortex

   C. the rubrospinal tract
   D. retriculospinal fibers
   E. the tectospinal tract

   A B C D E

3. Which statement concerning the ascending reticular activating system is <u>correct</u>?

   A. There is an uninterrupted pathway from the reticular for-
      mation of the brain stem to the cerebral cortex
   B. Impulses reaching the reticular formation from general
      sensory receptors have a significant role in determining
      levels of consciousness
   C. The ascending fibers originate in the lateral reticular
      area of the brain stem
   D. Stimulation derived from the special senses is irrelevant
      to the ascending activating system
   E. The reticular formation is included in a sensory pathway
      from receptors to the cerebral cortex which is comparable
      to lemniscal pathways with respect to awareness of sen-
      sory stimuli

   A B C D E

4. The projection from the lateral reticular area is to the

   A. hypothalamus
   B. spinal cord
   C. medial reticular area

   D. cerebral cortex
   E. thalamus

   A B C D E

5. Which source of impulses received by the reticular formation has a special relevance to a person's attention?

   A. Touch receptors
   B. Olfactory system
   C. Receptors in viscera

   D. Proprioceptors
   E. Cerebral cortex

   A B C D E

6. Which of the following thalamic nuclei receives afferents
   directly from the reticular formation?

   A. Ventral posterior
   B. Centromedian
   C. Lateral geniculate

   D. Ventral lateral
   E. Anterior

   A B C D E

ANSWERS, NOTES, AND EXPLANATIONS

1. A Of the sensory systems, only the dorsal column system, i.e., the
   fasciculus gracilis and fasciculus cuneatus, their corresponding nuclei,
   and the medial lemniscus, do not contribute afferents to the reticular
   formation. The senses of discriminative touch, proprioception, and

vibration are therefore not involved. Of the other systems listed, the spinothalamic tract of the spinal lemniscus contributes collateral branches to the lateral reticular area (parvicellular nucleus), olfac-totegmental fibers originating in olfactory cortical areas, nuclei on the central acoustic pathway, and fibers conveying visual data from the superior colliculi end in the central group of nuclei. However, impulses originating from the parietal lobe cortex are first relayed to the parvicellular reticular nuclei.

2. D There are abundant corticoreticular fibers from areas of cortex with motor functions. Reticulospinal fibers originate in the medial reticular area of the brain stem, especially the magnocellular reticular nucleus of the medulla and its extension into the dorsal pons as the caudal pontine reticular nucleus. The corticoreticular and reticulospinal connections, together with corticorubral fibers and the rubrospinal tract, are impor-tant components of the extrapyramidal motor system. The reticulospinal and rubrospinal fibers influence alpha and gamma motor neurons; in fact, the gamma reflex loop is an important aspect of muscular control by means of the extrapyramidal motor system. The reticular formation does not project directly to the corpus striatum, although the latter may be in-fluenced to some extent through a thalamic relay. Any influence on the primary motor cortex is likewise of a secondary nature, and the tecto-spinal tract is involved in visual and acoustic reflex responses.

3. B The reticular formation has an input from all types of sensory recep-tor, except for discriminative touch, proprioception, and vibration. The magnitude of input at any one time determines the level of generalized excitation of the cerebral cortex. The sensory modalities blend during transmission through the polysynaptic pathways of the reticular formation and the additional relays in the thalamus. Detailed awareness of specific sensory information depends on conduction through the lemniscal system. When the cortex is stimulated through the reticular activating system during sleep, the electroencephalogram changes from a synchronized, slow-wave pattern to the desynchronized, fast-wave pattern characteristic of the waking state. The projection to the thalamus, from which impulses are relayed to the cortex, comes from the medial reticular area of the brain stem. Impulses reaching the reticular formation from general sensory endings, especially those for touch, pressure, pain, and temperature, appear to be especially important in maintaining the waking state, whereas those of visual and acoustic origin, and from the cortex itself, are thought to sharpen one's attention to the experience of the moment.

4. C The lateral reticular area consists of the parvicellular reticular nuclei of the medulla and pons, the cuneiform and subcuneiform nuclei in the midbrain (the connections of which are as yet uncertain), and the pedunculopontine nucleus in the midbrain. Long axons of neurons in the central area proceed to the spinal cord, hypothalamus, and thalamus, and impulses are relayed to the cerebral cortex from the thalamus.

5. E Corticoreticular fibers originate in widespread areas of the cerebral cortex. They are considered to supply "psychic" stimuli that help to focus attention on whatever may be of special interest at the time. Visual and acoustic stimuli are also thought to be significant with re-respect to alertness and attention. Proprioceptors do not participate

in the function of the ascending activating sytem, and the other senses listed are involved mainly in its role as a factor determining levels of consciousness or transitions in the sleep-arousal cycle. Impulses of visceral origin reach the central reticular area from the spinal cord via the spinoreticular tract. Other sensory impulses (touch, pain, temperature, etc.) reach the same area by the same spinoreticular tract, where their axons branch profusely before terminating. In addition to spinal input, cranial nerve nuclei (spinal trigeminal nucleus, nucleus of the tractus solitarius, and vestibular nuclei), as well as collateral branches of axons of the auditory system, provide input to the central nuclei. Axons originating in olfactory cortical areas make up the olfactotegmental tract (a continuation from the medial forebrain bundle), and terminate in the central reticular nuclei in the tegmentum of the midbra midbrain.

6. B Most of the long ascending axons from the central reticular area terminate in the intralaminar thalamic nuclei, the largest of which is the centromedian nucleus. These nuclei have few direct cortical connections; however they send many fibers to surrounding nuclei of the thalamus which complete the pathway required for the ascending activating system by projecting to the cerebral cortex. Other ascending axons end in the midline thalamic nucleus and the hypothalamus.

M U L T I - C O M P L E T I O N   Q U E S T I O N S

DIRECTIONS: In each of the following questions or incomplete statements, one or more of the completions given is correct. At the lower right of each question, underline A if 1, 2, and 3 are correct; B if 1 and 3 are correct; C if 2 and 4 are correct; D if only 4 is correct; and E if all are correct.

----

1. Nuclei related functionally to neuronal aggregates designated as reticular nuclei include:

    1. Nuclei pontis
    2. Ventral tegmental nucleus in the midbrain
    3. Superior olivary nucleus in the pons
    4. Locus ceruleus in the pons   A B C D E

2. Certain general anesthetics probably exert their effects in part by suppression of neuronal activity in the

    1. general sensory relay nucleus of the thalamus
    2. cerebral cortex
    3. hippocampus of the limbic system
    4. reticular formation of the brain stem   A B C D E

3. Nuclei concerned exclusively with cerebellar function include:

    1. Paramedian reticular nucleus in the medulla
    2. Mesencephalic reticular nucleus
    3. Lateral reticular nucleus in the medulla
    4. Magnocellular reticular nucleus in the medulla A B C D E

A	B	C	D	E
1,2,3	1,3,	2,4	only 4	all correct

4. Visceral regions (centers) in the reticular formation include:

    1. A cardiovascular pressor area in the lateral area of the medulla
    2. An expiratory center in the lateral area of the medulla
    3. A cardiovascular depressor center in the central area of the medulla
    4. A "pneumotaxic" center in the midbrain   A B C D E

5. Items relevant to the ascending reticular activating system include:

    1. A slow-wave and a fast-wave pattern in the EEG
    2. Ascending fibers from the central reticular area to thalamic nuclei
    3. Depression by some anesthetics and tranquillizers
    4. Psychic stimuli of cortical origin for attention and general sensory stimuli for the sleep-arousal cycle   A B C D E

6. Which nuclei are included in the central reticular area?

    1. Ventral reticular nucleus of the medulla
    2. Pedunculopontine reticular nucleus
    3. Caudal pontine reticular nucleus
    4. Parvicellular reticular nuclei of the medulla and pons   A B C D E

ANSWERS, NOTES, AND EXPLANATIONS

1. C <u>2 and 4 are correct</u>. A ventral tegmental nucleus is present on each side of the midbrain, close to the central gray matter surrounding the cerebral aqueduct. It is considered to be a component of the reticular formation, along with the much larger aggregate of cells composing the pedunculopontine reticular nucleus. The locus ceruleus, at the rostral end of the floor of the fourth ventricle on each side, marks the position of a pontine nucleus, the neurons of which contain melanin pigment. The neurons of this nucleus contain large quantities of norepinephrine which they use as a transmitter substance. These neurons probably exert some rather general effect on the brain as a whole. A "neuromodalatory" action at synapses has also been suggested. The following nuclei are sometimes discussed in the context of the reticular formation, although largely for convenience: the area postrema in the medulla, and in the midbrain the interpeduncular nucleus, dorsal tegmental nucleus, interstitial nucleus of Cajal, nucleus of Darkschewitsch, and nucleus of the posterior commissure. The pontine nuclei (nucleus pontis) in the basal pons are on a pathway connecting a cerebral hemisphere with the opposite cerebellar hemisphere, whereas the superior olivary nucleus is on the acoustic pathway.

199

2. D <u>Only 4 is correct</u>. Cortical stimulation through the ascending reticular activating system is thought to be a major factor, although not necessarily the only one, in maintaining the conscious state. It is therefore not surprising that experimental evidence indicates that some general anesthetics produce unconsciousness by suppressing conduction through the polysynaptic pathways of the reticular formation. During anesthesia, conduction along the sensory lemnisci of the brain stem is unimpeded. The site of action of certain tranquillizing drugs may be the reticular formation.

3. B <u>1 and 3 are correct</u>. The paramedian reticular nucleus, adjacent to the median raphe of the medulla, is part of a feedback circuit involving the cerebellum, with which it has reciprocal connections. The lateral reticular nucleus in the medulla receives spinoreticular fibers, collaterals from the spinal lemniscus, and fibers from the red nucleus. This reticular nucleus sends fibers to the cerebellum via the inferior cerebellar peduncle. The pontine reticulotegmental nucleus is also a precerebellar nucleus, sending sensory data to the vermal and paravermal areas of the cerebellum via the inferior cerebellar peduncle. Fibers of cerebellar origin terminate in the central reticular area of the medulla and pons, for which this is only one of several sources of afferent fibers.

4. A <u>1, 2, and 3 are correct</u>. Electrical stimulation of the reticular formation in experimental animals reveals regions or "centers" in which neurons influence respiratory and cardiovascular functions through connections with neurons supplying the muscles of respiration, and autonomic nuclei for the heart and blood vessels. A "pneumotaxic" center in the dorsal pons controls the respiratory rhythm, and in the medulla there are inspiratory and expiratory centers in the region of the gigantocellular and parvicellular reticular nuclei, respectively. Cardiovascular centers are pressor, with acceleration of heart rate and raising of blood pressure, and depressor with the reverse effects. The pressor effect is obtained by stimulation in the region of the lateral reticular area of the medulla (parvicellular nucleus), and the depressor effect is obtained by stimulation in the region of the ventral and gigantocellular nuclei of the central reticular area of the medulla. Damage to the brain stem is hazardous to life because it contains neurons controlling the vital respiratory and cardiovascular functions.

5. E <u>All are correct</u>. The items listed are part of the evidence for the existence of an ascending activating system based on anatomical, physiological, and pharmacological studies. Anatomical and physiological investigations show the projection from the central area of the reticular formation to the intralaminar nuclei of the thalamus, and through relays in adjacent thalamic nuclei to the cerebral cortex. Similar studies show the corticoreticular connections that influence attention, and the general sensory afferents that are important in the sleep-arousal cycle. Physiological studies demonstrate the EEG changes on cortical stimulation through the activating system. The concept is reinforced by pharmacological investigation of anesthetic and tranquillizing agents; it explains the unconsciousness that results from damage to the brain stem. The sleep-arousal cycle is usually thought of as dependent on the amount of cortical stimulation received through the ascending activating system. However, pharmacological research indicates that there may be a dual

mechanism, in that induction of sleep may be an active, as well as a passive process.

6. B <u>1 and 3 are correct.</u> The parvicellular reticular nuclei of the medulla and pons comprise the lateral reticular area, also known as the sensory or association area. The lateral area sends axons to the central area which has afferents from additional sources and projects to the spinal cord and diencephalon. The central reticular area consists of the ventral reticular and gigantocellular reticular nuclei of the medulla, and the caudal and oral (rostral) pontine reticular nuclei. An appreciation of the histology of the lateral and central reticular areas is made difficult by the diffuse arrangement of the neurons, so that the constituent nuclei can be identified only by laborious research studies.

F I V E - C H O I C E   A S S O C I A T I O N   Q U E S T I O N S

DIRECTIONS: Each of the following groups of questions consists of a numbered list of descriptive words or phrases accompanied by a diagram with certain parts indicated by letters, or by a list of lettered headings. For each numbered word or phrase, SELECT THE LETTERED PART OR HEADING that matches it correctly and insert the letter in the space to the right of the appropriate number. <u>Each lettered heading may be selected once, more than once, or not at all.</u>

----

1. ____ Receives many fibers from the reticular formation

A. Reticulospinal fibers
B. Locus ceruleus
C. Gigantocellular reticular nucleus
D. Centromedian thalamic nucleus
E. Lateral reticular nucleus of medulla

2. ____ Supplements the pyramidal motor pathway
3. ____ Concerned exclusively with cerebellar function
4. ____ A component of the central area of the reticular formation
5. ____ Situated immediately beneath the rostral end of the floor of the fourth ventricle
6. ____ Receives numerous afferents from the lateral reticular area

7. ____ Receives olfactory impulses
8. ____ Lateral reticular area
9. ____ Rostral extension of the reticular formation

A. Zona incerta
B. Fast-wave EEG pattern
C. Mesencephalic reticular formation
D. Polysynaptic conduction
E. Parvicellular reticular nuclei

10. ____ Characteristic of transmission in the reticular formation
11. ____ Cortical stimulation by ascending activating system
12. ____ Located in the lateral region of the medulla and dorsal pons

ANSWERS, NOTES, AND EXPLANATIONS

1. D   The centromedian nucleus is the largest of the intralaminar nuclei of the thalamus. These nuclei are partially surrounded by a thin internal medullary lamina of white matter which divides the thalamus into three major nuclear groups. Fibers from the central reticular area of the brain stem terminate in the intralaminar thalamic nuclei. These nuclei project to surrounding thalamic nuclei, from which fibers proceed to widespread areas of the cerebral cortex. The foregoing connections complete the pathway for the ascending activating system and its effect on the sleep-arousal cycle and on alertness and attention. Axons from the central reticular area also terminate in the small midline nucleus of the thalamus and the hypothalamus. These connections are concerned with visceral and emotional responses on sensory stimuli reaching higher centers by way of the reticular formation.

2. A   Voluntary control of the musculature is exercised by the pyramidal motor system, consisting of the corticospinal and corticobulbar tracts, and by the extrapyramidal motor system. Corticorubral fibers and the rubrospinal tract, and corticoreticular and reticulospinal fibers, are important components of the extrapyramidal system. Reticulospinal fibers originate in the central reticular area, notably the gigantocellular nucleus in the medulla and its counterpart in the dorsal pons, the caudal pontine nucleus. The fibers descend in the ventral and lateral white columns of the spinal cord and the impulses thus conveyed influence alpha and gamma motor neurons.

3. E   The lateral reticular nucleus is situated near the lateral surface of the medulla, between the inferior olivary nucleus and the nucleus of the spinal trigeminal tract, and at the level of the caudal half of the inferior olivary nucleus. It is the only reticular nucleus that is sufficiently compact and discrete to be identifiable readily in sections. The principal afferents for the lateral reticular nucleus are spinoreticular fibers, collateral branches of fibers in the spinal lemniscus, and the red nucleus. Efferent fibers enter the cerebellum by way of the inferior cerebellar peduncle. (The lateral reticular nucleus is not to be confused with the lateral reticular area, composed of the parvicellular reticular nuclei of the medulla and pons.) Like the lateral reticular nucleus, the paramedian reticular nucleus of the medulla and the pontine reticulotegmental nucleus are concerned with cerebellar function. They are on a feed-back circuit based on reciprocal cerebellar connections. Regions of the central reticular area giving rise to reticulospinal fibers have afferents from the cerebellum, but they receive fibers from other sources as well.

4. C   The central area of the reticular formation consists of the ventral and gigantocellular reticular nuclei in the medulla and the caudal and oral (rostral) reticular nuclei in the dorsal pons. The central reticular area has afferents from diverse sources and efferents enter the diencephalon and spinal cord.

5. B   The locus ceruleus is a small dark area on each side of the rostral end of the fourth ventricle, marking the position of neurons containing melanin pigment. The locus ceruleus is thought to have a role in the

ascending activating system, and may act as a "neuromodulator" at synapses.

6. C The lateral reticular area, consisting of the parvicellular nuclei of the medulla and pons, receives sensory data from diverse sources. It is referred to as the sensory or association part of the reticular formation. It sends fibers to the central reticular area, which includes the gigantocellular nucleus of the medulla.

7. C Like other special senses, the olfactory system contributes afferents to the reticular formation and thereby has an influence on the ascending activating system. The fibers in question originate in olfactory cortical areas and are included in the medial forebrain bundle which traverses the lateral part of the hypothalamus. They continue as olfactotegmental fibers and terminate in the mesencephalic reticular formation.

8. E The lateral reticular area consists of the parvicellular nuclei in the medulla and pons. It is the recipient of cortical fibers from the parietal lobe and fibers conveying general and special sensory data. It projects to the medial reticular area.

9. A The zona incerta is a small region of gray matter in the subthalamus, bounded by the lenticular and thalamic fasciculi. It is continuous with the mesencephalic reticular formation in the tegmentum of the midbrain and an extension of the reticular formation into the diencephalon.

10. D Although long axons extend from the central area of the reticular formation to the diencephalon and spinal cord, these axons have many collateral branches which establish synaptic contact with neurons of the reticular formation. There is therefore much interaction between neurons and polysynaptic transmission of nerve impulses.

11. B Stimulation of cortical neurons through the ascending activating system in a state of sleep or drowsiness changes the slow-wave, synchronized pattern of the EEG to the fast-wave, desynchronized pattern of the waking and alert state. There is some pharmacological evidence of a dual process, in which the slow-wave pattern may be the result of an active, as well as a passive, process.

12. E The parvicellular nuclei of the medulla and pons consist of small neurons and along, with the midbrain reticular nuclei (cuneiform, subcuneiform, and pedunculopontine nuclei), compose the lateral area of the reticular formation. In the medulla, the parvicellular nucleus extends from the midolivary level to the rostral limit of the medulla, in the area beneath the vestibular nuclear complex, and rostrally as the parvicellular nucleus of the pons, which is situated in an area dorsal to the motor nucleus of the facial nerve and medial to the nucleus of the trigeminal spinal tract.

The Motor Systems

O B J E C T I V E S

BE ABLE TO:

*   Define the terms pyramidal system and extrapyramidal system.

*   Describe the origin, course, and termination of the corticobulbar and corticospinal tracts.

*   Discuss the main connections of the corpus striatum, subthalamic nucleus, and substantia nigra.

*   Describe how the red nucleus and the reticular formation of the brain stem participate in extrapyramidal motor pathways.

*   Distinguish between an upper motor neuron lesion and a lower motor neuron lesion.

*   Discuss briefly the motor disturbances resulting from lesions involving the corpus striatum, subthalamic nucleus, and substantia nigra.

F I V E - C H O I C E   C O M P L E T I O N   Q U E S T I O N S

DIRECTIONS: Each of the following questions or incomplete statements is followed by five suggested answers or completions. SELECT THE ONE BEST ANSWER OR COMPLETION in each case and underline the appropriate letter at the right.

----

1. The signs of a lower motor neuron lesion include:

    A. Spastic paralysis
    B. Diminished or absent tendon reflexes
    C. The sign of Babinski
    D. Slight atrophy of affected muscles
    E. All of the above   A B C D E

SELECT THE ONE BEST ANSWER OR COMPLETION

2. Which statement concerning the cell bodies of upper motor neurons is <u>correct</u>?

   A. All are situated in the cortex of the frontal and parietal lobes
   B. They include a significant number of cells in the globus pallidus
   C. They are in subcortical centers as well as in the cerebral cortex
   D. They are in the motor nuclei of cranial nerves
   E. They are restricted to motor areas of the frontal lobe   A B C D E

3. The corticospinal tract traverses the

   A. posterior limb of the internal capsule, the basis pedun-culi of the midbrain, and the pyramid of the medulla
   B. corona radiata, the dorsal pons, and the pyramid of the medulla
   C. genu of the internal capsule, the middle three-fifths of the basis pedunculi of the midbrain, and the basal portion of the pons
   D. Corona radiata, the tegmentum of the midbrain, and the basal portion of the pons
   E. Anterior limb of the internal capsule, the basal portion of the pons and the pyramid of the medulla   A B C D E

4. Athetoid movements are

   A. brisk and jerky
   B. an intention tremor
   C. referred to as "pill-rolling" movements
   D. sudden, gross, and flailing
   E. slow and sinuous   A B C D E

5. Corticobulbar fibers do NOT end in the

   A. motor nucleus of the facial nerve
   B. dorsal nucleus of the vagus nerve
   C. reticular formation
   D. abducens nucleus
   E. hypoglossal nucleus   A B C D E

6. The red nucleus is a relay station on a pathway between the

   A. dentate nucleus of the cerebellum and the lateral ventral nucleus of the thalamus
   B. globus pallidus and lower motor neurons
   C. substantia nigra and the thalamus
   D. cerebral cortex and lower motor neurons
   E. vestibular nuclei and ventral horn cells in the spinal cord

                               A B C D E

SELECT THE ONE BEST ANSWER OR COMPLETION

7. Which statement concerning the substantia nigra is <u>correct</u>?

   A. Its principal connections are with the red nucleus and
      the reticular formation
   B. It has neither direct nor indirect connections with the
      cerebral cortex
   C. Some of its efferent fibers terminate in the corpus striatum
   D. Certain constituent cells synthesize melanin which acts as a
      neurotransmitter substance
   E. Choreiform movements result from degeneration of its
      neurons   A B C D E

8. Which statement concerning the corticospinal tract is NOT
   correct?

   A. Its cells of origin are in the motor and premotor areas
      of the frontal lobe and in the general sensory area and
      the cortex posterior to it in the parietal lobe
   B. It traverses the posterior part of the posterior limb of
      the internal capsule
   C. About 85 percent of its fibers cross the midline in the
      decussation of the pyramids at the junction of the medulla
      and the spinal cord
   D. Most of its fibers are of large diameter because they are
      axons of giant pyramidal cells
   E. Impulses conveyed by most of its fibers reach lower motor
      neurons through small intercalated neurons   A B C D E

9. Fibers originating in the globus pallidus terminate mainly
   in the

   A. substania nigra
   B. ventral posteromedial and ventral posterolateral
      thalamic nuclei
   C. red nucleus and the reticular formation
   D. motor cortex of the frontal lobe
   E. ventral anterior and ventral lateral thalamic nuclei   A B C D E

10. Corticospinal fibers are interrupted in a lesion involving the

   A. basal or ventral pons
   B. genu of the internal capsule
   C. medulla dorsal to the inferior olivary nucleus
   D. dorsal portion of the pons
   E. tegmentum of the midbrain   A B C D E

ANSWERS, NOTES, AND EXPLANATIONS

1. B In addition to diminished or absent tendon reflexes, the signs of a
   lower motor neuron lesion include flaccid paralysis, decreased resistance

to passive movement, and progressive atrophy of the affected muscles. The other signs listed are characteristic of an upper motor neuron lesion that interrupts pyramidal and extrapyramidal pathways.

2. C Cell bodies of upper motor neurons are located in the cortex of the frontal and parietal lobes. Other cells located in subcortical nuclei give rise to the following fiber systems: rubrospinal tract, reticulospinal fibers, vestibulospinal tract, medial longitudinal fasciculus, tectospinal tract, and small descending fasciculi of minor importance.

3. A The corticospinal tract originates in the dorsal two-thirds of the precentral gyrus on the dorsolateral surface of the frontal lobe, the anterior part of the paracentral lobule on the medial aspect of the frontal lobe, and in adjoining areas of the frontal and parietal lobes. The corticospinal tract traverses the internal capsule well posterior to the genu, the middle three-fifths of the basis pedunculi in the midbrain, the basal portion of the pons, and the pyramid in the medulla. About 85 percent of the fibers then cross the midline to form the lateral corticospinal tract in the spinal cord; a few fibers enter the lateral corticospinal tract of the same side, and the remainder form the uncrossed ventral corticospinal tract.

4. E Each of the dyskinesias has a characteristic type of involuntary, purposeless movement. Athetoid and choreiform movements are associated with lesions involving the corpus striatum; the former being slow and sinuous, the latter brisk and jerky. Intention tremor, occurring at the end of a voluntary movement, is a sign of cerebellar dysfunction. The characteristic tremor of the fingers and thumb, as seen in paralysis agitans (Parkinson's disease), which results from neuronal degeneration in the substantia nigra, is referred to as the "pill-rolling" movement. The involuntary movements are sudden, gross, and flailing in hemiballismus, caused by a lesion in the subthalamic nucleus.

5. B Most corticobulbar fibers end in the reticular formation near the motor trigeminal nucleus, the motor facial nucleus, the nucleus ambiguus, and the hypoglossal nucleus. Several fibers make direct synaptic contacts with these cranial motor neurons. The dorsal nucleus of the vagus nerve is thereby excluded; it supplies smooth (but not cardiac muscle) and glandular cells of thoracic and abdominal viscera. The most important afferents to this nucleus originate in the hypothalamus, olfactory system, autonomic centers in the reticular formation, and the nucleus of the tractus solitarius.

6. D Corticorubral and rubrospinal fibers constitute a pathway of the extrapyramidal motor system. Fibers from the dentate nucleus of the cerebellum pass through and around the red nucleus en route to the ventral lateral nucleus of the thalamus. A pallidorubral connection is no longer thought to exist. Fibers pass directly from the substantia nigra to the ventral anterior and ventral lateral thalamic nuclei, as do fibers from vestibular nuclei to ventral horn cells in the spinal cord.

7. C The projection from the substantia nigra to the corpus striatum is of considerable physiological and clinical importance. Melanin-containing cells in the substantia nigra synthesize dopamine, which acts as a neurotransmitter substance at synapses in the neostriatum especially. L-dopa,

a metabolic precursor of dopamine, is used in the therapy of paralysis agitans because dopamine does not cross the blood-brain barrier. Some fibers from the substantia nigra end in the ventral anterior and ventral lateral thalamic nuclei, which in turn send fibers to motor areas of the cerebral cortex. Other fibers end in the amygdaloid body and superior colliculus of the midbrain. The main afferents to the substantia nigra arise from the caudate and lentiform nuclei; smaller numbers are from the subthalamic nucleus and the raphe nuclei of the midbrain and the pontine reticular formation. Choreiform movements are associated with neuronal degeneration in the corpus striatum, rather than in the substantia nigra.

8. D Only 3 percent of corticospinal fibers are of large diameter. They correspond numerically to the giant pyramidal or Betz cells in the part of the primary motor area (area 4 of Brodmann) from which corticospinal fibers originate. They are throught, therefore, to be axons of Betz cells, constituting a small proportion of rapidly conducting fibers in the corticospinal tract.

9. E Efferent fibers of the globus pallidus compose the lenticular fasciculus and the ansa lenticularis. Almost all the fibers terminate in the ventral anterior and ventral lateral nuclei of the thalamus, which in turn send fibers to motor areas of cortex in the frontal lobe. A few fibers from the globus pallidus end in a minor nucleus in the brain stem; this descending projection appears to be too small to be of appreciable functional significance.

10. A After traversing the posterior limb of the internal capsule, the corticospinal tract is situated in the ventral region of the brain stem. It traverses the basis pedunculi (crus cerebri) in the midbrain, the basal or ventral portion of pons, and the pyramid in the medulla.

M U L T I - C O M P L E T I O N   Q U E S T I O N S

DIRECTIONS: In each of the following questions or incomplete statements, one or more of the completions given is correct. At the lower right of each question, underline A if 1, 2, and 3 are correct; B if 1 and 3 are correct; C if 2 and 4 are correct; D if only 4 is correct; and E if all are correct.

----

1. An infarction in the posterior limb of the internal capsule could interrupt

    1. corticorubral fibers   3. corticospinal fibers
    2. thalamocortical fibers   4. corticoreticular fibers   A B C D E

2. The neotriatum is also referred to as the

    1. pallidum
    2. putamen and caudate nucleus
    3. lentiform nucleus
    4. striatum   A B C D E

	A	B	C	D	E
	1,2,3	1,3,	2,4	only 4	all correct

3. Which of the following receive fibers from the substantia
    nigra?

    1. Thalamus   3. Striatum
    2. Dentate nucleus   4. Lower motor neurons   A B C D E

4. The major connections of the subthalamic nucleus are with the

    1. red nucleus   3. thalamus
    2. reticular formation 4. globus pallidus   A B C D E

5. Which of the following influence spinal motor neurons either
    directly or with the intervention of small intercalcated
    neurons?

    1. Vestibular nuclei   3. Red nucleus
    2. Reticular formation 4. Corpus striatum   A B C D E

6. Lesions involving the corpus striatum are associated with

    1. Wilson's disease
    2. athetosis
    3. dystonia musculorum deformans
    4. chorea   A B C D E

7. Correct statements concerning the corticobulbar tract include:

    1. The most noticeable effect of interruption of the tract is
        voluntary paralysis of the contralateral lower facial muscles
    2. It originates in the inferior one-third of the primary motor
        area and the adjacent cortex
    3. It influences lower motor neurons associated with cranial
        nerves V, VII, IX, X, XI, and XII
    4. All its fibers cross the midline in the brain stem and end
        in motor nuclei of cranial nerves on the side opposite the
        hemisphere of origin   A B C D E

8. Which of the following signs occur ipsilaterally as a result of
    a lesion interrupting nerve fibers in the dorsal half of the
    lateral white column of the spinal cord?

    1. Flaccid paralysis
    2. Exaggerated tendon reflexes
    3. Progressive wasting of muscles
    4. Sign of Babinski   A B C D E

9. The main afferents to the paleostriatum are from the

    1. subthalamic nucleus 3. neostriatum
    2. thalamus   4. red nucleus
                                                           A B C D E

A	B	C	D	E
1,2,3	1,3,	2,4	only 4	all correct

10. Voluntary motor paralysis of the leg results from thrombosis involving the

    1. posterior cerebral artery
    2. posterior inferior cerebellar artery
    3. middle cerebral artery
    4. anterior cerebellar artery   A B C D E

ANSWERS, NOTES, AND EXPLANATIONS

1. E <u>All are correct</u>. Interruption of corticospinal, corticorubral, and corticoreticular fibers in the internal capsule results in signs of an upper motor lesion on the opposite side of the body, i.e., voluntary motor paralysis, hyperactive tendon reflexes, and the sign of Babinski. Interruption of thalamocortical fibers destined for the postcentral gyrus causes loss of general sensation on the opposite side of the body, with the exception that pain is still felt in a crude form.

2. C <u>2 and 4 are correct</u>. The corpus striatum consists of the lentiform nucleus and the caudate nucleus, the former being made up of the globus pallidus and putamen. The globus pallidus or pallidum is the paleostriatum, and the putamen and caudate nucleus compose the neostriatum or striatum.

3. B <u>1 and 3 are correct</u>. Fibers from the substantia nigra end in the ventral anterior and ventral lateral nuclei of the thalamus, and fibers from these nuclei project to motor areas of the cerebral cortex. The projection from the substantia nigra to the corpus striatum is especially important because degeneration of these neurons causes paralysis agitans, or Parkinson's disease. The substantia nigra has reciprocal connections with the red nucleus and reticular formation, but it does not send fibers to the cerebellum or to lower motor neurons.

4. D <u>Only 4 is correct</u>. The subthalamic fasciculus, running across the internal capsule, establishes reciprocal connections between the subthalamic nucleus and the globus pallidus of the lentiform nucleus. The subthalamic nucleus probably has other connections, but they are not well known.

5. A <u>1, 2, and 3 are correct</u>. Almost all efferent fibers from the globus pallidus of the corpus striatum travel to the ventral anterior and ventral lateral nuclei of the thalamus through two fasciculi, the lenticular fasciculus and the ansa lenticularis. There are only a very few descending fibers from the globus pallidus; these terminate in a small nucleus called the pedunculopontine nucleus, situated in the tegmentum of the brain stem at the junction of the midbrain and pons. In addition to the vestibulospinal, reticulospinal, and rubrospinal fibers mentioned, spinal motor neurons come under the control of corticospinal or pyramidal fibers. Still others include the tectospinal tract and two minor fasciculi, one originating in small nuclei in the midbrain and the other

in the nucleus of the tractus solitarius. The descending fibers influence both alhpa and gamma motorneurons. The gamma reflex loop is especially important with respect to components of the extrapyramidal motor system. Small intercalated neurons in the gray matter of the spinal cord frequently intervene between upper and lower motor neurons; this is almost the rule for corticospinal fibers.

6. E All are correct. Several dyskinesias are associated with pathological changes in the corpus striatum. The differences depend on the precise location of the lesion, its size, whether other parts of the brain are involved as well, and no doubt on other factors that are as yet poorly understood. In each instance the movements are involuntary and purposeless. Athetoid movements are slow and sinuous, involving the distal limb musculature especially, whereas choreiform movements are brisk and jerky, and involve the axial and proximal limb musculature preferentially. In Wilson's disease, there is spasticity and tremor; it is caused by a genetic error in copper metabolism and is also known as hepatolenticular degeneration because of concurrent cirrhosis of the liver. Dystonia musculorum deformans is a particularly disabling disorder because the involuntary athetoid movements are sustained, which leads to contracture of muscles.

7. A 1, 2, and 3 are correct. Corticobulbar fibers project to cranial nerve nuclei, except those cranial nuclei associated with extraocular muscles (III, IV, and VI) and the special sensory nerves (I, II, and VIII). In addition to the predominant contralateral cortical control of muscles of the head, there is significant ipsilateral control. The ventral half of the motor nucleus of the facial nerve receives only corticobulbar fibers from the opposite hemisphere, whereas the dorsal half of this nucleus receives corticobulbar fibers from the ipsilateral cortex as well as the contralateral cortex. As a result of an upper motor neuron lesion, therefore, the voluntary motor paralysis is most evident in the inferior facial muscles on the side opposite the lesion. The superior facial muscles are not significantly affected.

8. C 2 and 4 are correct. A lesion in the dorsal half of the lateral white column interrupts pyramidal fibers (the lateral corticospinal tract) and extrapyramidal fibers (the rubrospinal tract and some reticulospinal fibers). The resulting signs are therefore those of an upper motor lesion. Inferior to the level of the lesion, these are: spastic paralysis, exaggerated tendon reflexes, and a sign of Babinski (upturning of the great toe and spreading of toes on stroking the sole). Flaccid paralysis and progressive wasting of muscles are signs of a lower motor neuron lesion.

9. B 1 and 3 are correct. The paleostriatum or globus pallidus has reciprocal connections with the subthalamic nucleus by means of the subthalamic fasciculus. The subthalamic nucleus appears to have an inhibitory influence on the globus pallidus, as evidenced by the involuntary movements known as hemiballismus that occur when the subthalamic nucleus is involved in a lesion. By far the largest source of afferents to the paleostriatum is the neostriatum, i.e., the putamen and caudate nucleus. Corticopallidal and nigropallidal fibers have been described, but they are unimportant compared with fibers from the cerebral cortex and substantia nigra to the neostriatum.

10. D **Only 4 is correct.** The anterior cerebral artery supplies the superior portion of the motor area of the cerebral cortex, which is assigned to the contralateral leg. The remainder of the motor area is supplied by the middle cerebral artery. Thrombosis of the posterior cerebral artery is associated primarily with loss of vision in the contralateral visual field. Branches of the posterior inferior cerebellar artery supply the lateral area of the medulla, some distance from the pyramid.

F I V E - C H O I C E   A S S O C I A T I O N   Q U E S T I O N S

DIRECTIONS: Each of the following groups of questions consists of a numbered list of descriptive words or phrases accompanied by a diagram with certain parts indicated by letters, or by a list of lettered headings. For each numbered word or phrase, SELECT THE LETTERED PART OR HEADING that matches it correctly and insert the letter in the space to the right of the appropriate number. Each lettered heading may be selected once, more than once, or not at all.

A. Lenticular fasciculus
B. Hemiballismus
C. Corticospinal tract
D. Increased muscle tonicity
E. Corticostriate fibers

1. ____ Subthalamic nucleus
2. ____ Terminates in the putamen
3. ____ Controls independent use of the digits
4. ____ Globus pallidus
5. ____ Seen in an upper motor neuron lesion
6. ____ Traverses the subthalamus

A. Diminished tendon reflexes
B. Substantia nigra
C. Rubrospinal tract
D. Decussation of pyramids
E. Corticobulbar tract

7. ____ An extrapyramidal pathway
8. ____ Lower motor neuron lesion
9. ____ Paralysis agitans
10. ____ Motor nuclei of some cranial nerves
11. ____ Functionally related to the corpus striatum
12. ____ Corticospinal tract

ANSWERS, NOTES, AND EXPLANATIONS

1. B A lesion in the subthalamic nucleus results in hemiballismus, characterized by rapid, flailing movements involving muscles of the opposite side of the body.

2. E Corticostriate fibers originate in widespread areas of the cerebral cortex. They enter the putamen and caudate nucleus from the internal capsule, and the putamen from the external capsule. There are a few corticopallidal fibers as well.

3. C Both pyramidal and extrapyramidal pathways are responsible for voluntary motor action. The corticospinal tract is considered to confer speed and agility and to control such fine, nonstereotyped movements as individual use of the digits.

4. A Efferent fibers from the globus pallidus are contained in two fasciculi, the lenticular fasciculus and the ansa lenticularis. Almost all these fibers terminate in the ventral anterior and ventral lateral nuclei of the thalamus, from which fibers proceed to motor areas of cortex in the frontal lobe.

5. D The signs of an upper motor neuron lesion are produced by interruption of both pyramidal and extrapyramidal pathways. The tone of the muscles is increased. This phenomenon, known as spasticity, results from the continuous occurrence of the stretch reflex, which is normally suppressed by the activity of the descending tracts.

6. A The lenticular fasciculus passes medially from the globus pallidus; its fibers intersect the longitudinally running fibers of the internal capsule and traverse the subthalamus en route to the ventral anterior and ventral lateral nauclei of the thalamus.

7. C The red nucleus receives fibers from motor areas of cortex in the frontal lobe. The rubrospinal tract is therefore a component of an extrapyramidal pathway from the cortex to motor neurons in the spinal cord.

8. A The monosynaptic reflex arc for deep reflexes is interrupted in a lower motor neuron lesion; tendon reflexes that depend on the affected neurons are therefore diminished or absent.

9. B Paralysis agitans or Parkinson's disease is caused by degeneration of neurons projecting from the substantia nigra to the corpus striatum. Dopamine synthesized by these neurons is the neurotransmitter substance at their axon terminals and L-dopa, a metabolic precursor of dopamine, is used as a therapeutic agent in paralysis agitans.

10. E The corticobulbar tract is an important source of afferent fibers for motor nuclei of cranial nerves. Although control of muscles thus supplied is predominantly by the contralateral cortex, there is ipsilateral control as well, except for the inferior facial muscles. Paralysis of these muscles on the side opposite a lesion is therefore a prominent sign following interruption of the corticobulbar tract.

11. B Although physiological aspects of the projection from the substantia nigra to the corpus striatum are poorly understood, they are presumed to be important because of the disturbances of motor function resulting from degeneration of neurons in the substantia nigra.

12. D About 85 percent of the fibers of the corticospinal tract cross to the opposite side in the decussation of the pyramids and continue as the lateral corticospinal tract. The remainder constitute the uncrossed ventral corticospinal tract, except for a few that continue into the lateral corticospinal tract of the same side.

213

FIFTEEN

The Visual System

O B J E C T I V E S

BE ABLE TO:

* Discuss early development of the retina and the optic nerve.

* Describe and make a schematic drawing representing the four basic cellular layers of the retina.

* Explain binocular vision with the use of a diagram that shows projections from different parts of the retina on the lateral geniculate nucleus and the visual cortex.

* Discuss visual field representation in the retina, the lateral geniculate nucleus, and the visual cortex.

* State the blood supply to the retina, the optic chiasma and optic tract, the lateral geniculate body, and the visual cortex.

* Illustrate the visual pathway.

* Describe the pupillary light reflex and the accommodation reflex.

* Discuss the reflex or automatic responses to visual stimuli.

* Describe visual defects caused by interruptions in the visual pathway.

F I V E - C H O I C E   C O M P L E T I O N   Q U E S T I O N S

DIRECTIONS: Each of the following questions or incomplete statements is followed by five suggested answers or completions. SELECT THE ONE BEST ANSWER OR COMPLETION in each case and underline the appropriate letter at the right.

----

1. Visual impulses reaching the superior colliculus are concerned with

   A. reflex responses in the head   D. two of the above
   B. the accommodation reflex   E. all of the above
   C. the pupillary light reflex   A B C D E

SELECT THE ONE BEST ANSWER OR COMPLETION

2. Which combination of cells is best related to the neural layer of the retina?

   A. Pigmented epithelial, photoreceptor, ganglion
   B. Neuroglial, bipolar, pigmented epithelial
   C. Pigmented epithelial, neuroglial, ganglion
   D. Photoreceptor, association neurons, bipolar
   E. Ganglion, bipolar, photoreceptor, pigmented
      epithelial   A B C D E

3. Which statement about the retina is <u>correct</u>?

   A. The macula lutea is a depression in the fovea centralis
   B. The optic disc is the blind spot of the eye
   C. The functional retina terminates at the ora serrata
   D. The macula lutea is specialized for acuity of vision
   E. Rod cells and a capillary network are lacking in the
      center of the fovea   A B C D E

4. With respect to the visual field, which of the following statements is <u>correct</u>?

   A. The superior half of the field of vision is represented in
      in the lateral portion of the lateral geniculate nucleus
   B. The superior half of the field of vision is represented
      in the cortex of the lower lip of the calcarine sulcus
   C. The inferior half of the visual field is projected on the
      posterior portion of the lateral geniculate nucleus
   D. Two of the above
   E. All of the above   A B C D E

5. Which statement concerning the visual system is <u>false</u>?

   A. Fibers from the nasal half of each retina decussate in the
      optic chiasma
   B. Impulses conducted to the left hemisphere by the left optic
      tract are concerned with the left half of the field of vision
   C. Each optic nerve in the human is composed of about 1 million
      fibers
   D. The medial portion of the lateral geniculate body relays
      impulses from the inferior field of vision to the superior
      lip of the calcarine sulcus
   E. The optic tract winds around the rostral end of the cere-
      bral peduncle and ends at the lateral geniculate nucleus   A B C D E

6. Ablation of cortex around the left calcarine sulcus results in

   A. Blindness in the upper right visual field
   B. Blindness in the lower left visual field
   C. Blindness in the lower right visual field
   D. Two of the above
   E. All of the above   A B C D E

215

SELECT THE ONE BEST ANSWER OR COMPLETION

7. Which of the following statements concerning the lateral geniculate nucleus is <u>incorrect</u>?

    A. It produces a swelling inferior to the posterior projection of the pulvinar
    B. It is the site of termination of all optic nerve fibers
    C. It consists of six layers
    D. It receives fibers from both retinae
    E. Fibers from it terminate in the cortex adjacent to the calcarine sulcus   A B C D E

8. Which of the following statements about the accommodation reflex is <u>incorrect</u>?

    A. It includes ocular convergence and pupillary constriction
    B. Contraction of the ciliary muscle allows the lens to thicken
    C. Impulses from the visual association cortex reach the superior colliculus via the inferior brachium
    D. Synaptic relay of impulses is from the superior colliculus to the Edinger-Westphal nucleus, and then to the ciliary ganglion
    E. Impulses may pass from the motor cortex to the oculomotor nucleus via the corticobulbar tract   A B C D E

9. Which statement concerning the geniculocalcarine tract is <u>correct</u>?

    A. It takes the shortest possible route from the lateral geniculate nucleus to the visual cortex
    B. It traverses the retrolentiform and sublentiform parts of the posterior limb of the internal capsule
    C. Fibers constituting Meyer's loop terminate in the cortex inferior to the calcarine sulcus
    D. Two of the above
    E. All of the above   A B C D E

10. In the retina, which of the following statements concerning cone cells is <u>correct</u>?

    A. They are responsible for color vision
    B. They have a special role in peripheral vision
    C. They play a special role in discriminative and central vision
    D. Two of the above
    E. All of the above   A B C D E

ANSWERS, NOTES, AND EXPLANATIONS

1. D In the accommodation reflex, corticotectal connections are significant

216

in ocular responses to near objects; these consist of convergence of the eyes, thickening of the lens, and pupillary constriction. The pathway for the accommodation reflex includes corticotectal fibers from the visual association cortex traversing the superior brachium to reach the superior colliculus. Impulses are relayed to the Edinger-Westphal nucleus, the ciliary ganglion, and the ciliary and spincter pupillae muscles. Impulses reaching the superior colliculus directly from the retina are concerned with reflex responses through tectobulbar and tectospinal connections that allow turning of the eyes and head toward the source of a visual stimulus. If the stimulus is sudden and strong, in addition to the above movements, the eyelids may close and the arms may be raised as protection against an approaching object. For the pupillary light reflex, visual impulses from the retina impinge on the pretectal area, and are relayed to the Edinger-Westphal nucleus of the oculomotor complex, then to the ciliary ganglion in the orbit, and finally to the sphincter pupillae muscles in the iris. The pathways are separate for the light and accommodation reflexes, as indicated by the fact that they may be disassociated by disease processes. In syphilitic involvement of the central nervous system, for example, the light reflex may be abolished and the accommodation reflex retained. This is called the Argyll-Robertson pupil.

2. D The retina develops from the optic cup which consists of two separate layers in the embryo. The outer layer becomes the pigmented epithelium and the inner layer differentiates into the complex neural layer. The neural layer consists of the following cells: photorecptors (rod cells and cone cells), bipolar neurons, ganglion cells, association neurons (horizontal cells, interplexiform cells, and amacrine cells), and neuroglial cells.

3. A The macula lutea, the central area posteriorly in line with the visual axis, is a specialized region of the retina, abutting on the lateral edge of the optic disc. The fovea (or fovea centralis) is a depression in the center of the macula. Visual acuity is greatest at the fovea, the center of which contains only cone receptor cells. The retinal capillary network is absent in the center of the fovea. This visible fovea centralis is frequently referred to as the "macula" in opthalmoscopic examinations of the retina.

4. D There is a precise point-to-point projection from the retina to the lateral geniculate nucleus, and from this nucleus to the visual cortex in the occipital lobe. Fibers from the inferior retinal quadrants (representing the superior visual field) terminate in the lateral part of the lateral geniculate nucleus, and impulses are relayed to the anterior two-thirds of the visual cortex inferior to the calcarine sulcus. Fibers from the superior retinal quadrants (representing the inferior visual field) terminate in the medial part of the lateral geniculate nucleus, and impulses are relayed to the anterior two-thirds of the visual cortex superior to the calcarine sulcus. The macula projects to a relatively large posterior region of the lateral geniculate nucleus, which in turn sends fibers to the posterior one-third of the visual cortex in the region of the occipital pole.

5. B Fibers from the nasal or medial half of the right retina are concerned with the right half of the field of vision. They cross to the opposite side in the optic chiasma and join uncrossed fibers from the temporal or

lateral half of the left retina, which are concerned with the right half of the field of vision. The resulting left optic tract proceeds to the left lateral geniculate nucleus, which in turn projects to the left visual cortex. Therefore, impulses conducted to the left hemisphere are for the right field of vision.

6.   D   There is a detailed point-to-point projection of the retina on the lateral geniculate nucleus and the visual cortex. Fibers from the left halves of the two retinae (right visual field) terminate in the left lateral geniculate nucleus. Impulses are relayed to the visual cortex of the left hemisphere. Fibers from the superior quadrants (inferior field of vision) end in the medial part of the lateral geniculate nucleus, and impulses are relayed to the anterior two-thirds of the visual cortex superior to the calcarine sulcus. Fibers from the inferior quadrants (superior visual field) end in the lateral part of the lateral geniculate nucleus with a relay to the anterior two-thirds of the visual cortex inferior to the calcarine sulcus. Fibers from the macula lutea project to the posterior region of the lateral geniculate nucleus, which in turn sends fibers to the posterior one-third of the visual cortex. It is easy to understand the retinal and visual field projections on the lateral geniculate nucleus and the visual cortex, if you remember the following: (1) the field of vision, left or right, is represented in the contralateral side of the brain, and (2) 3 l's - fibers from the lower retina project to the lateral portion of the lateral geniculate nucleus, the fibers of which project to the lower lip of the calcarine sulcus.

7.   B   The lateral geniculate nucleus produces a small swelling, the lateral geniculate body, inferior to the posterior projection of the pulvinar of the thalamus. The nucleus is the site of termination of all optic tract fibers, except those which serve as afferent limbs of reflex arcs. These fibers enter the superior brachium and terminate in the pretectal nucleus and the superior colliculus of the midbrain.

8.   C   The accommodation reflex (accommodation-convergence reaction) consists of ocular convergence, pupillary constriction, and thickening of the lens. The pathway for the accommodation reflex is not fully understood, although it is thought to include the cerebral cortex. Impulses from the visual association cortex reach the midbrain through fibers in the superior brachium, probably being relayed to the oculomotor parasympathetic nucleus through the superior colliculus. Alternatively, impulses may pass from the visual association cortex to the motor cortex of the frontal lobe through association fibers of the hemisphere, and then reach the Edinger-Westphal nucleus via the corticobulbar tract.

9.   D   Fibers of the geniculocalcarine tract first traverse the retrolentiform and sublentiform parts of the posterior limb of the internal capsule. They then pass around the lateral ventricle, curving posteriorly toward their termination in the visual cortex. Some of the geniculocalcarine fibers travel anteriorly over the temporal horn of the lateral ventricle. These fibers, constituting the temporal or Meyer's loop, terminate in the visual cortex inferior to the calcarine sulcus.

10. D   Cone cells, although less numerous than rod cells, are especially important because of their role in visual acuity and color vision. The fovea centralis is specialized for visual acuity and contains mainly cone

cells. The proportion of cone cells to rod cells steadily decreases from the macula to the periphery of the retina. Cone cells contain a substance called iodopsin and photosensitive pigments that make them susceptible to differential stimulation of red, green, and blue light. Rod cells have a special role in peripheral vision and vision under conditions of low illumination.

M U L T I - C O M P L E T I O N   Q U E S T I O N S

DIRECTIONS: In each of the following questions or incomplete statements, one or more of the completions given is correct. At the lower right of each question, underline A if 1, 2, and 3 are correct; B if 1 and 3 are correct; C if 2 and 4 are correct; D if only 4 is correct; and E if all are correct.

---

1. Correct statements concerning cone cells in the retina include:

   1. They have a special role in peripheral vision
   2. They are responsible for detection of color
   3. They function in vision under low illumination
   4. They are necessary for central and discriminative vision   A B C D E

2. The macula lutea

   1. is in line with the visual axis
   2. abuts on the lateral edge of the optic papilla
   3. is a specialized region of the retina
   4. is pale pink in color when viewed through an ophthalmoscope   A B C D E

3. The optic radiation

   1. originates in the lateral geniculate nucleus
   2. consists of afferent projection fibers with respect to the cortex
   3. terminates in the calcarine cortex
   4. is supplied by the anterior cerebral artery   A B C D E

4. The left visual field is represented in the

   1. right lateral geniculate nucleus
   2. left lateral geniculate nucleus
   3. visual cortex of the right hemisphere
   4. visual cortex of the left hemisphere   A B C D E

5. Impulses from the inferior half of the retina project to the

   1. medial portion of the lateral geniculate nucleus
   2. lateral portion of the lateral geniculate nucleus
   3. superior lip of the calcarine sulcus
   4. inferior lip of the calcarine sulcus   A B C D E

A	B	C	D	E
1,2,3	1,3,	2,4	only 4	all correct

6. The visual cortex

    1. occupies the upper and lower lips of the calcarine
       sulcus
    2. is thin, heterotypical cortex of the granular type
    3. is marked by the line of Gennari
    4. receives a detailed point-to-point projection from
       the retina   A B C D E

7. In the pupillary light reflex,

    1. impulses reach the pretectal nucleus from the retina
    2. there is dilation of the pupil
    3. fibers from the Edinger-Westphal nucleus terminate
       in the ciliary ganglion
    4. impulses are relayed to the dilator pupillae muscle
       in the iris   A B C D E

8. When comparing cone cells with rod cells:

    1. The inner segment of a cone is thicker than the
       inner segment of a rod
    2. There is more endoplasmic reticulum in the inner
       segment of a cone than in that of a rod
    3. Iodopsin is present in cone cells and rhodopsin
       in rod cells
    4. There are approximately 1,000 membranous discs
       in the outer segment of cones and 700 discs in
       the outer segment of rods   A B C D E

9. Correct statements concerning the left optic nerve include:

    1. Damage to it causes blindness in the left field
       of vision
    2. It develops as an outgrowth from the telencephalon
    3. It is formed by fibers from the right nasal and left
       temporal retinae
    4. A lesion obstructing it causes blindness in the left
       eye   A B C D E

10. All fibers in the left optic tract

    1. end in the left lateral geniculate nucleus
    2. conduct impulses from the left field of vision
    3. originate in the left nasal retina and the right
       temporal retina
    4. are included in the tract as it winds around the
       rostral end of the cerebral peduncle   A B C D E

220

ANSWERS, NOTES, AND EXPLANATIONS

1. C 2 and 4 are correct. Cone cells have a special role in central discriminative vision and the detection of color, whereas rod cells are
responsible for peripheral vision and vision under conditions of low
illumination. Central vision with maximal acuity is provided by the
concentration of cone cells in the macula lutea and especially the fovea
centralis. The central part of the fovea is composed only of cone cells.
The proportion of cone cells to rod cells remains high through the macula
region, but steadily decreases from the macula to the periphery of the
retina. Photochemical properties of the outer cone segments permit
detection of colors.

2. A 1, 2, and 3 are correct. The macula lutea, an area at the posterior
pole of the eye in line with the visual axis, is a specialized region of
the retina 6 mm in diameter and abutting on the lateral edge of the optic
papilla. The macula is specialized for acuity of vision. The name macula
lutea or "yellow spot" is derived from the presence of diffuse yellow pigment (xanthophyll) among the neural elements of the macula. The yellow
pigment probably screens out much of the blue part of the visible spec-
trum, thereby protecting the photoreceptors from the dazzling effect of
strong light.

3. A 1, 2, and 3 are correct. Originating in the lateral geniculate nucleus, the geniculocalcarine tract or optic radiation first traverses the
retrolentiform and sublentiform parts of the posterior limb of the
internal capsule. The projection fibers spread out as a broad band bor-
dering the lateral ventricle. They then turn posteriorly into the occipital lobe and terminate in the visual cortex or area 17 of Brodmann.
Some fibers run anteriorly for a considerable distance in the temporal
lobe, superior to the inferior horn of the lateral ventricle; these fibers
constitute Meyer's loop. Branches of the posterior cerebral artery supply
the optic radiation.

4. B 1 and 3 are correct. There is a systematic segregation of fibers in
the optic chiasma to provide for binocular vision. Fibers from the medial
halves of the retinae decussate, so that the right optic tract contains
fibers from the lateral half of the right retina and the medial half of
the left retina. The right optic tract is therefore concerned with the
left field of vision. Fibers in the right optic tract terminate in the
right lateral geniculate nucleus, from which impulses are relayed through
the geniculocalcarine tract to the visual cortex (area 17) surrounding the
calcarine sulcus in the right cerebral hemisphere.

5. C 2 and 4 are correct. Fibers from the nasal or medial half of each
retina decussate in the optic chiasma and join uncrossed fibers from the
temporal or lateral half of the retina to form the optic tract. The optic
tract winds around the rostral end of the cerebral peduncle and ends in
the lateral geniculate nucleus of the thalamus. Fibers from the lateral
geniculate nucleus project to the visual cortex adjacent to the calcarine
sulcus via the geniculocalcarine tract. Fibers from the inferior half of
the retina end in the lateral portion of the lateral geniculate nucleus,
with a relay to the visual cortex in the anterior two-thirds of the
inferior lip of the calcarine sulcus. Impulses from the superior half of
the retina reach the medial portion of the lateral geniculate nucleus and

are relayed to the visual cortex in the anterior two-thirds of the superior lip of the calcarine sulcus.

6. E All are correct. The visual cortex occupies the superior and inferior lips of the calcarine sulcus on the medial surface of the hemisphere, and may extend slightly over the occipital pole. The visual cortex is thinner than cortex elsewhere, being only about 1.5 mm thick. This heterotypical, granular cortex is marked by the line of Gennari; it is therefore called the striate area. There is a detailed point-to-point projection of the retina on the lateral geniculate nucleus and the visual cortex.

7. B 1 and 3 are correct. In the pupillary light reflex, impulses from the retina reach the pretectal nucleus via the optic nerve, optic tract, and superior brachium. Impulses are relayed to the Edinger-Westphal nucleus of the oculomotor complex, then to the ciliary ganglion in the orbit, and finally to the sphincter pupillae muscle in the iris. Both pupils constrict in response to light entering one eye because the pretectal nucleus sends fibers to parasympathetic neurons supplying the sphincter pupillae muscles of both eyes.

8. E All are correct. There are approximately seven million cone cells compared to 130 rod cells. Like the rod cell, the cone cell consists of an outer portion or cone and an inner portion or cone fiber. The cone, like the rod, has outer and inner segments. The outer segment contains approximately 1000 double-layered discs compared to 700 in the rod cell. The chemistry of cones is different from rods: iodopsin is present in cones and rhodopsin in rods. The inner segment of a cone and the cone fiber is thicker than the corresponding parts of rod cells. In addition, the ellipsoid (region adjacent to the outer segment) is larger and there is more granular endoplasmic reticulum. Cone cells function in visual acuity and color vision; rod cells function in peripheral vision and in vision under conditions of low illumination (twilight or night vision).

9. D Only 4 is correct. The optic vesicles, precursors of the optic cups and optic stalks, evaginate from the prosencephalon of the embryonic brain at an early stage of development. The optic cups form the retinae and the optic stalks later become the optic nerves. The optic nerve contains about one million fibers that are axons of ganglion cells in the retina. A lesion affecting the optic nerve causes blindness in the corresponding eye. If the optic tract is damaged, the contralateral visual field is affected.

10. D Only 4 is correct. The optic tract winds around the rostral end of the cerebral peduncle and ends mainly in the lateral geniculate nucleus. A few fibers bypass this nucleus, enter the superior brachium, and end in the pretectal nucleus and the superior colliculus. The left optic tract is composed of fibers from the temporal half of the left retina and the nasal half of the right retina. It conducts impulses concerned with the right field of vision.

DIRECTIONS: Each of the following groups of questions consists of a numbered list of descriptive words or phrases accompanied by a diagram with certain parts ·indicated by letters, or by a list of lettered headings. For each numbered word or phrase, SELECT THE LETTERED PART OR HEADING that matches it correctly and insert the letter in the space to the right of the appropriate number. Each lettered heading may be selected once, more than once, or not at all.

A. Lateral portion of the
    lateral geniculate nucleus
B. Medial portion of the
    lateral geniculate nucleus
C. Posterior one-third of the
    lateral geniculate nucleus
D. Superior lip of the calcarine
    cortex
E. Inferior lip of the calcarine
    cortex

1. ____ Receives fibers from the macula lutea
2. ____ Receives fibers from the lateral portion of the lateral geniculate nucleus
3. ____ Receives fibers from the medial portion of the lateral geniculate nucleus
4. ____ Receives fibers from the inferior retinal quadrants
5. ____ Relays impulses for the most acute vision
6. ____ Receives fibers from the superior retinal quadrants

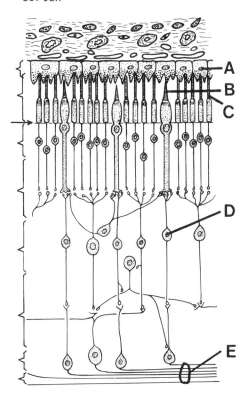

7. ____ Responsible for color vision

8. ____ Extend from the outer to the inner plexiform layers

9. ____ Form optic papilla

10. ____ Originates from outer layer of optic cup

11. ____ Contain rhodopsin

12. ____ Contain iodopsin

(From Barr, M.L. and Kiernan, J.A.: The Human Nervous System, 4th ed., 1983. Courtesy of Harper & Row, Publishers, Inc.)

ASSOCIATION QUESTIONS

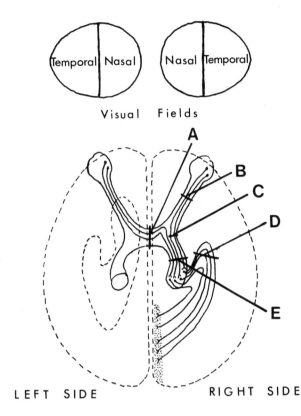

Visual Fields

LEFT SIDE   RIGHT SIDE

13. ____ Blindness in the right eye

14. ____ Left homonymous hemi-anopsia

15. ____ Bitemporal hemianopsia

16. ____ Nasal hemianopsia, right eye

17. ____ Loss of vision in the left upper visual field

18. ____ Damage to fibers from nasal retina (left eye) and temporal retina (right eye)

The drawing indicates lesions at different sites in the visual pathway. (Modified from Barr, M.L. and Kiernan, J.A.: The Human Nervous System, 4th ed., 1983. Courtesy Harper & Row, Publishers, Inc.)

ANSWERS, NOTES, AND EXPLANATIONS

1. C There is a point-to-point projection from the retina to the lateral geniculate nucleus, and from the latter to the visual cortex in the occipital lobe. Fibers from the macula lutea project to a relatively large posterior region of the lateral geniculate nucleus, which in turn sends fibers to the posterior one-third of the visual cortex in the region of the occipital pole. The portions of the lateral geniculate nucleus and visual cortex receiving fibers from the macula are disproportionately large because of the role of the macula in central vision with maximal discrimination.

2. D Fibers from the inferior half of the retina (superior visual field) terminate in the lateral portion of the lateral geniculate nucleus. The impulses are relayed via Meyer's loop of the geniculocalcarine tract to the anterior two-thirds of the visual cortex in the inferior lip of the calcarine sulcus.

3. E Fibers from superior retinal quadrants (representing the inferior visu-
    al field) terminate in the medial half of the lateral geniculate nucleus.
    The impulses are relayed to the anterior two-thirds of the visual cortex
    superior to the calcarine sulcus. Fibers from the inferior retinal quad-
    rants (representing the superior field of vision) terminate in the lateral
    half of the lateral geniculate nucleus. Impulses are relayed to the
    anterior two-thirds of the visual cortex, inferior to the calcarine
    sulcus.

4. A Fibers from the inferior retinal quadrants (superior field of vision)
    terminate in the lateral half of the lateral geniculate nucleus. The
    impulses are relayed via the geniculocalcarine tract to the anterior
    two-thirds of the visual cortex inferior to the calcarine sulcus.

5. C The posterior one-third of the lateral geniculate nucleus relays
    impulses for the most acute vision to the visual cortex of the occipital
    lobe via the geniculocalcarine tract. The portions of the lateral
    geniculate nucleus and visual cortex receiving fibers from the macula
    lutea are disproportionately largely because of the role of the macula in
    central vision with maximal discrimination.

6. B Fibers from the superior retinal quadrants (inferior field of vision)
    terminate in the medial portion of the lateral geniculate nucleus. The
    impulses are relayed to the anterior two-thirds of the visual cortex
    superior to the calcarine sulcus.

7. B Cone photoreceptors are especially important because of their role in
    visual acuity and color vision. The tapering outer segment of a cone con-
    sists of double layered discs. The chemistry of the membranous discs is
    of interest because they contain a substance called iodopsin. The pres-
    ence in separate cones of minute amounts of three photosensitive pigments
    is thought to provide differential stimulation by red, green, and blue
    light.

8. D Bipolar cells are true neurons interposed between photoreceptor cells
    and ganglion cells. In sections stained by a standard histological method
    such as H. & E., the cell body of a bipolar cell is located in the inner
    nuclear layer. Its dendrite extends into the outer plexiform layer, where
    it synapses with photoreceptor cells. Its axon synapses with ganglion
    cell dendrites in the inner plexiform layer.

9. E Ganglion cells form the last retinal link in the visual pathway. Their
    axons pass from all parts of the retina toward the posterior pole of the
    eye, where they converge to form the optic disc on the medial side of the
    macula lutea. The nerve fibers, which are heaped up slightly at the
    margin of the papilla, pass through the sclera or fibrous tunic to form
    the optic nerve. The optic disc is a blind spot because it contains no
    photoreceptor cells.

10. A Optic vesicles evaginate from the prosencephalon of the embryonic brain
    during the fourth week of development. The outer part of the optic
    vesicle invaginates to form an optic cup, consisting of two layers: an
    outer layer that becomes the pigment epithelium of the retina and an inner
    layer that differentiates into the neural layer of the retina. The neural
    layer is composed of photoreceptor, bipolar, and ganglion cells, as well

as association neurons and neuroglial cells.

11. C Rod cells consists of an outer portion, the rod, and an inner portion, the rod fiber. The rod consists of outer and inner segments; only the outer segment is light sensitive. The outer segment is occupied by double-layered membranous discs which include the pigment rhodopsin (visual purple). The photochemical properties of rhodopsin, together with the summation of excitation in the visual pathway through the retina, are responsible for the sensitivity of the rod system to low illumination.

12. B Cone cells, like rod cells, consist of an outer portion, the cone, and an inner portion, the cone fiber. The cone consists of outer and inner segments, the former being light sensitive. The outer cone segment, like the outer rod segment, is composed of double-layered .membranous discs. In cones they contain the pigment iodopsin, chemically related to the rhodopsin of rods. The cone cells function in visual acuity and color vision. The presence of three photosensitive pigments in separate cones provides differential stimulation by red, green, and blue light.

13. B The lesion involves the right optic nerve, interrupting all fibers from the retina of the right eye; thus, blindness results.

14. E If the right optic tract is damaged, fibers from the nasal half of the retina of the left eye (half of the left field of vision) and the temporal half of the retina of the right eye (half of the left field of vision) are interrupted, resulting in blindness in the left visual field. This visual defect is known as left homonymous hemianopsia. Hemianopsia means loss of vision for one-half of the visual field, and homonymous indicates that corresponding fields are affected for each eye.

15. A A lesion that interrupts fibers decussating in the optic chiasma results in a clinical condition known as bitemporal hemianopsia. Fibers from the nasal half of the retina cross the midline in the optic chiasma and join uncrossed fibers from the temporal half of the other eye to form the optic tract. The nasal half of the retina is concerned with the temporal field of vision because the retinal image is reversed as well as being inverted.

16. C When fibers on the lateral side of the optic chiasma are affected, as may happen when there is an aneurysm of the internal carotid artery in that location, nasal hemianopsia involving the right eye results. This is explained by the fact that the lateral area of the optic chiasma is composed of uncrossed fibers originating in the temporal half of the right retina. It is concerned with the nasal field of vision for the right eye.

17. D Some geniculocalcarine fibers travel anteriorly over the temporal horn of the lateral ventricle, before curving posteriorly toward the visual cortex. These fibers, constituting the temporal or Meyer's loop, terminate in the inferior lip of the calcarine sulcus. They conduct impulses from the inferior half of each retina, which is concerned with the superior field of vision, in this case the superior left visual field.

18. E Damage to the right optic tract interrupts fibers ending in the right lateral geniculate nucleus. They originate in the nasal or medial half of the left retina and the temporal or lateral half of the right retina. They are concerned with the left field of vision.

SIXTEEN

The Auditory System

OBJECTIVES

BE ABLE TO:

* Describe and make simple drawings of the cochlea, the cochlear duct, and the spiral organ (organ of Corti).

* Describe the histology of the spiral organ and the mechanism by which the hair cells are stimulated.

* Discuss the cochlear division of the eighth cranial nerve and the cochlear nuclei.

* Describe and make schematic drawings showing the auditory pathway to the cerebral cortex.

* Write brief notes on the efferent connections in the auditory system.

* List the effects of a unilateral lesion of the auditory cortex and of the cochlear division of the eighth cranial nerve.

F I V E - C H O I C E   C O M P L E T I O N   Q U E S T I O N S

DIRECTIONS: Each of the following questions or incomplete statements is followed by five suggested answers or completions. SELECT THE ONE BEST ANSWER OR COMPLETION in each case and underline the appropriate letter at the right.

----

1. Which statement concerning the spiral organ is correct?

    A. It includes cells specialized for a supporting role
    B. It is part of the scala tympani
    C. It includes sensory cells specialized for conversion of a mechanical stimulus into a nerve impulse
    D. Supporting cells contain bundles of tonofibrils
    E. Persistent exposure to excessively loud noises
       causes degenerative changes in the spiral organ   A B C D E

SELECT THE ONE BEST ANSWER OR COMPLETION

2. Which of the following statements concerning the cochlear ganglion is <u>correct</u>?

   A. It consists of cells grouped in a spiral arrangement at the periphery of the modiolus
   B. Axons of hair cells are in synaptic contact with neurons in the cochlear ganglion
   C. It consists of multipolar neurons
   D. Dendrites of ganglion cells enter the spiral organ through the spiral ligament
   E. Axons of ganglion cells enter the internal acoustic meatus from the apex of the cochlea   A B C D E

3. Which of the following combinations of structures are closest to, but not within, the cochlear duct?

   A. Modiolus, scala vestibuli, tectorial membrane
   B. Cochlear nerve, vestibular membrane, basilar membrane
   C. Scala vestibuli, osseous spiral lamina, scala tympani
   D. Phalangeal cells, tectorial membrane, hair cells
   E. Tectorial membrane, basilar membrane, scala tympani   A B C D E

4. Which cells are included in the spiral organ?

   A. Phalangeal cells   D. Two of the above
   B. Cells of Hensen   E. All of the above
   C. Pillar cells   A B C D E

5. The cochlear nuclei receive impulses from

   A. the membranous labyrinth   D. two of the above
   B. the cerebral cortex   E. all of the above
   C. the superior olivary nucleus   A B C D E

6. Most fibers of the lateral lemniscus terminate in

   A. the superior colliculus   D. two of the above
   B. the inferior colliculus   E. all of the above
   C. the medial geniculate body   A B C D E

7. In the spiral organ there are approximately___ inner hair cells and___ outer hair cells respectively.

   A. 7,000 and 25,000   D. 20,000 and   5,000
   B. 15,000 and 30,000   E. 50,000 and 100,000
   C. 1,000 and 10,000   A B C D E

8. Fibers from the ventral cochlear nucleus project to

   A. the contralateral inferior colliculus
   B. The contralateral superior olivary nucleus
   C. The contralateral nucleus of the lateral lemniscus
   D. Two of the above
   E. All of the above   A B C D E

228

SELECT THE ONE BEST ANSWER OR COMPLETION

9. Which statement concerning hair cells of the spiral organ
    is <u>correct</u>?

    A. A cilium is absent in hair cells of adults
    B. The tips of the hairs are embedded in the tectorial membrane
    C. There is a single row of inner hair cells
    D. Two are correct
    E. All are correct   A B C D E

10. Which of the following statements concerning efferent or des-
    cending auditory fibers is <u>incorrect</u>?

    A. Efferent fibers provide feedback circuits in the
        auditory pathway
    B. Descending fibers project from the auditory cortex to the
        inferior colliculus and the medial geniculate nucleus
    C. Efferent fibers terminate as synaptic end-bulbs on phalan-
        geal cells
    D. Descending fibers from the inferior colliculus proceed to
        the cochlear and superior olivary nuclei
    E. Efferent fibers leave the brain stem with the vestibular
        nerve and join the cochlear nerve in the internal
        acoustic meatus   A B C D E

ANSWERS, NOTES, AND EXPLANATIONS

1. B The spiral organ is part of the cochlear duct (scala media), which is
    the middle of three spiral spaces composing the cochlear canal.

2. A The spiral ganglion (cochlear ganglion) consists of cells grouped in a
    spiral arrangement at the periphery of the modiolus. These primary
    sensory neurons are bipolar, as are those in the vestibular ganglion.
    Bundles of dendrites enter the spiral organ through small apertures in
    the osseous spiral lamina. The axons traverse channels in the modiolus
    and enter the internal acoustic meatus from the base of the cochlea to
    form the cochlear division of the eighth cranial nerve.

3. C The cochlear duct takes the form of a spiral within the cochlear
    canal. The duct, which is triangular in transverse section, is separa-
    ted from the scala vestibuli by the thin vestibular membrane, and from
    the scala tympani by the osseous spiral lamina and the basilar membrane.
    The outer wall of the duct is in apposition with endosteum lining the
    cochlear canal of the bony labyrinth. The osseous spiral lamina is a
    spiral shelf extending from the modiolus. The cochlear nerve is located
    some distance from the cochlear duct in the internal acoustic meatus.
    The tectorial membrane, phalangeal cells, and hair cells are part of the
    spiral organ within the cochlear duct.

4. E The spiral organ consists of cells specialized for a supporting role
    and sensory cells specialized for conversion of mechanical stimuli into
    nerve impulses. There are two types of supporting cell, pillar cells

and phalangeal cells, in the spiral organ. Two rows of pillar cells, outer and inner, enclose the tunnel of Corti. Phalangeal cells are adjacent to and support the sensory hair cells. They have the same arrangement as hair cells, i.e., a single row of inner phalangeal cells located on one side of the tunnel of Corti, and from three to five rows of outer phalangeal cells on the other side. The spiral organ is completed on the inner side (toward the modiolus) by border cells and on the outer side by cells of Hensen.

5. E Axons of bipolar neurons in the spiral ganglion traverse channels in the modiolus, emerge from the base of the cochlea, and form the cochlear division of the eighth cranial nerve in the internal acoustic meatus. On emerging from the meatus, the fibers continue to the junction of the pons and medulla where they bifurcate, one branch synapsing on neurons in the dorsal cochlear nucleus and the other branch on neurons in the ventral cochlear nucleus. The cochlear nuclei receive feedback information form the auditory and adjacent cerebral cortex through relays in the medial geniculate body, inferior colliculus, and superior olivary nucleus. The cochlear nuclei receive most impulses from the membranous labyrinth and the cerebral cortex.

6. B Most fibers composing the lateral lemniscus synapse on neurons in the inferior colliculus. They reach the inferior colliculus with or without a synaptic relay in the nucleus of the lateral lemniscus. Fibers from the inferior colliculus traverse the inferior brachium and end on neurons in the medial geniculate body (nucleus). A few fibers of the lateral lemniscus may bypass the inferior colliculus and proceed directly through the inferior brachium to the medial geniculate nucleus. No fibers from the lateral lemniscus are known to course directly to the superior colliculus. Axons of neurons in the inferior colliculus project to neurons in the superior colliculus, from which axons in turn reach nuclei controlling the extraocular muscles and the neck muscles that are responsible for eye and head movements.

7. A The sensory cells are called hair cells, owing to the peculiar hair-like projections from their free ends. There is a single row of inner hair cells, numbering about 7,000. The outer hair cells, of which there are some 25,000, are arranged in three rows in the basal turn of the cochleal, increasing to five rows near the apex.

8. E Fibers from the ventral cochlear nucleus proceed to the region of the ipsilateral superior olivary nucleus, in which some fibers terminate. The majority of fibers continue across the pons with a slight anterior slope and, together with those from the superior olivary nucleus, constitute the trapezoid body. On reaching the contralateral side of the brain stem in the area of the superior olivary nucleus, the fibers either terminate in the superior olivary nucleus or turn abruptly superiorly in the lateral lemniscus to end mostly in the inferior colliculus. However, a few fibers terminate on neurons in the nucleus of the lateral lemniscus, which in turn ends on the inferior colliculus. Most of the fibers from the superior olivary nucleus join the lateral lemniscus and end on the inferior colliculus, or in the nucleus of the lateral lemniscus.

9. E Hairs project from the hair cell along a V- or W-shaped line, their tips being embedded in the tectorial membrane. The number of hairs per

cell varies from 50 to 150, the largest number being on hair cells at the base of the cochlea and the smallest number at the apex. The hairs are microvilli of an unusual shape. There is also a single cilium extending from a basal body, but it is no longer present in the adult. There is a single row of inner hair cells and three to five rows of outer hair cells, the number of rows increasing from the base to the apex of the cochlea. The inner and outer hair cells differ not only in their position, but also in certain details of ultrastructure and innervation.

10. C Efferent fibers, composing the olivocochlear bundle, leave the brain stem with the vestibular nerve, join the cochlear nerve in the internal acoustic meatus, and terminate as synaptic end-bulbs on hair cells of the spiral organ. These fibers, which are mainly crossed, originate in the superior olivary nucleus. They are part of a feedback circuit, causing inhibition of hair cells in regions of the spiral organ as required for sharpening auditory perception.

M U L T I - C O M P L E T I O N   Q U E S T I O N S

DIRECTIONS: In each of the following questions or incomplete statements, one or more of the completions given is correct. At the lower right of each question, underline A if 1, 2, and 3 are correct; B if 1 and 3 are correct; C if 2 and 4 are correct; D if only 4 is correct; and E if all are correct.

---

1. In the membranous labyrinth, scala media refers to

    1. the space between the bony and the membranous labyrinth
    2. part of the lumen of the membranous labyrinth
    3. a space in the cochlear duct that is filled with perilymph
    4. the cochlear duct   A B C D E

2. The spiral organ includes

    1. pillar cells   3. phalangeal cells
    2. hair cells   4. the tectorial membrane   A B C D E

3. The spiral ganglion

    1. consists of cell bodies of primary sensory neurons
    2. is located in the modiolus
    3. consists of bipolar neurons
    4. is intermingled with Scarpa's ganglion   A B C D E

4. The tectorial membrane

    1. consists of a gelatinous type of connective tissue
    2. is attached to the spiral limbus adjacent to the
       osseous spiral lamina
    3. is a ribbon-like structure
    4. extends over the spiral organ   A B C D E

5. The cochlear nerve

   1. runs in the internal acoustic meatus
   2. provides afferents for both cochlear nuclei
   3. contains efferents from the superior olivary nucleus
   4. originates from neurons in Scarpa's ganglion   A B C D E

6. The cochlear nuclei

   1. are located in the floor of the fourth ventricle on
      the surface of the pons
   2. are situated superficially in the rostral end of the
      lateral portion of the medulla
   3. receive fibers from Scarpa's ganglion
   4. receive fibers from the spiral ganglion   A B C D E

7. The lateral lemniscus

   1. consists of crossed and uncrossed fibers
   2. is composed of crossed fibers only
   3. receives fibers from the cochlear, superior olivary,
      and trapezoid nuclei
   4. terminates in the lateral geniculate body   A B C D E

8. The auditory system includes

   1. the external and middle ears
   2. the cochlea of the internal ear
   3. the auditory cortex
   4. pathways in the central nervous system   A B C D E

9. Destruction of the left medial geniculate nucleus causes

   1. complete deafness in the left ear
   2. great difficulty in judging the direction and
      distance of some sounds
   3. complete deafness in the right ear
   4. bilateral diminution of hearing   A B C D E

10. Exposure to loud and prolonged sounds may result in

   1. maximal vibration in a larger region of the basilar membrane
   2. degenerative changes in the spiral organ
   3. activation of more hair cells
   4. high tone deafness   A B C D E

ANSWERS, NOTES, AND EXPLANATIONS

1. C 2 and 4 are correct. The cochlear canal is divided by two partitions,
   the vestibular and basiliar membranes, into three spiral spaces. The

middle of these, the scala media, is the cochlear duct or that portion of the membranous labyrinth which is within the cochlea. The spiral spaces on each side of the cochlear duct are the scala vestibuli and the scala tympani. The lumen of the membranous labyrinth is continuous throughout and is filled with endolymph, whereas the interval between the membranous and bony labyrinths, i.e., the scala vestibuli and scala tympani in the cochlea, is filled with perilymph.

2. A 1, 2, and 3 are correct. The spiral organ (organ of Corti) consists of supporting cells and sensory or hair cells, and rests on the basilar membrane. Supporting cells containing bundles of tonofibrils are of two types, pillar cells and phalangeal cells. There are two rows of pillar cells, inner and outer, on each side of the tunnel of Corti, and phalangeal cells afford intimate support for the sensory cells. The sensory cells are called hair cells because of hair-like projections from their free ends. The tips of the hairs are embedded in the tectorial membrane, consisting of a gelatinous type of connective tissue. The tectorial membrane is attached to the spiral limbus on the osseous spiral lamina and extends over the spiral organ, but is not considered to be a part of it. The spiral organ is completed on the inner side by border cells and on the outer side by cells of Hensen. The tectorial membrane is usually excluded from the spiral organ by definition; however, it is a vital functional part of the acoustic mechanism.

3. A 1, 2, and 3 are correct. The spiral ganglion (cochlear ganglion) consists of cells arranged in a spiral configuration at the periphery of the modiolus. These primary sensory neurons are bipolar, as are those of the vestibular ganglion. The peripheral processes enter the spiral organ through minute channels in the osseous spiral lamina. The central processes traverse channels in the modiolus and enter the internal acoustic meatus from the base of the cochlea to form the cochlear division of the eighth cranial nerve. The vestibular (Scarpa's ganglion) located at the bottom of the internal acoustic meatus, is completely separated from the spiral ganglion.

4. E All are correct. The tectorial membrane is a ribbon-like structure consisting of a gelatinous type of connective tissue, composed primarily of protein with similarities to epidermal keratin. It is attached to the spiral limbus and extends over the spiral organ. The tips of the hairs of the sensory cells are embedded in the membrane.

5. A 1, 2, and 3 are correct. The cochlear nerve consists mainly of axons of bipolar neurons in the spiral ganglion. The myelinated axons traverse the internal acoustic meatus as the cochlear division of the vestibulochlear nerve. At the junction of the medulla and pons, the fibers bifurcate and end in the dorsal and ventral cochlear nuclei. The relatively small number of efferent fibers leave the superior olivary nucleus as the olivocochlear bundle of Rasmussen, travel with the vestibular nerve initially, and join the cochlear nerve in the internal acoustic meatus. They terminate as synaptic end-bulbs on hair cells. Axons of cells in Scarpa's ganglion, located at the bottom of the internal acoustic meatus, form the vestibular division of the eighth cranial nerve.

6. C 2 and 4 are correct. Axons of bipolar neurons in the spiral ganglion traverse channels in the modiolus, emerge from the base of the cochlea, and enter the internal acoustic meatus as the cochlear division of the eighth cranial nerve. On leaving the meatus, the fibers continue to the junction of the pons and medulla, where they bifurcate and synapse with cells in the dorsal and ventral cochlear nuclei. The dorsal cochlear nucleus is situated superficially and immediately adjacent to the base of the inferior cerebellar peduncle, in the floor of the lateral recess of the fourth ventricle well out laterally where it forms a prominence called the tuberculum acousticum. The ventral cochlear nucleus is immediately ventral to and continuous with the dorsal nucleus.

7. B 1 and 3 are correct. The lateral lemniscus consists mainly of efferent fibers of the dorsal and ventral cochlear nuclei. Fibers from the ventral cochlear nucleus proceed to the region of the ipsilateral superior olivary nucleus, in which some of them terminate. The majority of fibers continue across the pons, with a slight anterior slope and, together with fibers contributed by the superior olivary nucleus, constitute the trapezoid body. On reaching the superior olivary nucleus of the contralateral side, the fibers either turn rostrally in the lateral lemniscus or terminate in the superior olivary nucleus, from which fibers are added to the lateral lemniscus. Cells scattered among the trapezoid fibers constitute the nucleus of the trapezoid body, whose connections are similar to those of the superior olivary nucleus. Fibers from the dorsal cochlear nucleus pass obliquely to the region of the contralateal superior olivary nucleus, most of them continuing in the lateral lemniscus.

8. E All are correct. The auditory system consists of the auricle, the external acoustic meatus, and the tympanic membrane of the external ear; the ossicles, maleus, incus, and stapes, of the middle ear; the cochlear duct and spiral organ of the internal ear; the auditory pathways to the inferior colliculus, medial geniculate nucleus, and auditory area of the cerebral cortex.

9. D Only 4 is correct. Interruption of a cochlear nerve or destruction of cochlear nuclei causes complete deafness on the affected side. Because the secondary acoustic pathways are both crossed and uncrossed, lesions involving the lateral lemniscus, inferior colliculus, medial geniculate body, or auditory cortex cause bilateral diminution of hearing, more marked in the contralateral ear. Removal of one temporal lobe impairs the ability to discern the direction and distance of the source of sounds.

10. E All are correct. Vibration of the basilar membrane begins at the base of the cochlea and travels along the membrane with increasing magnitude to a point determined by the pitch or tone. An increase in the intensity of sound causes maximal vibration in a larger region of the basilar membrane, thereby activating more hair cells and neurons. Persistent exposure to excessively loud sounds is known to cause degenerative changes in the spiral organ at the base of the cochlea. This results in high tone deafness, which is common in workers who are exposed to loud sounds from various types of engine.

FIVE-CHOICE ASSOCIATION QUESTIONS

DIRECTIONS: Each of the following groups of questions consists of a numbered list of descriptive words or phrases accompanied by a diagram with certain parts indicated by letters, or by a list of lettered headings. For each numbered word or phrase, SELECT THE LETTERED PART OR HEADING that matches it correctly and insert the letter in the space to the right of the appropriate number. Each lettered heading may be selected once, more than once, or not at all.

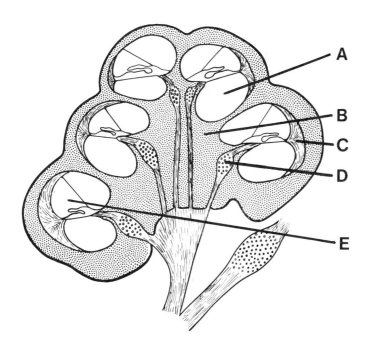

(From Barr, M.L. and Kiernan, J.A., The Human Nervous System, 4th ed., 1983. Courtesy of Harper & Row Publishers Inc.)

1. ____ Membranous labyrinth
2. ____ Consists of bipolar neurons
3. ____ Located the in outer wall of the cochlear canal
4. ____ Perilymph
5. ____ Reissner's membrane
6. ____ Bony pillar or core
7. ____ Lumen of bony labyrinth

ASSOCIATION QUESTIONS

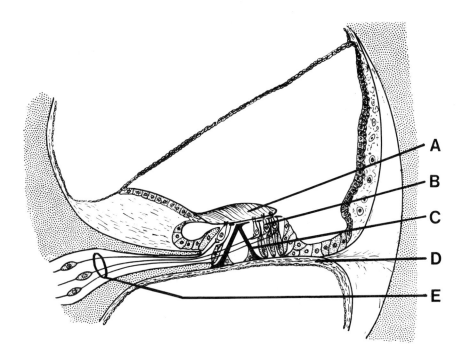

(From Barr, M.L. and Kiernan, J.A., 4th ed., 1983. Courtesy of Harper & Row Publishers Inc.)

8. ____Consists of connective tissue and squamous cells
9. ____Neuroepithelial cell
10. ____Composed of gelatinous connective tissue
11. ____Derived from neurons in the spiral ganglion
12. ____Microvilli
13. ____Consists of a compact bundle of tonofibrils
14. ____Attached to the spiral limbus

ANSWERS, NOTES, AND EXPLANATIONS

1. E The scala media or cochlear duct is the middle of three spiral spaces in the cochlear canal; it is continuous with the saccule in the vestibule of the bony labyrinth through a narrow channel called the ductus reuniens. The lumen of the membranous labyrinth is continuous throughout and is filled with endolymph produced in the stria vascularis in the outer wall of the cochlear duct. The other spiral spaces of the cochlea, the scala vestibuli and the scala tympani, contain perilymph.

2. D The spiral ganglion consists of cells in a spiral arrangement at the periphery of the modiolus. These primary sensory neurons are bipolar, as are those of the vestibular ganglion. Bundles of dendrites traverse fine channels in the osseous spiral lamina and enter the spiral organ where they make synaptic contact with hair cells.

3. C The spiral ligament consists of a thickening of the endosteum along the external wall of the cochlear canal. The outer edge of the basilar membrane is attached to this ligament, whereas its inner edge is attached to the osseous spiral lamina.

4. A The scala tympani and the scala vestibuli are spiral spaces that lie on each side of the cochlear duct within the cochlea. The osseous spiral lamina and the basilar membrane separate the cochlear duct from the scala tympani, and the vestibular membrane separates it from the scala vestibuli.

5. E Reissner's membrane, an alternative name for the vestibular membrane, consists of two layers of simple squamous epithelium separated by a trace of connective tissue.

6. B The cochlea has the shape of a snail's shell, in which there are two and three-quarters turns around a conical pillar of bone called the modiolus. The base of the modiolus forms the deep end of the internal acoustic meatus. Blood vessels and fibers belonging to the cochlear division of the eighth cranial nerve pass through numerous openings at the bottom of the meatus into the modiolus. The cell bodies of bipolar neurons compose the spiral ganglion which is disposed spirally along the base of the osseous spiral lamina. The dendrites of these cells enter the spiral organ and end on the hair cells.

7. A The scala tympani and the scala vestibuli are spiral spaces that lie on each side of the cochlear duct within the cochlea. The osseous spiral lamina and the basilar membrane separate the cochlear duct from the scala tympani, and the vestibular membrane separates it from the scala vestibuli.

8. D The basilar membrane of the cochlear duct is made up of collagen fibers and sparse elastic fibers embedded in a ground substance, with most of the fibers being directed across the membrane. The surface facing the scala tympani consists of a thin layer of connective tissue covered by squamous cells of mesenchymal origin. The cells of the spiral organ cover the surface facing the cochlear duct. In comparison, the vestibular membrane consists of two layers of simple squamous epithelium separated by a small amount of connective tissue.

9. B As in the vestibular system, hair cells in the spiral organ are modified epithelial cells that have certain properties of nerve cells; thus they are classified as neuroepithelial cells. When stimulated, a wave of action potential passes over the surface of a hair cell and continues as a nerve impulse along a bipolar sensory neuron to the cochlear nuclei.

10. A The tectorial membrane is a ribbon-like structure attached to the spiral limbus or endosteal thickening on the osseous spiral lamina. It consists of a gelatinous type of connective tissue composed primarily of

a protein having certain similarities to epidermal keratin. The tectorial membrane extends over the spiral organ. The tips of the hairs of the sensory hair cells are embedded in it.

11. E The spiral organ is supplied by peripheral processes of bipolar neurons that are grouped in a spiral arrangement to form the spiral ganglion at the periphery of the modiolus. Bundles of dendrites enter the spiral organ through small apertures in the osseous spiral lamina and make synaptic contact with the hair cells.

12. B Sensory cells are called hair cells because of the hair-like projections from their free ends. The hairs, which are microvilli of an unusual type, project from the cell along a V- or W-shaped line and their tips are embedded in the tectorial membrane. The number of hairs per cell varies from 50 to 150, the largest number being on hair cells at the base of the cochlea and the smallest number on cells at the apex. There is also a single true cilium, but it is absent in the adult.

13. C In the spiral organ there are two types of supporting cell containing tonofibrils, pillar, and phalangeal cells. There are two rows of pillar cells, inner and outer, on each side of the tunnel of Corti. Each pillar cell consists mainly of a compact bundle of tonofibrils (the pillar), extending from the basilar membrane to the free surface of the spiral organ. The tonofibrils appear as compact arrays of microtubules in electron micrographs. The inner and outer pillars converge and each ends in a flange directed outward. The nucleus of the pillar cell is in a cytoplasmic region in the acute angle between the pillar and the basilar membrane.

14. A The tectorial membrane, a ribbon-like structure consisting of a gelatinous type of connective tissue, is attached to the spiral limbus adjacent to the osseous spiral lamina.

SEVENTEEN

The Vestibular System

OBJECTIVES

BE ABLE TO:

* Differentiate between the static and kinetic labyrinths and discuss the role of the vestibular system in the maintenance of equilibrium and the coordination of eye and head movements.

* Describe the vestibular components of the bony and membranous labyrinths.

* Describe the histology of the sensory areas of the utricle and saccule and the mechanism by which hair cells are stimulated.

* Discuss the vestibular division of the eighth cranial nerve, the vestibular nuclear complex, and projections from the vestibular nuclei to the cerebellum, spinal cord, and nuclei in the brain stem.

* Discuss the transmission of vestibular impulses to the cerebral cortex.

* List the signs elicited by strong vestibular stimulation and discuss clinical tests for determining the integrity of the vestibular system.

FIVE-CHOICE COMPLETION QUESTIONS

DIRECTIONS: Each of the following questions or incomplete statements is followed by five suggested answers or completions. SELECT THE ONE BEST ANSWER OR COMPLETION in each case and underline the appropriate letter at the right.

----

1. In the membranous labyrinth, the word "macula" refers to

    A. a connection between the saccule and the cochlear duct
    B. the sensory epithelium in the semicircular ducts
    C. a specialized area where endolymph is produced
    D. the sensory epithelium in the utricle and saccule
    E. an aperture in the vestibule of the bony labyrinth   A B C D E

SELECT THE ONE BEST ANSWER OR COMPLETION

2. The vestibular nuclear complex receives fibers from

    A. the cerebellum   D. two of the above
    B. the spinal cord   E. all of the above
    C. the membranous labyrinth   A B C D E

3. Which combination of structures is related to the kinetic
    labyrinth?

    A. Crista ampullaris, semicircular duct, cupula
    B. Semicircular canal, otolithic membrane, ampulla
    C. Cupula, saccule, semicircular duct
    D. Vestibule, crista ampullaris, ampulla
    E. Macula utriculi, macula sacculi, otolithic membrane   A B C D E

4. Vestibulocerebellar fibers terminate in the

    A. paleocerebellar cortex
    B. fastigial nuclei and archicerebellar cortex
    C. neocerebellar cortex
    D. cortex of the flocculonodular lobe only
    E. fastigial nuclei only   A B C D E

5. Which statement concerning a vestibular projection to the
    cerebral cortex is correct?

    A. There is a vestibular area on the basal surface of the
        temporal lobe
    B. A thalamic nucleus relays vestibular data to the medial
        surface of the parietal lobe
    C. There is no such cortical area because impulses of vesti-
        bular origin do not reach the cerebrum
    D. There is evidence for a vestibular area on the dorso-
        lateral surface of the parietal lobe
    E. Although the existence of a vestibular cortical area
        is suspected, there is no evidence to indicate its
        location   A B C D E

6. Which statement about the vestibulospinal tract is correct?

    A. It originates in the lateral vestibular nucleus and
        crosses to the opposite side of the brain stem,
        rostral to the pyramidal decussation
    B. It is an ipsilateral tract originating in all vesti-
        bular nuclei
    C. It is an uncrossed tract originating in the lateral
        vestibular nucleus
    D. With cell bodies restricted to the lateral vestibu-
        lar nucleus, the axons terminate in cervical segments
        of the spinal cord only
    E. It originates from more than one nucleus of the vesti-
        bular complex and terminates ipsilaterally throughout
        the spinal cord   A B C D E

SELECT THE ONE BEST ANSWER OR COMPLETION

7. In the hair cells of the crista ampullaris, the true cilium is situated

   A. on the side of the hairs toward the utricle
   B. in the center of the hairs
   C. haphazardly at the periphery of the hairs
   D. on the side of the hairs away from the utricle
   E. according to A and D in about equal numbers   A B C D E

8. Neural structures involved prominently in the maintenance of equilibrium include:

   A. Cristae of the semicircular ducts and the ascending portion of the medial longitudinal fasciculus
   B. Vestibulocerebellar fibers ending in neocerebellar cortex
   C. Lateral vestibular nucleus and vestibulospinal tract
   D. Maculae of the utricle and saccule and the ascending portion of the medial longitudinal fasciculus
   E. Lateral vestibular nucleus and the descending portion of the medial longitudinal fasciculus   A B C D E

ANSWERS, NOTES, AND EXPLANATIONS

1. D The maculae are about 2 x 3 mm in size; one on the floor of the utricle and the other on the medial wall of the saccule. They include sensory hair cells, the hairs (microvilli) of which are embedded in an otolithic membrane. The short connection between the saccule and the cochlear duct (the acoustic portion of the membranous labyrinth) is called the ductus reuniens. The sensory areas of the semicircular ducts are known as cristae. The endolymph is produced in the stria vascularis of the cochlear duct. The fenestra vestibuli and fenestra cochleae in the vestibule of the bony labyrinth are concerned with acoustic mechanisms.

2. E Fibers from the fastigial nucleus and the cortex of the archicerebellum reach the vestibular nuclei by way of the medial area of the inferior cerebellar peduncle. Most fibers of the vestibular nerve convey impulses from sensory areas of the vestibular labyrinth and end in the vestibular nuclear complex; the remainder enter the cerebellum to end in the archicerebellar cortex or in the fastigial nucleus.

3. A The kinetic labyrinth is defined as that part of the membranous labyrinth which reponds only to movements of the head. It consists of the three semicircular ducts enclosed in the semicircular canals of the bony labyrinth, with perilymph intervening. Each semicircular duct has an ampulla at one end in which the sensory area (crista ampullaris) is situated. This sensory area consists of specialized epithelium containing hair cells from which hairs project into a cupula composed of gelatinous connective tissue. The semicircular ducts are affected by movement, especially changes in direction of movement called angular movement or angular rotation, accompanied by acceleration or deceleration. Such movement in or near the plane of a duct is accompanied by endolymphatic flow,

241

with deflection of the cupula and bending of the hairs. The utricle and saccule enclosed by the vestibule of the bony labyrinth, together with their sensory areas composed of a macula and otolithic membrane, compose the static labyrinth.

4. B The three functional divisions of the cerebellum are the vestibulo-cerebellum, spinocerebellum, and pontocerebellum, so named because of the source of certain of their afferent fibers. They are also known as the archicerebellum, paleocerebellum, and neocerebellum respectively, because of their order of appearance in vertebrate evolution. The archicerebellum consists mainly of the flocculonodular lobe and its associated nuclei, the fastigial nuclei. These, therefore, are the principal sites of termination of fibers entering the cerebellum directly from the vestibular nerve or indirectly from the vestibular nuclei.

5. D There is experimental and clinical evidence for the existence of a vestibular area on the dorsolateral surface of the parietal lobe, just posterior to the inferior part of the general sensory or somesthetic area. Axons of cells in the vestibular nuclei appear to run rostrally close to the medial lemniscus, and there is a relay in the posterior ventral nucleus of the thalamus. Vestibular data reaching the cerebral cortex combine with proprioceptive data in supplying information for motor regulation and spatial orientation. On the basis of clinical observations, a vestibular area has been postulated in the superior temporal gyrus of the temporal lobe anterior to the auditory area. The significance of the latter observations vis-a-vis vestibular projections to the cortex has yet to be clarified.

6. C The lateral vestibular nucleus (Deiters' nucleus) includes large multipolar neurons; it is the sole source of the vestibulospinal tract. The constituent fibers descend in the medulla dorsal to the inferior olivary complex and continue into the ventral white column of the spinal cord. The fibers of the uncrossed vestibulospinal tract terminate on alpha and gamma motor neurons throughout the spinal cord, although in largest numbers in the cervical and lumbosacral enlargements. The descending portion of the medial longitudinal fasciculus, consisting of crossed and uncrossed fibers from the medial and inferior vestibular nuclei, is included in the sulcomarginal fasciculus of the ventral white column. It terminates in cervical segments of the spinal cord. The vestibulospinal tract and the descending portion of the medial longitudinal fasciculus are sometimes called the lateral and medial vestibulospinal tracts, respectively.

7. A The crista ampullaris is situated adjacent to the opening of a semi-circular duct into the utricle. The hairs of the sensory hair cells are bent toward or away from the utricle, depending on the direction of flow of endolymph and displacement of the cupula. Because the hair cells are activated when the hairs are bent in the direction of the cilium, which is consistently on the side of the hairs toward the utricle, movement of the cupula in that direction is excitatory. Movement in the opposite direction suppresses the low-level, tonic discharge from the hair cells. In the maculae of the utricle and saccule, on the other hand, the position of the cilium with respect to the hairs differs from one region of the macula to another. This accounts for the difference in the specific hair cells that are stimulated (or inhibited) according to the direction of displacement of the otolithic membrane by gravity.

8. C The functions of the static and kinetic labyrinths overlap to a considerable degree. However, the static labyrinth has a special relevance to the maintenance of balance or equilibrium, and the kinetic labyrinth to eye movements during movements of the head as required to maintain appropriate visual fixation. With respect to maintaining balance, the lateral vestibular nucleus receives data directly via the vestibular nerve and indirectly from the archicerebellum (vestibulocerebellum). The lateral vestibular nucleus gives rise to the large vestibulospinal tract.

M U L T I - C O M P L E T I O N   Q U E S T I O N S

DIRECTIONS: In each of the following questions or incomplete statements, one or more of the completions given is correct. At the lower right of each question, underline <u>A if 1, 2, and 3</u> are correct; <u>B if 1 and 3</u> are correct; <u>C if 2 and 4</u> are correct; <u>D if only 4</u> is correct; and <u>E if all</u> are correct.

----

1. The vestibular nerve

    1. runs in the internal acoustic meatus
    2. provides afferents for all the nuclei in the
        vestibular complex
    3. includes some fibers that enter the cerebellum
    4. contains a few efferent fibers   A B C D E

2. The descending portion of the medial longitudinal
    fasciculus

    1. consists of both crossed and uncrossed fibers
    2. is included in the fasciculus sulcomarginalis of the
        spinal cord
    3. originates in the medial and inferior vestibular
        nuclei
    4. extends the length of the spinal cord   A B C D E

3. The static labyrinth

    1. contains areas of sensory epithelium known as cristae
    2. responds mainly to changes in direction of head
        movement
    3. depends on the flow of endolymph
    4. needs otolithic membranes to function
        appropriately   A B C D E

4. The vestibular nuclear complex

    1. is situated deep to the lateral area
        of the rhomboid fossa
    2. is located entirely in the pons
    3. consists of four nuclei
    4. is located entirely in the medulla   A B C D E

A	B	C	D	E
1,2,3	1,3,	2,4	only 4	all correct

5. The kinetic labyrinth

   1. consists of the semicircular ducts
   2. contains sensory areas called cristae
   3. responds to movements of the head
   4. receives nerve fibers from the spiral ganglion   A B C D E

6. The ascending portion of the medial longitudinal fasciculus

   1. terminates mainly in the reticular formation
   2. originates in all vestibular nuclei
   3. is difficult to identify because it consists of
      unmyelinated fibers
   4. runs close to the abducens, trochlear, and oculo-
      motor nuclei   A B C D E

7. The vestibular ganglion

   1. consists of cell bodies of primary sensory neurons
   2. is intermingled with the spiral ganglion
   3. consists of bipolar neurons
   4. is situated at the medial opening of the internal
      acoustic meatus   A B C D E

8. Strong stimulation of the vestibular system may result
in a transitory

   1. deviation from a straight line in walking
   2. nystagmus
   3. feeling of turning
   4. deviation of a finger from an object at which it
      is pointed   A B C D E

ANSWERS, NOTES, AND EXPLANATIONS

1. E <u>All are correct</u>. The vestibulocochlear nerve occupies the internal acoustic meatus along with the facial nerve and the labyrinthine vessels. The vestibular division of this nerve penetrates the rostral end of the medulla, deep to the root of the inferior cerebellar peduncle. Most of its fibers terminate in the nuclei composing the vestibular complex; the remainder enter the cerebellum. The vestibular nerve contains a few efferent fibers originating in the vestibular nuclei and perhaps in the fastigial nucleus of the cerebellum. They terminate on hair cells of the maculae and cristae, on which they have an inhibitory effect. The cochlear nerve contains a larger number of efferent fibers that inhibit the hair cells of the spiral organ (organ of Corti).

2. A <u>1, 2, and 3 are correct</u>. The descending portion of the medial longitudinal fasciculus, which does not extend beyond the cervical region of the spinal cord, consists of crossed and uncrossed fibers from the

medial vestibular nucleus. The fibers are included in the fasciculus sulcomarginalis of the ventral white column of the spinal cord, along with reticulospinal fibers and others from small nuclei in the midbrain. The principal role of the descending portion of the medial longitudinal fasciculus appears to be the adjustment of the tonus of neck muscles as required for changing positions of the head.

3. D <u>Only 4 is correct</u>. The static labyrinth, consisting of the utricle and saccule, provides data concerning the orientation of the head with respect to gravity. The sensory epithelium consists of a macula in the floor of the utricle and another in the medial wall of the saccule. Each macula has an otolithic membrane which is deflected by gravity, thereby bending the hairs of hair cells in one or another direction. The otolithic membrane is also deflected by quick tilting movements and by linear acceleration or deceleration. In this respect the utricle and saccule have a kinetic as well as a static role in vestibular function.

4. B <u>1 and 3 are correct</u>. The vestibular nuclear complex consists of superior, lateral, medial, and inferior nuclei, identified on the basis of cytoarchitecture and neural connections. They lie lateral to the sulcus limitans in the lateral area of the rhomboid fossa in the floor of the fourth ventricle. This area is known as the vestibular area. The superior nucleus is in the pons and the other nuclei are in the medulla.

5. A <u>1, 2, and 3 are correct</u>. The kinetic portion of the membranous labyrinth consists of the anterior, posterior, and lateral semicircular ducts, which open at each end into the utricle. Movement of the head in or near the plane of a duct causes a flow of endolymph within the duct. This deflects the cupula and bends the hairs of the hair cells in the crista ampullaris. The nerve fibers ending on hair cells come from the vestibular ganglion; those coming from the spiral ganglion end on hair cells in the spiral organ in the cochlea.

6. C <u>2 and 4 are correct</u>. The ascending portion of the medial longitudinal fasciculus, consisting of crossed and uncrossed fibers, originates in all nuclei of the vestibular complex. The fasciculus runs rostrally close to the midline, beneath the floor of the fourth ventricle and just ventral to the central gray matter surrounding the cerebral aqueduct of the midbrain. This position brings the fasciculus close to the abducens, trochlear, and oculomotor nuclei, in which its fibers terminate. These nerve fibers are myelinated and the compact bundle stands out clearly in sections stained for white matter.

7. B <u>1 and 3 are correct</u>. Unlike primary sensory neurons elsewhere, those of the vestibular and spiral ganglia are bipolar, as in embryonic stages before other primary sensory neurons become unipolar (pseudounipolar). The two ganglia of the eighth cranial nerve are separate and distinct; the vestibular ganglion is situated at the bottom of the internal acoustic meatus and the spiral ganglion is located in the modiolus of the cochlea.

8. E <u>All are correct</u>. All the effects listed result when a person is rotated and the rotation is stopped suddenly. In the caloric test used clinically, the external acoustic meatus is irrigated with warm or cool water, setting up convection currents in the endolymph, especially in the lateral semicircular duct. Strong vestibular stimulation may produce

nausea and even vomiting in susceptible persons. Motion sickness is thought to be caused by prolonged vestibular stimulation involving the macula utriculi especially, although in this instance psychic and emotional factors play an important role.

F I V E - C H O I C E   A S S O C I A T I O N   Q U E S T I O N S

DIRECTIONS: Each of the following groups of questions consists of a numbered list of descriptive words or phrases accompanied by a diagram with certain parts indicated by letters, or by a list of lettered headings. For each numbered word or phrase, SELECT THE LETTERED PART OR HEADING that matches it correctly and insert the letter in the space to the right of the appropriate number. Each lettered heading may be selected once, more than once, or not at all.

A. Medial longitudinal fasciculus (ascending portion)
B. Vestibulocerebellar fibers
C. Lateral vestibular nucleus
D. Vestibulospinal tract
E. Medial longitudinal fasciculus (descending portion)

1. _____ Origin of vestibulospinal tract
2. _____ Coordination of head and eye movements
3. _____ To cervical segments of spinal cord only
4. _____ Principal pathway for maintaining balance
5. _____ Included in the inferior cerebellar peduncle
6. _____ Runs throughout the spinal cord

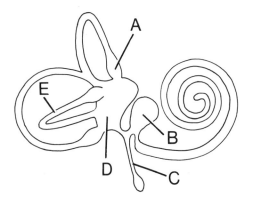

7. _____ Absorption of endolymph

8. _____ Contains the macula utriculi

9. _____ Endolymph flow in horizontal rotation

10. _____ Contains a crista

11. _____ Contains the macula sacculi

12. _____ End of anterior vertical

(From Barr, M.L. and Kiernan, J.A.: The Human Nervous System, 4th ed., 1983. Courtesy of Harper & Row, Publishers, Inc.)

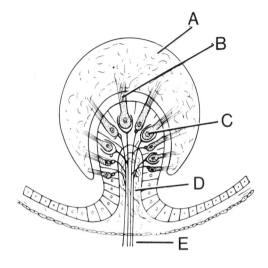

A

B

C

D

E

13. ____Ridge of connective tissue

14. ____Included in the crista

15. ____From vestibular ganglion

16. ____Neuroepithelial cell

17. ____Gelatinous connective tissue

18. ____Microvilli

(From Barr, M.L. and Kiernan, J.A.: The Human Nervous System, 4th ed., 1983. Courtesy of Harper & Row, Publishers, Inc.)

ANSWERS, NOTES, AND EXPLANATIONS

1. C The lateral vestibular nucleus (Deiters' nucleus) contains the cell bodies for all the fibers constituting the vestibulospinal tract. This large tract, which is uncrossed, descends in the medulla dorsal to the inferior olivary complex and continues in the ventral white column of the spinal cord. Fibers of the vestibulospinal tract terminate on motor neurons throughout the length of the spinal cord, predominantly in the cervical and lumbosacral enlargements.

2. A The ascending portion of the medial longitudinal fasciculus originates in all vestibular nuclei and ends in the abducens, trochlear, and oculomotor nuclei. This connection provides for movement of the eyes during movement of the head as required to maintain visual fixation. The medial longitudinal fasciculus also contains internuncial fibers connecting the three nuclei that control extraocular muscles, augmenting synchronization of eye movements as required for biocular vision.

3. E Composed of axons, both crossed and uncrossed, of cells in the medial vestibular nucleus, the descending portion of the medial longitudinal fasciculus is included in the fasciculus sulcomarginalis in the ventral white column of the spinal cord. The fibers end on motor neurons in cervical segments of the spinal cord. Among other possible roles, this connection provides for changes in the tonus of neck muscles as appropriate for various positions of the head. The descending portion of the medial longitudinal fasciculus and the much larger vestibulospinal tract are also known as the medial and lateral vestibulospinal tracts, respectively.

4. D The vestibulospinal tract, originating in the lateral vestibular nucleus and running ipsilaterally the length of the cord, is the principal vestibular pathway in the central nervous system for the maintenance of balance or equilibrium. Although data received from both the static and kinetic labyrinths contribute to this function, the former is more

important. This kinetic labyrinth has a special relevance to the control of eye movements.

5.   B Fibers from the superior, medial, and inferior vestibular nuclei enter the cerebellum via the medial area of the inferior cerebellar peduncle. They terminate in archicerebellar cortex, composed mainly of the flocculo-nodular lobe, and in the fastigial nucleus. There is also a smaller complement of vestibulocerebellar fibers that come directly from the vestibular nerve.

6.   D The vestibulospinal tract runs throughout the spinal cord sending fibers to all segments, especially those related to the limbs, whereas fibers of the descending portion of the medial longitudinal fasciculus terminate in cervical segments only.

7.   C The sketch is an anterolateral view of the right membranous labyrinth. The labyrinth is filled with endolymph produced in the stria vascularis of the cochlear duct. The endolymphatic duct, arising from the communication between the utricle and the saccule, occupies a channel in the petrous part of the temporal bone. It runs to its posterior surface, where a terminal expansion, the endolymphatic sac, is embedded in the dura mater. This sac is surrounded by venules, into which endolymph is absorbed.

8.   D The macula utriculi, situated on the floor of the utricle, is about 2 x 3 mm in size. Except when the macula is horizontal, the otolithic membrane is deflected by gravity and the hairs of the hair cells are bent in one or another direction. There is a cilium at the periphery of the hairs, the location differing from one part of the macula to another. The hair cells are stimulated or inhibited, depending on whether the hairs are bent toward or away from the cilium. The pattern of nerve impulse conduction by fibers of the vestibular nerve varies according to the direction in which the otolithic membrane is defected.

9.   E Flow of endolymph in the lateral semicircular duct is maximal when rotation of the head is approximately in the horizontal plane. The flow results from inertia or momentum of the endolymph at the beginning or end of rotation, respectively. The ampulla is at the lateral end of the left and right lateral semicircular ducts, so that at the beginning of rotation the flow of endolymph through the ampulla is toward the adjacent utricle on one side and away from it on the other side. The direction of flow in the ducts is reversed when rotation stops. The same principles hold for the vertical semicircular ducts. The consequent pattern of nerve impulse conduction provides the brain with accurate information concerning movements of the head.

10. A The ampulla of the anterior semicircular duct, like the ampullae of the other two ducts, contains a crista in which there are sensory hair cells. This duct is transverse to the long axis of the petrous temporal bone, in a plane that is at right angles to the posterior vertical semicircular duct. The anterior and posterior ducts of the two sides form functional pairs because they are in the same plane of space. The two lateral semicircular ducts, which slope inferoposteriorly at an angle of 30 degrees from the horizontal, likewise form a functional pair.

11. B The macula of the saccule has the same structural and functional

characteristics as the macula of the utricle; however the macula is vertically disposed on the medial wall of the saccule and horizontal on the floor of the utricle.

12. A The ampulla of the anterior semicircular duct is at one end of the duct and therefore adjacent to the utricle. The same position applies to the other semicircular ducts. Both ends of each duct open into the utricle in order that there may be endolymphatic flow; this takes place through a common stem at one end of the vertical ducts.

13. D The sketch illustrates the structure of the sensory area (crista) of a semicircular duct. A ridge of connective tissue, derived from the lamina propria of the duct, projects into the ampulla; this transverse septum supports the sensory epithelium.

14. C The crista ampullaris, like the maculae of the utricle and saccule, consists of hair cells surrounded by columnar supporting cells. The maculae of the utricle and saccule are flat, disk-like areas of sensory epithelium, whereas each crista is folded over the surface of the transverse septum.

15. E The sensory areas of the semicircular ducts, utricle, and saccule are supplied by peripheral processes of cells in the vestibular ganglion (Scarpa's ganglion), located at the bottom of the internal acoustic meatus These fibers (functional dendrites) make synaptic contact with hair cells in end-bulb and chalice-like configurations.

16. C Hair cells are epithelial cells modified to provide certain properties of nerve cells; they therefore come under the heading of neuroepithelial cells. When stimulated, a wave of action potential passes over the surface of a hair cell and continues as a nerve impulse along a neuron, the axon of which is one of the many fibers of the vestibular nerve.

17. A The cupula consists of gelatinous connective tissue without the otoliths characteristic of the otolithic membrane. Instead of being displaced by gravity, as in the case of the otolithic membrane, the cupula moves in response to the flow of endolymph in the semicircular duct. Depending on the plane in which the head is moving, and whether movement is be- ginning or ending, the cupula "swings like a door" toward or away from the opening of the ampulla into the utricle.

18. B The hairs embedded in the cupula are essentially microvilli, i.e., cytoplasmic processes projecting from the hair cells. A true cilium also projects from the hair cells at the periphery of the hairs. It is always on the side of the hairs toward the utricle. The sensory cells are excited when the hairs are bent in the direction of the cilium and inhibited when bent in the opposite direction. Flow of endolymph and displacement of the cupula toward the utricle are therefore excitatory, whereas flow of endolymph and displacement of the cupula away from the utricle are inhibitory.

EIGHTEEN

The Limbic and Olfactory Systems

OBJECTIVES

LIMBIC SYSTEM

BE ABLE TO:

* List the regions of gray matter and the tracts that are included in the limbic system.

* Describe the hippocampal formation and its connections.

* Make a simple diagram illustrating the fornix and the source and terminations of its fibers.

* Discuss in general terms, the functional aspects of the limbic system.

OLFACTORY SYSTEM

BE ABLE TO:

* Give a brief account of the components of the olfactory system, using a simple diagram to illustrate the olfactory mucosa, bulb, tract, and trigone.

* Point out the olfactory cortical areas in the brain and discuss briefly the effects of projections from them to autonomic centers and the limbic system.

LIMBIC SYSTEM

F I V E - C H O I C E   C O M P L E T I O N   Q U E S T I O N S [1]

DIRECTIONS: Each of the following questions or incomplete statements is followed by five suggested answers or completions. SELECT THE ONE BEST ANSWER OR COMPLETION in each case and underline the appropriate letter at the right.

----

1. The fimbria of the hippocampus continues as the

    A. alveus
    B. body of fornix
    C. crus of fornix
    D. mamillary body
    E. claustrum

                                                     A B C D E

SELECT THE ONE BEST ANSWER OR COMPLETION

2. Which statement about the hippocampus is <u>incorrect</u>?

   A. It is a phylogenetically old region of the cortex
   B. Its cortex consists of only three layers
   C. It forms a curved elevation in the floor of the tem-
      poral horn of the lateral ventricle
   D. The expanded anterior end of the hippocampus is known
      as the parahippocampal gyrus
   E. Its efferent fibers first form the alveus and then
      accumulate as the fimbria   A B C D E

3. Which of the following is NOT a part of the limbic system?

   A. Cingulate gyrus   D. Mamillary body
   B. Amygdaloid nucleus   E. Claustrum
   C. Hippocampal formation   A B C D E

4. Select the <u>incorrect</u> statement about the fornix.

   A. Partially conceals the dorsal surface of the diencephalon
   B. Ends mainly in the hippocampus of the temporal lobe
   C. Consists of a robust bundle of myelinated axons of cells
      in the hippocampus
   D. Is the main efferent tract of the hippocampal formation
   E. Includes both projection and commissural fibers   A B C D E

5. Which statement about the stria terminalis is FALSE?

   A. Follows the curvature of the tail of the caudate nucleus
   B. Mainly terminates in the septal area and hypothalamus
   C. Originates in the amygdaloid nucleus
   D. Is a robust afferent bundle of fibers
   E. Divides in the region of the interventricular foramen   A B C D E

6. There is no good evidence that the limbic system is involved
   with

   A. behavior related to preservation of the individual
   B. conscious appreciation of smell
   C. brain mechanisms for recent memory
   D. visceral responses associated with emotion
   E. emotions associated with sexual behavior   A B C D E

7. Select the <u>incorrect</u> statement about the anterior nucleus
   of the thalamus.

   A. Forms part of the limbic system of the brain
   B. Gives rise to the projection of the thalamus known
      as the pulvinar
   C. With the fornix, it bounds the interventricular foramen
   D. Has main connections with the mamillary body
   E. Communicates with the cortex of the cingulate gyrus   A B C D E

SELECT THE ONE BEST ANSWER OR COMPLETION

8. Which of the following gyri is NOT a cortical area of the
    limbic system?

    A. Hippocampal   D. Superior temporal
    B. Dentate   E. Parahippocampal
    C. Cingulate   A B C D E

ANSWERS, NOTES, AND EXPLANATIONS

1. C   The fornix contains myelinated axons of cells located in the hippo-
    campus. The fibers first form the alveus, a thin layer of white matter on
    the ventricular surface of the hippocampus; they then accumulate as the
    fimbria along the medial edge of the hippocampus.

2. D   The expanded anterior end of the hippocampus is known as the pes hippo-
    campus because of its resemblance to an animal's paw (L. pes, the foot).
    Part of the parahippocampal gyrus is in direct continuity with the
    hippocampus.

3. E   The claustrum is a thin sheet of gray matter of unknown significance,
    situated between the lentiform nucleus and the insula. It is not part of
    the limbic system.

4. B   Most of the fibers of the fornix end in the mamillary body, with a
    small number ending in the ventromedial hypothalamic nucleus. Some fibers
    leave the column of the fornix immediately inferior to the interventricu-
    lar foramen, and turn posteriorly into the anterior nucleus of the thala-
    mus. Other fibers separate from the fornix and are distributed to the
    septal area and the anterior region of the hypothalamus.

5. D   The stria terminalis, a fiber bundle of the limbic system, is a slender
    strand of fibers running along the medial side of the tail of the caudate
    nucleus. Most of its fibers originate in the amygdaloid nucleus and end
    in the septal area and the hypothalamus.

6. B   Although the hippocampal formation receives olfactory information, it
    presumably elicits emotional responses to odors and aromas. There is no
    good evidence that the hippocampal formation or the limbic system is
    concerned with the conscious appreciation of smell.

7. B   The anterior nucleus of the thalamus is responsible for the anterior
    tubercle of the thalamus and forms part of the gray matter included in the
    limbic system of the brain. The other diencephalic component of this
    system is the hypothalamus, especially the mamillary body. The pulvinar
    is the posterior projection of the thalamus over the rostral end of the
    midbrain.

8. D   The cortical areas of the limbic system consist of the hippocampus, the
    dentate gyrus, the parahippocampal gyrus (all in the temporal lobe), and
    the cingulate gyrus on the medial surface of the cerebral hemisphere
    superior to the corpus callosum.

MULTI-COMPLETION QUESTIONS

DIRECTIONS: In each of the following questions or incomplete statements, one or more of the completions given is correct. At the lower right of each question, underline A if 1, 2, and 3 are correct; B if 1 and 3 are correct; C if 2 and 4 are correct; D if only 4 is correct; and E if all are correct.

---

1. Which regions of gray matter are included in the limbic system of the brain?

   1. Cingulate gyrus   3. Amygdala
   2. Hippocampal formation   4. Mamillary bodies   A B C D E

2. The principal fiber bundles of the limbic system are the

   1. anterior thalamic radiation   3. posterior commissure
   2. mamillothalamic tract   4. fornix   A B C D E

3. The hippocampal formation consists of the

   1. dentate gyrus   3. parahippocampal gyrus
   2. hippocampus   4. cingulate gyrus   A B C D E

4. The limbic lobe of the cerebral hemisphere consists of the

   1. cingulate gyrus   3. parahippocampal gyrus
   2. dentate gyrus   4. fusiform gyrus   A B C D E

5. Correct statements about the hippocampus include:

   1. Develops by a process of continuing expansion of the
      medial edge of the temporal lobe
   2. Occupies the floor of the temporal horn of the lateral
      ventricle
   3. Is an extension of the parahippocampal gyrus on the
      external surface of the cerebral hemisphere
   4. Has a C-shaped outline in a coronal section through the
      hippocampal formation   A B C D E

6. Bilateral removal of the temporal lobes in man results in the Kluver-Bucy syndrome, characterized by

   1. docility   3. a memory defect
   2. a voracious appetite 4. decreased sexual activity   A B C D E

7. Which parts of the limbic system are located in the temporal lobe of the cerebral hemisphere?

   1. Cingulate gyrus   3. Mamillary body
   2. Dentate gyrus   4. Amygdaloid nucleus   A B C D E

A	B	C	D	E
1,2,3	1,3,	2,4	only 4	all correct

8. Which of the following fiber bundles is associated with the
    limbic system?

    1. Fornix
    2. Cingulum
    3. Mamillothalamic tract
    4. Stria terminalis   A B C D E

ANSWERS, NOTES, AND EXPLANATIONS

1. E All are correct. In addition to the regions listed, the parahippo-
    campal gyrus and the anterior nucleus of the thalamus are part of the gray
    matter of the limbic system. This system is concerned with basic
    emotional drives of importance to the preservation of the individual and
    the species. It also has a significant role in the memory mechanisms of
    the brain.

2. C 2 and 4 are correct. The mamillothalamic tract establishes reciprocal
    connections between the mamillary body and the anterior nucleus of the
    thalamus. This nucleus also has reciprocal connections with the cortex of
    the cingulate gyrus. The fornix projects from the hippocampus to the
    hypothalamus, mostly ending in the mamillary body. In addition to the two
    main fiber bundles of the limbic system listed, there is the stria
    terminalis. This slender efferent fiber bundle of nerve fibers arises
    from the amygdaloid nucleus and terminates mainly in the septal area and
    the anterior portion of the hypothalamus.

3. A 1, 2, and 3 are correct. The hippocampal formation consists of the
    hippocampus, the dentate gyrus, and the portion of the parahippocampal
    gyrus that is in direct continuity with the hippocampus. The cingulate
    gyrus on the medial surface of the cerebral hemisphere is included in the
    limbic system, but it is not part of the hippocampal formation.

4. B 1 and 3 are correct. The cingulate and parahippocampal gyri are con-
    nected by a narrow isthmus inferior to the splenium of the corpus callosum
    forming the limbic lobe of the cerebral hemisphere. This is part of the
    gray matter associated with the limbic system; other regions of gray
    matter similarly associated are: the hippocampal formation, a large part
    of the amygdaloid nucleus, the hypothalamus (especially the mamillary
    bodies), and the anterior nucleus of the thalamus.

5. E All are correct. *The hippocampus is a particularly important structure.*
    It consists of a three-layered archicortex compared to the phylogeneti-
    cally newer, six-layered neocortex of the parahippocampal gyrus. There is
    considerable evidence indicating that the hippocampus may be concerned
    with memory, particularly recent memory. Relatively large bilateral
    lesions of the hippocampus are associated with profound impairment of
    memory for recent events, associated with mild behavioral changes.

6. A 1, 2, and 3 are correct. Removal of the temporal lobes, including the
    hippocampus, dentate gyrus, and amygdaloid nucleus, is characterized by
    a voracious appetite, increased (sometimes perverse) sexual activity, and
    docility. There is also a loss of recognition of people and impairment of

memory, particularly recent memory.

7. C <u>2 and 4 are correct</u>. All the structures listed are parts of the limbic system, but only the dentate gyrus and the amygdaloid nucleus are located in the temporal lobe of the cerebral hemisphere. The parahippocampal gyrus and the hippocampus of the limbic system are also located in the temporal lobe. The cingulate gyrus begins inferior to the genu of the corpus callosum and continues superior to the corpus callosum, as far as the splenium. The mamillary body, part of the limbic system, is a small swelling on the basal surface of the hypothalamus.

8. E <u>All are correct</u>. The fornix is the efferent tract of the hippocampus, arching over the thalamus and terminating mainly in the mamillary body. There are reciprocal connections between the mamillary body and the anterior thalamic nucleus through the readily demonstrable fiber bundle known as the mamillothalamic tract. The cingulate gyrus on the medial surface of the cerebral hemisphere, extending into the white matter of the parahippocampal gyrus. These fibers bring the cortex of the parahippocampal and cingulate gyri into communication. The stria terminalis is a slender bundle of fibers that begins in the amygdaloid nucleus and 'ends mainly in the septal area and the hypothalamus.

F I V E - C H O I C E   A S S O C I A T I O N   Q U E S T I O N S

DIRECTIONS: Each of the following groups of questions consists of a numbered list of descriptive words or phrases accompanied by a diagram with certain parts indicated by letters, or by a list of lettered headings. For each numbered word or phrase, SELECT THE LETTERED PART OR HEADING that matches it correctly and insert the letter in the space to the right of the appropriate number. <u>Each lettered heading may be selected once, more than once, or not at all.</u>

A. Amygdaloid nucleus

B. Limbic lobe

C. Fornix

D. Mamillothalamic tract

E. Alveus

1. ____ Thin layer of white matter covering the ventricular surface of the hippocampus

2. ____ Formed by the cingulate and parahippocampal gyri

3. ____ Gives rise to the stria terminalis

4. ____ Mamillothalamic tract

5. ____ Major efferent fiber bundle from the hippocampus

6. ____ Its body adheres to the inferior surface of the corpus callosum

ASSOCIATION QUESTIONS

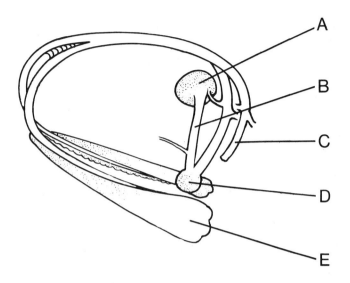

7. ____ Efferent tract of the hippocampus
8. ____ Carries fibers connecting the mamillary body and the anterior thalamic nucleus
9. ____ Responsible for the anterior tubercle of the thalamus
10. ____ Produces an elevation on the temporal horn of the lateral ventricle
11. ____ Part of the hypothalamus
12. ____ Anterior thalamic nucleus

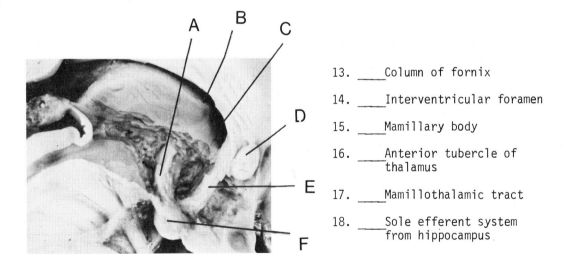

13. ____ Column of fornix

14. ____ Interventricular foramen

15. ____ Mamillary body

16. ____ Anterior tubercle of thalamus

17. ____ Mamillothalamic tract

18. ____ Sole efferent system from hippocampus

(The above diagram and photograph are from Barr, M.L. and Kiernan, J.A.: The Human Nervous System, 4th ed.., 1983, Courtesy of Harper & Row, Publishers, Inc.)

ANSWERS, NOTES, AND EXPLANATIONS

1. E Fibers of cells in the hippocampus first form the alveus on its ventricular surface. The fibers then accumulate as the fimbria along the medial edge of the hippocampus. The fimbria continues as the crus of the fornix.

2. B The cingulate and parahippocampal gyri are connected by a narrow isthmus inferior to the splenium of the corpus callosum, forming the limbic lobe of the cerebral hemisphere. This is a C-shaped configuration of cortex on the medial surface of the cerebral hemisphere.

3. A A large part of the amygdaloid nucleus is included with the limbic system. It gives rise to a slender efferent bundle called the stria terminalis which follows the curve of the tail of the caudate nucleus onto the dorsal surface of the thalamus. Most of its fibers terminate in the septal area and the anterior part of the hypothalamus. The remaining fibers reach the habenular nucleus through the stria medullaris thalami.

4. D The mamillothalamic tract is sometimes called the bundle of Vicq d'Azyr in honor of a French comparative anatomist who lived during the eighteenth century. The mamillothalamic tract projects from the mamillary body to the anterior nucleus of the thalamus, which in turn projects to the cingulate gyrus.

5. C The fornix is the main efferent fiber bundle from the hippocampus. Most of its fibers project through the hypothalamus to the mamillary body. The fornix (L. arch) passes over the thalamus and separates into two columns.

6. C The body of the fornix, formed by the convergence of the two crura (L. legs) of the fornix, adheres to the inferior surface of the corpus callosum. The body of the fornix separates into two columns, each of which curves ventrally anterior to the interventricular foramen.

7. C The fornix, a column of which is labeled, constitutes a large and discrete efferent pathway of the hippocampus. It arches over the thalamus as the crus and body and then divides into two columns which continue through the hypothalamus, dividing it into medial and lateral areas. Most fibers terminate in the mamillary body, but a few end in the ventromedial hypothalamic nucleus.

8. C There are reciprocal connections between the mamillary body and the anterior thalamic nucleus through the mamillothalamic tract, which can be easily demonstrated by gross dissection.

9. A The anterior thalamic nucleus is responsible for the anterior tubercle of the thalamus which, with the fornix, bounds the interventricular foramen. This nucleus is included in the limbic system of the brain and has reciprocal connections with the mamillary body and the cortex of the cingulate gyrus.

10. E The hippocampus develops during the fetal period by a process of expansion and folding of the medial edge of the temporal lobe. It does so in such a way that the gyrus comes to occupy the floor of the temporal horn

of the lateral ventricle. In the mature brain, therefore, the parahippocampal gyrus on the external surface is continuous with the hippocampus along the medial edge of the temporal lobe.

11. D The mamillary bodies are part of the hypothalamus; they form swellings on its basal surface. They are also part of the limbic system of the brain. There are reciprocal connections between the mamillary body and the anterior thalamic nucleus (labeled A) through the mamillothalamic tract (labeled B).

12. A The anterior nucleus of the thalamus is included in the limbic system because its principal connections are with the mamillary body and the cingulate gyrus. The limbic system is concerned with basic emotional drives of importance to preservation of the individual and the species. It also has a significant role in memory mechanisms of the brain.

13. E In addition to a few afferent fibers from the septal (medial olfactory) area, the fornix constitutes the sole efferent system from the hippocampus. These efferent fibers are axons of cells in the hippocampus; they converge to form the fimbria.

14. C The interventricular foramen is the communication between the lateral and third ventricles of the brain. Each column of the fornix curves ventrally, anterior to the foramen, on its way to the hypothalamus.

15. F The mamillary body is a nipple-like swelling on the basal surface of the hypothalamus. Most fibers of the column of the fornix terminate in the mamillary body, with a small number ending in the ventromedial hypothalamic nucleus.

16. B The anterior tubercle of the thalamus is formed by the anterior thalamic nucleus. Note that this tubercle and the column of the fornix bound the interventricular foramen. The anterior thalamic nucleus is included in the limbic system of the brain. Its principal connections are with the mamillary body and the cingulate gyrus.

17. A The mamillary body gives rise to the mamillothalamic tract, a large fiber bundle of the limbic system. This tract ascends and terminate in the anterior thalamic nucleus.

18. E This large bundle of white fibers, one of two columns of the fornix, forms as the body of the fornix separates. The fornix constitutes the sole efferent fiber system of the hippocampus, and the main efferent fiber system of the hippocampal formation (hippocampus, dentate gyrus, and the portion of the parahippocampal gyrus that is in direct continuity with the hippocampus)

F I V E - C H O I C E   C O M P L E T I O N   Q U E S T I O N S

DIRECTIONS: Each of the following questions or incomplete statements is followed by five suggested answers or completions. SELECT THE ONE BEST ANSWER OR COMPLETION in each case and underline the appropriate letter at the right.

----

1. Which statement concerning olfactory cells is <u>incorrect</u>?

    A. Sensory cells are located in the olfactory epithelium
    B. Bipolar neurons are modified to serve as sensory receptors
    C. They are supported by pseudostratified columnar epithelium
    D. They are the functional cells with regard to smell
    E. Axons from these cells form the olfactory tract   A B C D E

2. The main region for awareness of olfactory stimuli is the

    A. olfactory mucosa   D. Intermediate olfactory
    B. lateral olfactory area   area
    C. medial olfactory area   E. septal area   A B C D E

3. Which of the following is an <u>incorrect</u> statement about the medial olfactory area?

    A. Known alternatively as the septal area
    B. Located on the medial aspect of the frontal lobe
    C. Includes the uncus of the temporal lobe
    D. Closely integrated with the limbic system
    E. Connected with the other olfactory areas by the
        diagonal band of Broca   A B C D E

4. One of the following statements about the human olfactory tract is FALSE. Which is it?

    A. Extends rostrally from its attachment to the brain
    B. Expands caudally into a prominent olfactory trigone
    C. The olfactory bulb appears as a slight expansion of it
    D. Passes towards the anterior perforated substance
    E. Divides into lateral and medial olfactory striae   A B C D E

5. All the statements below about the lateral olfactory area are TRUE <u>except</u>:

    A. Includes the uncus of the temporal lobe
    B. Is the main region for the awareness of olfactory stimuli
    C. Site of termination of afferents from the olfactory bulb
    D. Includes part of the amygdaloid nucleus
    E. Closely integrated with the limbic system   A B C D E

SELECT THE ONE BEST ANSWER OR COMPLETION

6. Which statement about the olfactory bulb is <u>incorrect</u>?

    A. Lies on the cribriform plate of the ethmoid bone
    B. Develops as a diverticulum from the forebrain
    C. Receives the central processes of the olfactory cells in the nasal mucosa
    D. Gives rise to about 20 bundles of olfactory nerve fibers
    E. Contains many large, characteristically-shaped mitral cells

                                                                    A B C D E

ANSWERS, NOTES, AND EXPLANATIONS

1. E The axons of olfactory cells converge to form the olfactory nerves, which pass through the foramina in the cribriform plate of the ethmoid bone and terminate in the olfactory bulb. Axons of cells in the olfactory bulb form the olfactory tract. The functional cells with respect to smell are the olfactory cells in the olfactory mucosa. They serve as sensory receptors as well as conducting neurons (neuroepithelial cells).

2. B The lateral olfactory area is the principal region for the awareness of olfactory stimuli. It is therefore called the primary olfactory area. The name septal area is an alternative designation for the medial olfactory area, a part of the limbic system. The septal area is described as an area on the medial surface of the frontal lobe, inferior to the genu and rostrum of the corpus collosum. It consists of the cortex and collections of neurons (septal nuclei) deep to the cortex, the septal nuclei extending as scattered neurons in the septum pellucidum. The intermedial olfactory area is rudimentary in man.

3. C The uncus of the temporal lobe is part of the lateral olfactory area, the primary olfactory area. The three-layered paleocortex of the uncus merges into the six-layered neocortex of the parahippocampal gyrus. The anterior part of this gyrus is called the entorhinal area and functions as olfactory association cortex.

4. B In lower animals, the well-developed olfactory tract expands caudally into a prominent olfactory trigone, from which the lateral and medial striae (gyri) continue to the cortex of the olfactory system. The olfactory trigone and striae are poorly represented in the human brain and may not be obvious on casual inspection.

5. E The medial olfactory area is more closely integrated with the limbic system than other olfactory areas. It is also concerned with the emotional aspects of behavior. It receives afferents from the olfactory bulb through the medial stria. The lateral olfactory area is the primary olfactory area, receiving afferents from the olfactory bulb through the lateral stria.

6. D The olfactory nerve fibers are central processes (axons) of the bipolar olfactory cells in the nasal mucosa. They converge and collect into about 20 bundles which pass through the foramina in the cribriform plate. They continue to enter the inferior surface of the olfactory bulb.

260

MULTI-COMPLETION QUESTIONS

DIRECTIONS: In each of the following questions or incomplete statements, one or more of the completions given is correct. At the lower right of each question, underline A if 1, 2, and 3 are correct; B if 1 and 3 are correct; C if 2 and 4 are correct; D if only 4 is correct; and E if all are correct.

---

1. The primary olfactory area includes the

   1. olfactory bulb and tract
   2. uncus of the temporal lobe
   3. anterior perforated substance
   4. dorsomedial portion of the amygdaloid nucleus   A B C D E

2. Correct statements about the human olfactory system include:

   1. It triggers autonomic responses
   2. Disorders of this system are rarely encountered in
      clinical neurology
   3. Loss of the ability to appreciate odors is not a
      serious disability
   4. Olfactory hallucinations may indicate the presence of
      a temporal lobe lesion   A B C D E

3. The olfactory receptor cells are

   1. bipolar neurons
   2. primary sensory neurons
   3. components of the olfactory mucosa
   4. commonly called mitral cells   A B C D E

4. The medial olfactory area is

   1. also known as the septal area
   2. the principal region for the awareness of
      olfactory stimuli
   3. on the medial aspect of the frontal lobe
   4. situated between the olfactory trigone and the
      optic tract   A B C D E

5. Main projections from olfactory areas include:

   1. Diagonal band of Broca   3. Lateral olfactory stria
   2. Stria medullaris thalami   4. Medial forebrain bundle   A B C D E

6. The anterior perforated substance is

   1. situated between the olfactory trigone and the optic tract
   2. designated as the intermediate olfactory area
   3. caudal to the point of attachment to the olfactory tract
   4. pierced by many central arteries supplying deep
      structures   A B C D E

261

ANSWERS, NOTES, AND EXPLANATIONS

1. **C** <u>2 and 4 are correct.</u> The lateral olfactory area is called the primary olfactory area because it is the main region for the awareness of olfactory stimuli. This area includes the uncus of the temporal lobe, the entorhinal area (anterior part of the parahippocampal gyrus), the region of the limen insulae, and part of the amygdaloid nucleus. The dorsomedial portion of this nucleus is part of the olfactory system, whereas the ventromedial portion is concerned with the limbic system.

2. **E** <u>All are correct.</u> It is well known that the olfactory system triggers autonomic responses, such as salivation, when there is a pleasing aroma connected with food. Disorders of the olfactory system are not common, but when present they may have considerable diagnostic importance. For example, a tumor in the floor of the anterior cranial fossa may interfere with the sense of smell by putting pressure on the olfactory bulb, or tract, or both. Also, a lesion involving the uncus may cause a false sense of disagreeable odors.

3. **A** <u>1, 2, and 3 are correct.</u> Mitral cells are the most prominent cellular component of the olfactory bulb. The bipolar olfactory cells of the olfatory mucosa are modified neurons, functioning both as sensory cells and as primary sensory neurons. A modified dendrite extends to the surface, ending as an exposed bulbous enlargement bearing cilia. An axon ends in the olfactory bulb.

4. **B** <u>1 and 3 are correct.</u> Although the septal area receives olfactory fibers through the medial olfactory stria, it is doubtful that it makes a significant contribution to the sense of smell at the conscious level. The septal area appears to be more closely related to the limbic system. However, fibers originating in the septal area and included in the stria terminalis and medial forebrain bundle are important in bringing about visceral responses to olfactory stimuli.

5. **C** <u>2 and 4 are correct.</u> The stria medullaris thalami is a bundle of nerve fibers running along the dorsomedial border of the thalamus and ending in the habenular nucleus. These fibers are part of the pathway from olfactory areas to autonomic nuclei (parasympathetic) in the brain stem. The medial forebrain bundle traverses the lateral area of the hypothalamus, giving off fibers to the hypothalamic nuclei and continues to the brain stem. The olfactory system triggers autonomic responses, such as salivation, via these connections.

6. **E** <u>All are correct.</u> The anterior perforated substance derives its name from the perforations formed when the central arteries are torn off during removal of the brain. The thin paleocortex at this site receives fibers from the olfactory trigone and is designated as the intermediate olfactory area. It is doubtful that this area makes a significant contribution to the sense of smell at the conscious level.

DIRECTIONS: Each of the following groups of questions consists of a numbered list of descriptive words or phrases accompanied by a diagram with certain parts indicated by letters, or by a list of lettered headings. For each numbered word or phrase, SELECT THE LETTERED PART OR HEADING that matches it correctly and insert the letter in the space to the right of the appropriate number. Each lettered heading may be selected once, more than once, or not at all.

A. Intermediate olfactory area
B. Diagonal band of Broca
C. Lateral olfactory area
D. Medial forebrain bundle
E. Medial olfactory area

1. ____ Uncus
2. ____ Anterior perforated substance
3. ____ Septal area
4. ____ Connects different regions of olfactory cortex
5. ____ Primary olfactory area
6. ____ Projection fibers from olfactory areas

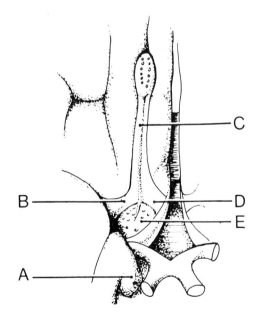

7. ____ Receives afferents through the lateral stria
8. ____ Attached to the brain anterior to the anterior perforated substance
9. ____ Anterior perforated substance
10. ____ A lesion at this site may produce olfactory halluc- inations
11. ____ Ends in the primary olfactory area
12. ____ Carries fibers to the septal area

ANSWERS, NOTES, AND EXPLANATIONS

1. C The uncus is part of the lateral olfactory area; other parts are the limen insulae, the entorhinal area (anterior part of the parahippocampal gyrus), and the dorsomedial part of the amygdaloid nucleus. These regions compose the primary olfactory area and, in contrast to areas of cortex for sensations other than smell, fibers reach them without synapsing in the thalamus.

2. A The anterior perforated substance is designated as the intermediate olfactory area. It receives olfactory fibers from the olfactory trigone. When the brain is removed, the small central arteries entering the brain break off and their paths form the perforations from which this region derives its name.

3. E The medial olfactory area on the medial aspect of the frontal lobe is often referred to as the septal area. It lies inferior to the genu and rostrum of the corpus callosum, and anterior to the lamina terminalis. Although the septal area receives olfactory fibers, it is not considered important as far as the conscious appreciation of smell is concerned. It appears to be more closely integrated with the limbic system, sharing the function of the limbic system with respect to emotions.

4. B The diagonal band of Broca consists of a band of fibers deep to the cortex, immediately anterior to the optic tract. This fasciculus connects the different regions of olfactory cortex.

5. C The lateral olfactory area, consisting of the uncus of the temporal lobe, the entorhinal area (anterior part of the parahippocampal gyrus), the limen insulae, and the dorsomedial portion of the amygdaloid nucleus, is the principal region for the awareness of olfactory stimuli. It is therefore called the primary olfactory area.

6. D The medial forebrain bundle is one of the two main projections from the olfactory areas; the other is the stria medullaris thalami. Although all olfactory areas contribute to these tracts, most of the fibers originate in the medial olfactory area. The medial forebrain bundle traverses the lateral area of the hypothalamus, giving off fibers to hypothalamic nuclei, and then continues to the brain stem. The stria medullaris thalami is part of another pathway to autonomic nuclei in the brain stem.

7. A The uncus of the temporal lobe receives afferent fibers from the olfactory bulb via the lateral olfactory stria. It is part of the lateral olfactory area, the principal region for the awareness of olfactory stimuli.

8. C The olfactory tract is a narrow band of fibers that originates in the olfactory bulb and extends posteriorly. It is attached to the cerebrum in the area of the anterior perforated substance. Most of its fibers are axons of mitral cells in the olfactory bulb.

9. E The anterior perforated substance, located between the olfactory trigone and the optic tract, derives its name from the penetration of many small blood vessels (central arteries) into the brain in this region. This region, called the intermediate olfactory area, does not make a

significant contribution to the sense of smell at a conscious level.

10. A   A lesion in the temporal lobe in the region of the uncus may cause olfactory hallucinations, usually of disagreeable odors. This is the principal region for awareness of olfactory stimuli. The olfactory aura is usually part of an uncinate fit and precedes a seizure, if the lesion is epileptogenic in nature.

11. B   The lateral olfactory stria ends in the lateral olfactory area consisting of the uncus of the temporal lobe, the entorhinal area (anterior part of the parahippocampal gyrus), the region of the limen insulae, and the amygdaloid nucleus. The lateral olfactory area is the principal region for the awareness of olfactory stimuli and is therefore called the primary olfactory area.

12. D   A few olfactory fibers in the medial olfactory stria terminate in the medial olfactory area (septal area), from which there are projections to the hypothalamus and brain stem for visceral responses to odors and aromas. The septal area is closely integrated with the limbic system; it is doubtful that it makes a significant contribution to the sense of smell at the conscious level.

NINETEEN

The Autonomic Nervous System and Visceral Afferents

BE ABLE TO:

* Explain what is meant by the name autonomic nervous system.

* Discuss the two divisions of the autonomic nervous system, briefly describing their functions.

* Make a diagram illustrating efferent pathways of the sympathetic and parasympathetic systems.

* Describe, with aid of a diagram, the general plan of the sympathetic trunk and its rami communicantes.

* State the embryological origin of preganglionic and postganglionic neurons in the sympathetic and parasympathetic systems.

* Discuss the sympathetic disturbance known as Horner's syndrome.

F I V E - C H O I C E   C O M P L E T I O N   Q U E S T I O N S

DIRECTIONS: Each of the following questions or incomplete statements is followed by five suggested answers or completions. SELECT THE ONE BEST ANSWER OR COMPLETION in each case and underline the appropriate letter at the right.

----

1. Select the incorrect statement.

    A. Cardiac muscle receives fibers from both autonomic divisions
    B. Sympathetic responses are dramatically expressed during stress situations
    C. The medulla of the suprarenal gland is supplied directly by preganglionic sympathetic neurons
    D. The parasympathetic system has a diffuse effect causing a mass reaction throughout the body   A B C D E

2. Preganglionic parasympathetic neurons are located in the
    _____nucleus/nuclei.

    A. Edinger-Westphal   D. sacral parasympathetic
    B. superior salivatory   E. all of the above
    C. lacrimal

3. Which statement about the thoracolumbar outflow is FALSE?

    A. Consists of preganglionic sympathetic fibers
    B. Arises from all thoracic and lumbar segments
    C. Passes through the white rami communicantes
    D. Gives rise to the various splanchnic nerves
    E. Originates in the intermediolateral cell columns   A B C D E

4. The white communicating rami contain _____fibers.

    A. parasympathetic postganglionic
    B. preganglionic sympathetic
    C. postsynaptic sympathetic
    D. parasympathetic preganglionic
    E. postganglionic sympathetic   A B C D E

5. Select the <u>correct</u> statement concerning preganglionic sympa-
    thetic neurons.

    A. The cells of the lateral horn of gray matter are motor-
        type cells
    B. Their axons leave the spinal cord with the motor roots
        of spinal nerves
    C. Reach the sympathetic trunk by way of the white com-
        municating rami
    D. Synapse with many postganglionic neurons in the ganglia
        of the sympathetic trunk
    E. All of the above   A B C D E

6. <u>Incorrect</u> statements about preganglionic parasympathetic
    neurons include:

    A. Have long axons which leave the brain in the third,
        seventh, ninth, and tenth cranial nerves
    B. Are located in nuclei of the brain stem and in the
        sacral region of the spinal cord
    C. Synapse with postganglionic neurons in the chain of
        ganglia situated on each side of the vertebral column
    D. Each neuron synapses with a limited number of post-
        ganglionic neurons
    E. All of the above   A B C D E

SELECT THE ONE BEST ANSWER OR COMPLETION

7. The major controlling and integrating center for the autonomic system is the

    A. hypothalamus
    B. reticular formation
    C. limbic system
    D. amygdala
    E. Edinger-Westphal nucleus   A B C D E

8. Which of the following functions is NOT caused by activity of the parasympathetic system?

    A. Constriction of the pupil
    B. Erection of the penis
    C. Reduction of the rate of the heart beat
    D. Stimulation of gastric secretion
    E. Vasoconstriction of cutaneous vessels   A B C D E

9. Which of the following ganglia does not contain postganglionic parasympathetic neurons?

    A. Celiac   D. Submandibular
    B. Ciliary   E. Pterygopalatine
    C. Otic   A B C D E

10. A lesion of the first thoracic segment of the spinal cord results in a number of signs typical of Horner's syndrome. Which sign is atypical?

    A. Ptosis of the upper eyelid
    B. Pupillary constriction
    C. Recession of the eye
    D. Narrowing of the palpebral fissure
    E. Prominence of the eyeball   A B C D E

11. Which statement is <u>incorrect</u>?

    A. The heart is supplied with pain afferents which course centrally in the middle and inferior cervical branches and thoracic cardiac branches of the sympathetic trunk
    B. Pain impulses from a distended gallbladder pass centrally in the greater splanchnic nerve on the right side and enter the spinal cord through the seventh and eighth thoracic roots
    C. Pain is referred to the inferior chest wall when the central area of the diaphragm is irritated by a diseased gallbladder
    D. Pain of duodenal origin is referred to the anterior abdominal wall just superior to the umbilicus
    E. Afferent fibers from the appendix are included in the lesser splanchnic nerve and impulses enter the tenth thoracic segment of the spinal cord   A B C D E

SELECT THE ONE BEST ANSWER OR COMPLETION

12. The viscera are insensitive to

    A. touch   D. cold
    B. cutting   E. all of the above
    C. heat   A B C D E

ANSWERS, NOTES, AND EXPLANATIONS

1. D Unlike the sympathetic system, the parasympathetic system is a
   discretely functioning system. It acts in localized regions rather than
   causing a mass reaction throughout the body. This discrete function
   results from two factors: (1) each preganglionic neuron synapses with a
   few postganglionic neurons which end on a limited number of effector
   cells, and (2) acetylcholine, the chemical mediator at the synapses
   between preganglionic and postganglionic neurons and at the contacts
   between postganglionic terminals and effector cells, is rapidly in-
   activated by cholinesterase. Thus each parasympathetic discharge is of
   short duration.

2. E Preganglionic parasympathetic neurons are located in the nuclei of
   several cranial nerves (III, VII, IX, and X) and sacral nerves (2, 3, and
   possibly 4). These neurons have long axons (preganglionic fibers) which
   synapse on postganglionic cells in ganglia, or on neurons scattered in the
   walls of the pelvic viscera in the case of the sacral outflow.

3. B The thoracolumbar outflow (sympathetic) originates in the intermediolateral cell columns of all thoracic spinal segments and the superior two
   or three lumbar segments. In some individuals the intermediolateral
   columns begin in the eighth cervical segment.

4. B The preganglionic (presynaptic) sympathetic fibers pass from all the
   thoracic and the superior two or three lumbar spinal segments. These
   fibers are axons of preganglionic neurons located in the intermediolateral
   column which forms the lateral horn of gray matter. They reach the sympathetic trunk by way of the corresponding ventral roots and white communicating rami.

5. E All the statements about preganglionic sympathetic neurons are correct.
   Preganglionic fibers for abdominal and pelvic viscera continue through the
   sympathetic trunk without synapsing and enter the splanchnic nerves. The
   fibers terminate on postganglionic neurons located in plexuses surrounding
   the main branches of the abdominal aorta, notably the celiac and superior
   and inferior mesenteric plexuses.

6. C Preganglionic parasympathetic neurons synapse with postganglionic parasympathetic neurons in: (1) one of the four autonomic ganglia of the
   head, or (2) in autonomic ganglia close to or within the walls of the
   viscera. For example, *in the head*, preganglionic fibers from the Edinger-
   Westphal nucleus are carried by the ocular nerve to the orbit, where they
   synapse with neurons in the ciliary ganglion. *In the abdomen*, pregang-

269

lionic fibers from the dorsal vagal nucleus are carried by the vagus nerve to the gastrointestinal tract, where they synapse with neurons in Auerbach's and Meissner's plexuses, as far as the left colic flexure.

7. A The hypothalamus is the major controlling and integrating center for the autonomic system. Centers in the reticular formation and visceral afferent nuclei are also important. The autonomic system comes under a wide range of influences which act via the hypothalamus, including those of the limbic system and the amygdala.

8. E Sympathetic stimulation causes vasoconstriction of cutaneous blood vessels and vasodilation of blood vessels in skeletal muscle. The smooth muscle and secretory cells of viscera and cardiac muscle come under the dual influence of the sympathetic and parasympathetic divisions of the autonomic system. They are functionally antagonistic to one another and a delicate balance between them maintains a more or less constant level of visceral activity (homeostasis).

9. A The celiac is a prevertebral ganglion containing postganglionic sympathetic neurons. Sympathetic fibers which did not synapse in the paravertebral ganglia synapse in prevertebral ganglia. Parasympathetic preganglionic fibers do not synapse in the prevertebral ganglia because these are sympathetic ganglia.

10. E Prominence of the eyeball (exophthalmos) does not result from interruption of the sympathetic supply to the eye; however (1) pupillary constriction (miosis) resulting from paralysis of the dilator pupillae muscle; (2) drooping of the upper eyelid (ptosis) caused by paralysis of the tarsal muscle of the levator palpebrae superioris muscle; and (3) slight recession of the eye into the orbit (enophthalmos) resulting from paralysis of Muller's orbital muscle result from interruption of the sympathetic supply to the eye. In some cases of Horner's syndrome, there is vasodilation of cutaneous blood vessels in the face causing a red flush, and there may be a lack of sweating of the face. Horner's syndrome may occur following a lesion at almost any point in the sympathetic pathway in the brain stem, cervical spinal cord, cervical sympathetic trunk, and in the postganglionic sympathetic fibers from the superior cervical ganglion.

11. C The pain is referred to the inferior chest wall if the periphery of the diaphragm is irritated by disease of the liver or gallbladder. When the central area of the diaphragm is irritated, the pain is referred to the right shoulder because this area is supplied by the phrenic nerve which originates from the third, fourth, and fifth cervical segments.

12. E Because the viscera are insensitive to cutting, operations may be performed on visceral structures under local anesthesia. However, the pain endings are stimulated by the presence of abnormal function or disease. Most commonly pain is caused by distention of hollow viscera, e.g., of the gallbladder when the cystic duct is obstructed by a gallstone.

MULTI-COMPLETION QUESTIONS

DIRECTIONS: In each of the following questions or incomplete statements, one or more of the completions given is correct. At the lower right of each question, underline A if 1, 2, and 3 are correct; B if 1 and 3 are correct; C if 2 and 4 are correct; D if only 4 is correct; and E if all are correct.

----

1. Which of the following structures come under the dual influence of the sympathetic and parasympathetic divisions of the autonomic nervous system?

   1. Lungs   3. Stomach
   2. Heart   4. Peripheral blood vessels   A B C D E

2. Which of the following functions results from parasympathic innervation?

   1. Pupillary constriction
   2. Stimulation of salivary secretion
   3. Reduction of the rate and force of the heart beat
   4. Bronchoconstriction   A B C D E

3. Sources of preganglionic parasympathetic neurons include:

   1. Dorsal motor nucleus of the vagus
   2. Sacral autonomic nucleus
   3. Edinger-Westphal nucleus
   4. Intermediolateral cell nuclei (columns)   A B C D E

4. The parasympathetic division of the autonomic nervous system includes the

   1. ciliary ganglion
   2. dorsal motor nucleus of CN X
   3. superior salivatory nucleus
   4. pelvic splanchnic outflow   A B C D E

5. Structures containing preganglionic sympathetic fibers include:

   1. Gray communicating ramus (ramus communicans)
   2. Ventral roots of all thoracic spinal nerves
   3. Pelvic splanchnic nerves
   4. Greater splanchnic nerve   A B C D E

6. Sympathetic ganglia are found in which of the following regions:

   1. Cervical   3. Lumbar
   2. Thoracic   4. Sacral   A B C D E

A	B	C	D	E
1,2,3	1,3,	2,4	only 4	all correct

7. The sympathetic disturbance known as Horner's syndrome results from

    1. hemisection of the cervical region of the spinal cord
    2. sectioning of the white communicating ramus to the cervicothoracic ganglion
    3. excision of the inferior cervical and superior two thoracic sympathetic ganglia
    4. sectioning of the ventral root of the first thoracic spinal nerve   A B C D E

8. True statements about preganglionic parasympathetic fibers include:

    1. Come from the nuclei of the IIIrd, VIIth, IXth, and Xth cranial nerves
    2. Are axons of neurons in the Edinger-Westphal nucleus
    3. Form the pelvic splanchnic nerves
    4. Are short processes that synapse in the brain stem   A B C D E

9. Postganglionic sympathetic neurons are

    1. derived from the neural crest of the embryo
    2. located in the intermediolateral cell column in the thoracolumbar region
    3. found in plexuses surrounding the main branches of the abdominal aorta
    4. generally "cholinergic" because they form acetylcholine   A B C D E

10. Correct statements about the autonomic nervous system include:

    1. Also called the visceral afferent system
    2. The neurotransmitter between preganglionic and post-ganglionic neurons is acetylcholine
    3. The parasympathetic system is said to be "adrenergic"
    4. The transmitter substance between postganglionic sympathetic terminals and effector cells is norepinephrine   A B C D E

11. Correct statements include:

    1. The respiratory centers for the automatic control of respiration are located in the reticular formation of the medulla
    2. Inspiration is initiated by stimulation of neurons in the inspiratory center by carbon dioxide of the circulating blood
    3. The inspiratory center is located medially in the medulla
    4. A pneumotaxic center is located laterally in the medulla   A B C D E

A	B	C	D	E
1,2,3	1,3,	2,4	only 4	all correct

12. <u>Correct</u> statements include:

1. Visceral afferents in the glossopharyngeal and vagus nerves are important in the maintenance of normal arterial blood pressure
2. Baroreceptors are located in the arch of the aorta and the carotid sinus.
3. Terminal dendritic branches in the arch of the aorta and the carotid sinus signal changes in arterial pressure
4. Baroreceptors are sensitive to stretching of the walls of the structures in which they are located   A B C D E

ANSWERS, NOTES, AND EXPLANATIONS

1. A <u>1, 2, and 3 are correct.</u> The smooth muscle and secretory cells of visera and cardiac muscle come under the dual influence of the sympathetic and parasympathetic divisions of the autonomic system. They are functionally antagonistic to one another and a delicate balance between them maintains a more or less constant level of visceral activity (homeostasis) under normal conditions. The smooth muscle in the walls of peripheral blood vessels, sweat glands, and arrector pili muscles are controlled only by the sympathetic division of the autonomic nervous system.

2. E <u>All are correct.</u> Stimulation of parasympathetic neurons has a more local action than stimulation of sympathetic neurons, and generally the effect is to sustain energy sources by promoting glandular secretion and maintaining a steady heart rate and respiration. The two divisions of the autonomic nervous system are functionally antagonistic to one another.

3. A <u>1, 2, and 3 are correct.</u> The intermediolateral cell columns (nuclei) are the source of preganglionic sympathetic fibers. They form the small lateral horns of gray matter extending from segment T1 through L2 or L3 segments of the spinal cord. Similar cells in the base of the ventral horn in segments S2 through S4 constitute the sacral autonomic nucleus, from which the preganglionic fibers of the sacral portion of the parasympathetic division arise.

4. E <u>All are correct.</u> The ciliary ganglion is a small peripheral ganglion of the parasympathetic system, situated near the apex of the orbit. It contains postganglionic neurons with which preganglionic fibers from the Edinger-Westphal nucleus synapse. Postganglionic fibers from this ganglion innervate the sphincter pupillae and ciliary muscles of the eye through the short ciliary nerves.

5. C <u>2 and 4 are correct.</u> The preganglionic fibers (axons of preganglionic neurons in the intermediolateral column in thoracolumbar segments of the cord) reach the sympathetic trunk by way of the corresponding ventral roots and white communicating rami. Splanchnic fibers are preganglionic fibers that do not synapse in ganglia of the sympathetic trunk (paravertebral), but synapse in prevertebral ganglia, e.g., celiac. The various

splanchnic nerves (greater, lesser, and least splanchnics) arise from the inferior intermediolateral cell columns, synapse in paravertebral plexuses (e.g., celiac), and then proceed to various organs (e.g., smooth muscle of a sphincter). The pelvic splanchnic nerves are derived from the sacral parasympathetic nuclei in spinal cord segments S2 - S4 and synapse directly on neurons in the plexuses in the walls of pelvic organs.

6. E All are correct. The preganglionic fibers pass from all thoracic and the superior two or three lumbar segments (T1 to L2 or L3) to the sympathetic chain of ganglia. Preganglionic sympathetic fibers which synapse in the cervical ganglia course superiorly through the sympathetic trunk. Similarly, preganglionic sympathetic fibers to inferior lumbar, sacral, and coccygeal ganglia course inferiorly through the sympathetic trunk.

7. E All are correct. Hemisection of the cervical region of the spinal cord interrupts descending autonomic fibers in the lateral white column which convey impulses from higher centers (mainly the hypothalamus) to preganglionic sympathetic neurons in the intermediolateral column in the thoracolumbar region of the spinal cord. Sectioning of the white ramus communicans interrupts preganglionic sympathetic fibers passing to the cervicothoracic ganglion. Excision of the inferior cervical and superior two thoracic ganglia, and cutting of the ventral root of the first thoracic nerve, also interrupts the preganglionic sympathetic fibers to the eye, resulting in Horner's syndrome.

8. A 1, 2, and 3 are correct. Preganglionic parasympathetic neurons have long processes that synapse with postganglionic neurons in peripheral or terminal ganglia, near or within the structure being innervated. Each preganglionic fiber synapses with a limited number of postganglionic neurons, which synapse on a limited number of effector cells. Hence, the parasympathetic system acts in localized and discrete regions rather than causing a mass reaction throughout the body.

9. B 1 and 3 are correct. Preganglionic sympathetic neurons are located in the intermediolateral cell column of all thoracic spinal segments and the superior two or three lumbar segments. Axons of these neurons constitute the thoracolumbar or sympathetic outflow. The neurotransmitter substance between pre- and postganglionic sympathetic neurons is acetylcholine. However the transmitter substance between postganglionic terminals and effector cells is norepinephrine (noradrenalin). The sympathetic system is therefore "adrenergic", except for the sympathetic supply to sweat glands which is "cholinergic".

10. C 2 and 4 are correct. The autonomic nervous system, the motor or efferent supply of smooth muscle, cardiac muscle, and gland cells, is sometimes referred to as the visceral efferent system. Acetylcholine is the media- tor at synapses between preganglionic and postganglionic neurons of the autonomic nervous system and at terminals of postganglionic parasympathetic fibers. The parasympathetic neurons, fibers, and synapses are classified as "cholinergic" because they form, transport, and release acetylcholine, the chemical mediator of nervous activity across the synapse.

11. A 1, 2, and 3 are correct. A pneumotaxic center is located in the pontine reticular formation. It regulates the rhythmicity of inspiration and

10   expiration.

12.   E <u>All are correct</u>. Baroreceptors are sensory nerve endings in the walls
      of the atria of the heart, the vena cava, the arch of the aorta, and the
      carotid sinus. The cells bodies of neurons supplying terminal dendritic
      branches in the arch of the aorta are located in the inferior ganglion of
      the vagus nerve, whereas those for the carotid sinus are located in the
      inferior ganglion of the glossopharyngeal nerve.

F I V E - C H O I C E   A S S O C I A T I O N   Q U E S T I O N S

DIRECTIONS: Each of the following groups of questions consists of a
numbered list of descriptive words or phrases accompanied by a diagram with
certain parts indicated by letters, or by a list of lettered headings. For
each numbered word or phrase, SELECT THE LETTERED PART OR HEADING that
matches it correctly and insert the letter in the space to the right of the
appropriate number. <u>Each lettered heading may be selected once, more than</u>
<u>once, or not at all.</u>

A. Sacral autonomic nucleus

B. Intermediolateral cell column

C. Acetylcholine

D. Neural crest cells

E. Norepinephrine

1. _____ Location of preganglionic parasympathetic neurons
2. _____ Extends from spinal cord segment T1 through L2 or 3
3. _____ Source of preganglionic sympathetic fibers
4. _____ Sacral segments S2 through S4 of the spinal cord
5. _____ Released from synaptic vesicles
6. _____ Liberated at postganglionic sympathetic terminals
7. _____ Forms lateral horn of gray matter in spinal cord
8. _____ Give rise to postganglionic autonomic neurons

A. Parasympathetic

B. Sympathetic

C. Baroreceptor

D. Reticular formation

E. Special visceral afferent

9. _____ Smell
10. _____ Decreases glandular secretion
11. _____ Constriction of the pupil
12. _____ Cardiovascular centers
13. _____ Cardiac inhibition
14. _____ Activated by hypotension

275

ASSOCIATION QUESTION

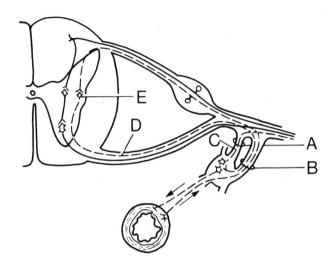

15. ____White ramus communicans

16. ____Source of preganglionic sympathetic fibers

17. ____Preganglionic sympathetic fiber

18. ____"Adrenergic" fiber

19. ____Gray ramus communicans

20. ____Contains visceral afferent and efferent fibers

ANSWERS, NOTES, AND EXPLANATIONS

1. A The sacral autonomic nucleus (parasympathetic), located in the base of the ventral horn in segments S2 through S4, consists of motor-type cells. These neurons give rise to the preganglionic fibers of the sacral portion of the parasympathetic system.

2. B The intermediolateral cell column (nucleus) forms the small lateral horn of gray matter in the spinal cord, which extends from segment T1 through L2 or L3. It consists of motor-type cells that give rise to pre-

ganglionic sympathetic fibers. These neurons receive stimuli from visceral afferents or the dorsal roots, and from autonomic centers in the brain by way of fibers in the lateral white column.

3. B The source of preganglionic sympathetic fibers is the neurons in the intermediolateral column, which forms the lateral horn of gray matter in the spinal cord. These fibers come from all thoracic segments and the superior two or three lumbar segments. Hence they constitute the thoracolumbar outflow. In some people, the intermediolateral cell column begins in the eighth cervical segment.

4. The sacral autonomic or parasympathetic nucleus extends from spinal cord segments S2 through S4. The fibers from these neurons form the sacral portion of the parasympathetic system. These long axons synapse with postganglionic neurons scattered in the walls of the pelvic viscera.

5. C Acetylcholine is the chemical mediator at the synapses between preganglionic and postganglionic autonomic neurons, and also at the contacts between postganglionic parasympathetic neurons and effector cells of the organs innervated. Acetylcholine is formed in the cell bodies of neurons and is carried along the fibers for storage in synaptic vesicles. The acetylcholine is released from the synaptic vesicles by a nerve impulse traveling along the axons.

6. E In the sympathetic division of the autonomic nervous system, norepin-

    ephrine (noradrenalin) is the transmitter substance between postganglionic terminals and effector cells. It is liberated at these terminals and is also secreted by the medulla of the suprarenal gland (adrenal gland), when it is stimulated by preganglionic sympathetic fibers. Cells of the suprarenal medulla, like postganglionic sympathetic neurons, are derived from neural crest cells.

7. B The intermediolateral column forms the small lateral horn of gray matter in the spinal cord, extending from segment T1 through L2 or L3. Its constituent neurons are motor type cells that give rise to preganglionic sympathetic fibers, many of which synapse on neurons in ganglia of the sympathetic trunk (paravertebral ganglia). The fibers of the various splanchnic nerves pass without interruption through the paravertebral ganglia and synapse in the prevertebral ganglia (e.g., the celiac).

8. D Neural crest cells, derived from the embryonic neural crest, give rise to spinal ganglia, sensory ganglia of cranial nerves, and all autonomic ganglia. The cells also give rise to cells in the medulla of the suprarenal gland with which preganglionic sympathetic neurons synapse. The suprarenal medullary cells are dependent upon neural input (acetylcholine) for release of the catecholamines norepinephrine and epinephrine (adrenalin).

9. E The sense of smell and taste (special senses eliciting visceral responses) come under the heading of special visceral afferents.

10. B Postganglionic sympathetic fibers, distributed to glands, cause vaso-constriction which decreases secretion.

11. A Postganglionic parasympathetic fibers from the ciliary ganglion are distributed to the constrictor pupillae and the ciliary muscles of the eye through short ciliary nerves. These impulses cause pupillary constriction.

12. D The cardiovascular centers are located in the reticular formation of the brain stem. These centers are connected with the dorsal vagal nucleus and the intermediolateral column of the spinal cord by reticulospinal fibers.

13. A Reduction of the rate and force of the heart beat is brought about by the parasympathetic system.

14. C The baroreceptors in the arch of the aorta and the carotid sinus signal changes in arterial blood pressure. They are activated by a fall in blood pressure (hypotension).

15. B Preganglionic fibers (axons of preganglionic neurons) from thoracic and superior lumbar segments of the spinal cord traverse the corresponding ventral roots and white communicating rami (rami communicantes). They synapse on neurons in ganglia of the sympathetic chain, or pass uninter-rupted through them to synapse on neurons in a prevertebral ganglion found in the celiac and the superior or inferior mesenteric plexuses.

16. E The source of preganglionic sympathetic neurons is the intermedio-lateral cell column (nucleus), extending from segment T1 through L2 or L3

of the spinal cord. This collection of neurons forms the small lateral horn of gray matter visible in these regions of the cord.

17. D The preganglionic sympathetic fiber is the axon of a preganglionic neuron in the intermediolateral column of the spinal cord. It is the first of the two neurons that take part in transmission of impulses from the central nervous system to the viscera. This nerve fiber reaches the sympathetic trunk by way of the corresponding ventral root and the white communicating ramus.

18. C The postganglionic sympathetic fiber is "adrenergic" because norepine-phrine (noradrenalin) is the transmitter substance between its terminal and the effector cells of the organ innervated. The sympathetic system is "adrenergic" *except* for the sympathetic supply to sweat glands, cutaneous blood vessels, and the arrector pili muscles, which is "cholinergic".

19. A For the body wall, postganglionic fibers are distributed by way of gray rami communicantes and spinal nerves to blood vessels, arrector pili muscles, and sweat glands.

20. B The white communicating ramus contains both visceral afferent and visceral efferent fibers. The sensory neurons for pain of visceral origin are associated with the sympathetic division of the autonomic nervous system. The cell bodies of the primary sensory neurons are in the spinal

ganglia of the thoracic and superior two or three lumbar spinal nerves. The dendrites of these neurons reach the sympathetic trunk by way of the white communicating rami. Preganglionic sympathetic fibers of neurons in the intermediolateral column of the spinal cord reach the sympathetic trunk by way of corresponding ventral roots and white rami communicantes.

TWENTY

Review Examination of the Nervous System

INTRODUCTORY NOTE: *The following 38 questions are based on the material covered in all chapters of this Study Guide and Review Manual. The questions are typical of multiple-choice examinations such as those of the National Board of Medical Examiners. You should be able to answer them in 25 - 30 minutes.*

Before beginning, tear out the answer sheet from the back of this book and read the directions on how to use it. The key to the correct responses is on page 286.

F I V E - C H O I C E   C O M P L E T I O N   Q U E S T I O N S

DIRECTIONS: Each of the following questions or incomplete statements is followed by five suggested answers or completions. SELECT THE ONE BEST ANSWER OR COMPLETION in each case and underline the appropriate letter at the right.

----

1. Which statement about the retina is <u>incorrect?</u>

    A. The functional retina terminates at the ora serrata
    B. The optic disc is the blind spot of the eye
    C. The macula lutea is a depression in the fovea centralis
    D. The macula lutea is specialized for acuity of vision
    E. Rod cells and a capillary network are lacking in the center of the fovea

2. Which cells are included in the spiral organ?

    A. Pillar cells   D. Hair cells
    B. Cells of Hensen   E. All of the above
    C. Phalangeal cells

3. Which statement about the thoracolumbar outflow is FALSE?

    A. Consists of preganglionic sympathetic fibers
    B. Gives rise to the various splanchnic nerves
    C. Passes throuigh the white rami communicantes
    D. Arise from all thoracic and lumbar segments
    E. Originates in the intermediolateral cell columns

SELECT THE ONE BEST ANSWER OR COMPLETION

4. Which of the following is NOT a part of the limbic system?

A. Claustrum
B. Amygdaloid nucleus
C. Hippocampal formation
D. Mamillary bodies
E. Cingulate gyrus

5. Which statement concerning the vestibulospinal tract is correct?

A. It originates in the lateral vestibular nucleus and crosses to the opposite side of the brain stem, rostral to the pyramidal decussation
B. It originates from more than one nucleus of the vestibular complex and terminates ipsilaterally throughout the spinal cord
C. It is an uncrossed tract originating in the lateral vestibular nucleus
D. With cells bodies restricted to the lateral vestibular nucleus, the axons terminate in cervical segments of the spinal cord only
E. It is an ipsilateral tract originating in all vestibular nuclei

6. Myelin sheaths in the central nervous sytem are formed by

A. astrocytes
B. Schwann cells
C. fibroblasts
D. oligodendrocytes
E. microglial cells

7. Concerning the histology of a peripheral nerve, which of the following constitutes a sheath surrounding a bundle or fascicle of nerve fibers?

A. Perineurium
B. Endoneurium
C. Axolemma
D. Neurolemma
E. Epineurium

8. Choose the incorrect statement.

A. The dorsal spinocerebellar tract originates in the nucleus dorsalis
B. The intermediolateral cell column extends through the whole length of the cord
C. The fasciculus proprius is present in all the funiculi
D. On entering Lissauer's zone, dorsal root fibers divide into short ascending and descending branches
E. The spinothalamic tract for pain and temperature is especially important clinically

SELECT THE ONE BEST ANSWER OR COMPLETION

9. In the midbrain the tract for conduction of light touch sensation from the left side of the face is located in the

   A. right cerebral peduncle   D. left tectal region
   B. right tectal region   E. none of the above
   C. left cerebral peduncle

10. Preganglionic fibers ending in the ciliary ganglion originate in the

   A. pons   D. medulla
   B. midbrain   E. thoracic and lumbar
   C. thalamus   cord

11. Which statement concerning the human cerebellum is incorrect?

   A. Has a cortex of gray matter
   B. Has three pairs of central nuclei
   C. Contains a medullary center of white matter
   D. Three pairs of peduncles connect it to the brain stem
   E. Consists of a vermis and two cerebellar hemispheres

12. With which of the following does the hypothalamus have important efferent connections?

   A. Spinal cord   D. Brain stem
   B. Hypophysis cerebri   E. All of the above
   C. Cerebrum

13. The corpus striatum influences the motor and premotor cortical areas via

   A. the subthalamic fasciculus, ventral thalamic nuclei, and thalamocortical fibers
   B. striatocortical fibers in the internal and external capsules
   C. pallidothalamic fibers, ventral lateral and ventral anterior thalamic nuclei, and thalamocortical fibers
   D. the lenticular fasciculus, medial thalamic nucleus, and thalamocortical fibers
   E. the ansa lenticularis, intralaminar thalamic nuclei, and a thalamocortical projection

14. Identify the numbered area of Brodmann that is NOT sensory cortex.

   A. 3   D. 41
   B. 8   E. 43
   C. 17

15. The frontal meningeal artery is a branch of the ____artery.

   A. middle meningeal   D. vertebral
   B. ophthalmic   E. accessory meningeal
   C. occipital

SELECT THE ONE BEST ANSWER OR COMPLETION

16. Which structure is NOT included in the floor of the central part
    of a lateral ventricle?

    A. Vena terminalis   D. Tail of the caudate nucleus
    B. Stria terminalis   E. Lateral surface of the thalamus
    C. Body of the fornix

        M U L T I - C O M P L E T I O N   Q U E S T I O N S

    DIRECTIONS: In each of the following questions or incomplete statements,
    one or more of the completions given is correct. At the lower right of each
    question, underline A if 1, 2, and 3 are correct; B if 1 and 3 are correct;
    C if 2 and 4 are correct; D if only 4 is correct; and E if all are correct.
    ----

17. The forepart of the roof of the fourth ventricle is formed by the

    1. superior medullary velum   3. superior cerebellar peduncle
    2. middle cerebellar peduncle   4. superior vermis

18. The dorsolateral fasciculus in the spinal cord consists of

    1. long, thickly myelinated fibers
    2. group A and group C fibers
    3. descending motor fibers
    4. fibers for pain and temperature

19. Modalities of general sensation conducted ipsilaterally in the
    spinal cord include:

    1. Vibration   3. Two-point touch discrimination
    2. Muscle, joint, and tendon sense 4. Coolness and warmth

20. Nuclei concerned exclusively with cerebellar function include:

    1. Lateral reticular nucleus in the medulla
    2. Nucleus raphe pallidus
    3. Paramedian reticular nucleus in the medulla
    4. Gigantocellular reticular nucleus in the medulla

21. The main afferents to the paleostriatum are from the

    1. thalamus   3. red nucleus
    2. subthalamic nucleus   4. neostriatum

22. The major connection of the subthalamic nucleus is with the

    1. red nucleus   3. reticular formation
    2. thalamus   4. globus pallidus

283

23. Lesions involving the corpus striatum are associated with

    1. chorea
    2. athetosis
    3. Wilson's disease
    4. dystonia musculorum deformans

24. In the pupillary light reflex,

    1. fibers from the Edinger-Westphal nucleus terminate in the ciliary ganglion
    2. there is dilation of the pupil
    3. impulses reach the pretectal nucleus from the retina
    4. impulses are relayed to the dilator pupillae muscle in the iris

25. All fibers in the left optic tract

    1. originate in the left nasal retina and the right temporal retina
    2. conduct impulses from the left field of vision
    3. end in the left lateral geniculate nucleus
    4. are included in the tract as it winds around the rostral end of the cerebral peduncle

26. The lateral lemniscus

    1. is composed of crossed fibers only
    2. consists of crossed and uncrossed fibers
    3. terminates in the lateral geniculate body
    4. receives fibers from the cochlear, superior olivary, and trapezoid nuclei

27. The kinetic labyrinth

    1. responds to movements of the head
    2. contains sensory areas called cristae
    3. consists of the semicircular ducts
    4. receives nerve fibers from the spiral ganglion

DIRECTIONS: Each of the following groups of questions consists of a numbered list of descriptive words or phrases accompanied by a diagram with certain parts indicated by letters, or by a list of lettered headings. For each numbered word or phrase, SELECT THE LETTERED PART OR HEADING that matches it correctly and insert the letter in the space to the right of the appropriate number. Each lettered heading may be selected once, more than once, or not at all.

A. Corticostriate fibers

B. Sign of Babinski

C. Corticospinal tract

D. Hemiballismus

E. Lenticular fasciculus

28. ____ Traverses the subthalamus

29. ____ Subthalamic nucleus

30. ____ Globus pallidus

31. ____ Controls independent use of digits

32. ____ Observed in an upper motor neuron lesion

33. ____ Terminate in the putamen

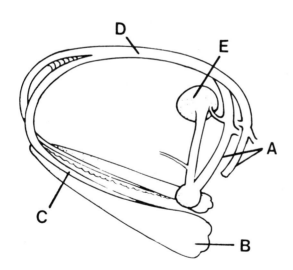

34. ____ Columns of the fornix

35. ____ Anterior nucleus of the thalamus

36. ____ Fimbria

37. ____ Hippocampus

38. ____ Body of fornix

KEY TO CORRECT RESPONSES

1. C	9. A	17. B	25. D	33. A
2. E	10. B	18. C	26. C	34. A
3. D	11. B	19. A	27. A	35. E
4. A	12. E	20. B	28. E	36. C
5. C	13. C	21. C	29. D	37. B
6. D	14. B	22. D	30. E	38. D
7. A	15. A	23. E	31. C	
8. B	16. E	24. B	32. B	

INTERPRETATION OF YOUR SCORE

Number of Correct Responses	Level of Performance
30 - 38	Excellent - Exceptional
26 - 37	Superior - Very Superior
20 - 25	Average - Above Average
16 - 19	Poor - Marginal
15 or less	Very Poor - Failure

ANSWER SHEET

DIRECTIONS: Indicate your answer by
blackening between the guidelines as
shown in the sample.

Sample

A ==== B ▃▃▃ C ==== D ==== E ====

1 A ===B===C===D===E===   2 A ===B===C===D===E===   3 A ===B===C===D===E===

4 A ===B===C===D===E===   5 A ===B===C===D===E===   6 A ===B===C===D===E===

7 A ===B===C===D===E===   8 A ===B===C===D===E===   9 A ===B===C===D===E===

10 A ===B===C===D===E===   11 A ===B===C===D===E===   12 A ===B===C===D===E===

13 A ===B===C===D===E===   14 A ===B===C===D===E===   15 A ===B===C===D===E===

16 A ===B===C===D===E===   17 A ===B===C===D===E===   18 A ===B===C===D===E===

19 A ===B===C===D===E===   20 A ===B===C===D===E===   21 A ===B===C===D===E===

22 A ===B===C===D===E===   23 A ===B===C===D===E===   24 A ===B===C===D===E===

25 A ===B===C===D===E===   26 A ===B===C===D===E===   27 A ===B===C===D===E===

28 A ===B===C===D===E===   29 A ===B===C===D===E===   30 A ===B===C===D===E===

31 A ===B===C===D===E===   32 A ===B===C===D===E===   33 A ===B===C===D===E===

34 A ===B===C===D===E===   35 A ===B===C===D===E===   36 A ===B===C===D===E===

37 A ===B===C===D===E===   38 A ===B===C===D===E===

NOTES

NOTES

NOTES

NOTES

NOTES